NEW MEDICAL CHALLENGES DURING THE SCOTTISH ENLIGHTENMENT

THE WELLCOME SERIES IN THE HISTORY OF MEDICINE

Forthcoming:

Medicine by Post in Eighteenth-Century Britain: The Changing Rhetoric of Illness in Doctor–Patient Correspondence and Literature
Wayne Wild

The Wellcome Series in the History of Medicine series editors are
V. Nutton, C.J. Lawrence and M. Neve.
Please send all queries regarding the series to Michael Laycock,
The Wellcome Trust Centre for the History of Medicine at UCL,
210 Euston Road, London NW1 2BE, UK.

NEW MEDICAL CHALLENGES DURING THE SCOTTISH ENLIGHTENMENT

Guenter B. Risse

Rodopi

Amsterdam – New York, NY 2005

First published in 2005
by Editions Rodopi B. V., Amsterdam – New York, NY 2005.

Design and Typesetting by Michael Laycock,
The Wellcome Trust Centre for the History of Medicine at UCL.
Printed and bound in The Netherlands by Editions Rodopi B.V.,
Amsterdam – New York, NY 2005.

Index by Indexing Specialists (UK) Ltd.

British Library Cataloguing in Publication Data
A catalogue record for this book is available from the British Library
ISBN 90-420-1814-3

'New Medical Challenges during the Scottish Enlightenment' –
Amsterdam – New York, NY:
Rodopi. – ill.
(Clio Medica 76 / ISSN 0045-7183;
The Wellcome Series in the History of Medicine)

Front cover:

Scottish student facing a board of medical examiners at Surgeons' Hall. Coloured aquatint by J. Stadler, 1800, after S. Collings after T. Smollett.
Courtesy: *Wellcome Library*, London.

Printed in The Netherlands

All titles in the Clio Medica series (from 1999 onwards) are available to download from the IngentaConnect website: http://www.ingentaconnect.com

Contents

In Memory of Lester S. King and Roy S. Porter
Mentors, Colleagues, and Personal Friends

Preface

Forty years ago Lester King, then a lecturer at the University of Chicago, introduced me to the eighteenth century. A pathologist by training, Dr. King was an avid philosopher and historian who had already published *The Medical World of the Eighteenth Century* (1958) and *The Growth of Medical Thought* (1963). Both books featured extensive chapters concentrating on modern medical rationalism and classification. His enthusiasm for these subjects was contagious. When time came to select a topic for a Ph.D. dissertation, my 'Lehrer' suggested a broad but largely unexamined topic in Anglo–Saxon history of science: 'Naturphilosophie', where I was expected to take advantage of my fluency in the German language – my mother tongue. However, a perusal of primary sources, especially the works of the philosopher Friedrich W.J. Schelling (1775–1854) disclosed the deep medical roots of this philosophy of nature. Indeed, Schelling's ideas were based on notions of vitality proposed by the Scottish physician, John Brown (1735–88), a former student of William Cullen, one of the eighteenth-century luminaries of the Edinburgh Medical School. My revised proposal to study Brown's medical system in Germany towards the end of the century was initially received with scant enthusiasm in an era when Whig history and notions of medical progress still held considerable sway. To write the evolution of a 'failed' theory and practice created by an iconoclastic alcoholic and opium addict that was soon consigned to the junk heap of history seemed somewhat wasteful, even irrelevant. Employing what King characterised as a 'small residue of Prussian arrogance and aggressiveness' I eventually prevailed and with his grudging support was able to submerge myself in the world of eighteenth-century medical systems and their therapeutical implications. Following approval of my still unpublished thesis in 1971 titled 'The History of John Brown's Medical System in Germany During the Years 1790–1806', my subsequent scholarly research brought me frequently to Edinburgh, where I was able to access the rich manuscript collections located at the Royal College of Physicians, the Edinburgh University Library, and Scottish Record Office, among others. Numerous articles and my book *Hospital Life in Enlightenment Scotland: Care and Teaching at the Royal Infirmary of Edinburgh* (Cambridge University Press, 1986) followed. Roy Porter not only favourably refereed my hospital manuscript, but also continued to provide invaluable suggestions and encouragement for my involvement in what he had termed 'medical history from below'.

This collection of revised and unpublished articles may well signal the end of my involvement with the field of eighteenth-century Scottish medicine, although I still harbour some hope to revamp and extend my original work on John Brown. I want to express once more my gratitude to Joan P.S. Ferguson, former Librarian of the Royal College of Physicians, Edinburgh, for her kindness and generosity, allowing me to peruse the valuable archival collection of student notebooks and lecture notes. Similar thanks go to the personnel at Special Collections, Edinburgh University Library, and its former Medical Archive Centre. In the United States, Dorothy T. Hanks at the History of Medicine Division, National Library of Medicine, and Richard J. Wolfe, Curator of Rare Books at the Boston Medical Library helped to locate further student notebooks. For his part, James T. Goodrich provided another set of lecture notes and casebooks that are now in my personal archival collection. Stephanie Blackden, Michael Barfoot, and Christopher Lawrence shared their expertise, patiently introducing an odd medical doctor of German extraction from Argentina to Scottish social history. Over the years, several colleagues contributed their knowledge and experience to make these essays possible. Among them I would like to acknowledge the late Lloyd G. Stevenson and William Coleman, as well as William Bynum, Rosemary Stevens and Dorothy Porter. Malcolm Nicholson originally solicited one of the articles on the charitable aspects of the Edinburgh Infirmary, Robert Jütte organised a meeting on the history of clinical cases and also prompted me to concentrate on Cullen's role as health advisor for the 1999 meeting of the International Association for the History of Medicine and Health, while Fiona MacDonald co-ordinated a symposium where I had planned to discuss lead mining. My involvement with the history of malaria stems from a stint as Fulton Fellow at Yale University, arranged by my former student, John Harley Warner. Among former graduate students helping to gather materials for these papers were Caroline Acker, Rebecca Ratcliffe, Andrea Richardson, and Deirdre O'Reilly in San Francisco. Last, but not least, I would like to thank both my daughter Alisa and my wife Sandy for their valuable editorial assistance and the Wellcome Trust Centre for the History of Medicine at UCL referees for their editorial suggestions.

Seattle,
September 2004.

Introduction

The Scottish Enlightenment continues to attract the attention of historians.[1] Situated at the dawn of the Industrial Revolution, consumer society and rise of the middle class, this period offers fascinating opportunities for detailed studies dealing with the effects of a new urban and commercial world.[2] As pointed out by Paul Wood and Charles W.J. Withers in their recent historiographical essay, studies centred on science and medicine reached maturity in the 1970s and flourished in subsequent decades.[3] Authors such as John Christie, J.B. Morell, and Anand Chitnis were among the first to draw the intellectual and social contours of knowledge pertaining to the 'natural' world.[4] Subsequent contributions by Roger Emerson, Thomas L. Hankins and Christopher Lawrence placed science and medicine at the very centre of Scotland's ideology of improvement,[5] a notion currently under challenge. In a recent essay, Richard B. Sher has attempted to define the Scottish Enlightenment as a broad cultural movement that includes all branches of polite learning, including scientific and medical aspects.[6] Such a framework allows for a better integration of future studies in this field. Moreover, both Withers and Wood conclude their review by suggesting that work on all topics should continue to address different levels of historical analysis and contribute to a better interpretation of the Enlightenment's belief in the unity and utility of knowledge.

This collection of original essays aims to further enrich our understanding of the place and nature of Scottish health, science, and medicine. Recent authors have stressed the linkages between sites and ways of knowing.[7] The primary focus is on Edinburgh, and the topics selected for study are expressions of its local scientific culture.[8] Each chapter constitutes a particular window into specific aspects of the medical past based on hitherto seldom-tapped documentation: book manuscripts, consultation letters, hospital registration and management records, as well as student essays, lecture notes, and notebooks. Printed materials, including books, legal documents, and newspaper reports, supplement these sources. The resulting portraits review a number of social and scientific practices. They include charitable endeavours, debates between members of a learned society, vivisection experiments, disease construction and classification, as well as clinical management and teaching. The images conjured also display a number of common characteristics. Subjected to greater magnification, the selected topics expose the anxieties of Scotland's affluent class, its preoccupation with health and the quest for moral and social recognition through charitable endeavours. Other pictures cover a sector of the population that has often remained silent in history: the 'deserving' poor. Yet, their presence and incorporation into the eighteenth-century medical world had a profound impact on the construction of theories, clinical practices, and institutional arrangements.

The second goal and common thread of this book is to document basic ambiguities and contradictions surrounding health-related issues in eighteenth-century Scotland. Commercial society created work and wealth but threatened virtue and health. Luxurious lifestyles as well as poverty took their toll on debilitated bodies, triggering disease. Migrant farm workers toiling in the notoriously unhealthy English fens imported a disabling fever only to see their fortunes reversed as the new Scottish agriculture cleared swamps and created jobs at home. Because of the growing economic importance of metal extraction, the hitherto disposable lives of miners acquired greater importance and prompted rehabilitation efforts. Thanks to the richness of the extant sources, and employing an anti-Whiggish approach to the subject, the essays expose a world of uncertainty, confusion, and paradox. Frequent quotations from some of the protagonists aim to rediscover their distinct voices and meanings. To place medical ideas and practices into a proper context, each chapter also offers extensive background information, often returning to the ancient roots of a featured medical problem. In spite of the fashionable veneer of nerves and sensibility used for explaining the workings of human body and mind, medical practitioners continued to rely on older notions of bodily behaviour based on classical humoralism to treat their patients. Prominent physicians such as William Cullen (1710–90), frequently depicted all clinical phenomena as occurring under 'ambiguities', including patients' stories, disease classifications and the actions of particular remedies.

The first three essays deal with several aspects of institutional history, illuminating new forms of public activity in eighteenth-century urban centres. Much has been written about the creation of a 'public sphere' of social intercourse instrumental in creating identity and culture for bourgeois members of civil society.[9] The notion has found wide acceptance as an empirical phenomenon and analytical tool for discussions concerning science in the Enlightenment,[10] and eighteenth-century Scotland in particular.[11] Two public Edinburgh spheres are featured: a charitable organisation created for the purpose of erecting and managing a hospital, and a society for medical students attending the local university. Both the

Edinburgh Infirmary and the Royal Medical Society were essential to the success of the Edinburgh Medical School.[12]

The first chapter deals with the meaning and rewards of charitable giving specifically directed towards the care of the sick. The focus is on the voluntary hospital movement in Enlightenment Britain and, in particular, the creation of a philanthropic community in Edinburgh planning to establish an infirmary for the care of poor patients. While the current historiography of private charity is broadening, the aim remains largely on the actions and perceived motives of donors.[13] This study, however, attempts to present a more balanced view by including the recipients of charity – hospitalised patients – as well as their caregivers. To accomplish its goals, this philanthropic movement employed a religious and humanistic rhetoric of good works and sympathy to unify urban elites and build impressive testimonials to their devotions and entrepreneurial spirit. Like with all gifts, benefactors expected proper social acknowledgement of their generosity in the form of greater moral, political, and cultural status. Using the example of the famous Edinburgh Infirmary, the paper focuses on its foundation, governance, and economy.[14] Fuelling this particular philanthropic effort were a number of local concerns and national agendas. These are analysed in some detail. The result was an institution that became the pride of a city and nation.

More importantly, the story revisits some of the managerial and financial aspects of running such an enterprise and reviews the expectations and duties of charitable patienthood. Medicine's professional interests were not neglected. In Britain's competitive health-related market, voluntary hospital positions enhanced professional status and reputation based in part on the acquisition of clinical skills and therapeutic knowledge. The latter derived from multiple drug trials, exposing the tensions between charitable and scientific objectives. In the end, hospital practice exposed new fault lines regarding physician relationships with poor patients and other colleagues, notably surgeons, forcing the establishment of new ethical guidelines and educational standards.[15]

A broad survey of the activities carried out at the Royal Medical Society of Edinburgh with special attention to the last two decades of the eighteenth century follows in Chapter 2. This organisation was the oldest Scottish medical institution exclusively run and devoted to medical students attending the local university. True to the Enlightenment tenets, the Society's stated objective was 'the improvement of medical knowledge'.[16] The Society was initially designed as a finishing school for budding medical gentlemen. Like other clubs and societies, it was a public space, a forum where students could hone their rhetorical and debating skills necessary for engaging with future colleagues and private patients. For this purpose, the students admitted for membership were required to write and present papers at monthly sessions, which were followed by lively discussions. The Society's activities expose the students' ambiguous position as independent agents running their own learned society while continuing to show deference to their academic teachers and university authorities. This is the first attempt to explore and present the broad range of surviving student dissertations collected by the Society. They offer a valuable window into the making of medical science in Edinburgh.

The papers cover an important period in the Society's life when membership nearly doubled and the debates often became intense and contentious. Key topics examined by students ranged from epistemological issues such as system-building and scientific methodology, general studies of the physical and human environment in other cultures, chemistry, physiology and clinical subjects.[17] Particular attention is given to the motivations, planning and execution of experiments. With support from the Society's leadership, students expressed a willingness to engage in problem-solving by conducting trials on themselves as well as on animals. Despite the cruelty inherent in their vivisections, members revealed genuine scientific curiosity, ingenuity and a desire to advance knowledge. Both research and clinical experiences fostered new approaches to existing theoretical and practical issues. Pedagogical demands for greater access to hospital patients revealed a desire to supplement book knowledge with bedside experiences. Behind a façade of didactic exercises, the Society gradually shifted from an elite debating club into an institution adopting new epistemological foundations for medical knowledge.

Chapter 3 returns to Edinburgh's Royal Medical Society and considers in detail a series of events that took place in this institution during the years 1778–90. At that time, dissension and factionalism engulfed the Society, shattering its earlier framework of polite disputation. The main cause for this rift was the growing antagonism between supporters of rival medical theories and practices. Many students supported the system of William Cullen, the celebrated representative of Edinburgh medicine, while others were sympathisers of Cullen's former student, John Brown, an occasional extramural lecturer. Brown's open rejection of Cullen's ideas in 1778 and the publication of his own medical system two years later deeply influenced the Society's activities, transforming the meetings into bitter confrontations between the 'Cullenians' and 'Brunonians'.[18] At stake were fundamental epistemological issues as well as a stinging critique of the traditional 'antiphlogistic' or depleting therapies based on bleeding and purging.

This chapter is partially based on a unique source of documentation from the Scottish Record Office: a bundle of newspapers and set of legal petitions. The story provides a unique and fascinating window into the influence of Brunonianism in Edinburgh, packed with colourful events, including raucous debates of rival student papers and duelling threats. When accounts of the rather contentious proceedings appeared in a local tabloid, the Society leadership, citing issues of professional privacy, filed a lawsuit involving the most famous lawyers in Edinburgh. In an attempt to control medical knowledge, members were prohibited from divulging details of the weekly deliberations under threat of expulsion. The episode brought into sharp relief the tensions between the need for professional secrecy and the public's desire to share health-related knowledge – after all, the Enlightenment was at its core an educational movement. In fact, both Brown's own views and the student debates reveal a clear tendency to simplify, and thus, demystify medicine. Moreover, this incident confirmed the fragile nature of medicine's professional authority and the growing powers of print media to reach, inform, and influence broad sectors of the public.

Section II features several studies on the topics of health and disease. Chapter 4 concentrates on the Enlightenment's optimism about human power to reshape the world and the assumption of responsibility for individual physical and moral health. Taking advantage of Britain's consumer revolution among the upper and 'middling' layers of society, new forms of advertising and marketing techniques as well as fashionable cures encouraged health promotion. Besides random self-help, medical advice offered a more structured and traditional rationale to reach this goal. Mastery over this knowledge and its professional delivery lent moral legitimacy as well as social and economic advantage to British physicians competing for patronage. The inquiry exposes the recommendations made by the Scottish physician William Cullen (1710–90) to improve the lifestyle and health of his mostly affluent patients. Responding to contemporary concerns, this prominent representative of Enlightenment medicine functioned as 'hygienist', defined as a physician attempting to regulate health and prevent illness.[19] Given his professional reputation, Cullen was ideally positioned to play such a role of advisor and educator, particularly since prudent living became an important virtue in eighteenth-century Scottish culture. In condemning the world of luxury and indulgence spawned by modern commercialism, physicians like Cullen played the role of moral crusaders still yearning for the simplicity, frugality, and probity of earlier times. His advice reveals a critical cultural shift away from traditional notions that equated bodily vigour with stoutness and hearty living.

Cullen's ideas, summarised in unpublished essays as well as consultation letters proffered through the mails, focused on his clients' temperament, constitution, environment, diet and lodgings, as well as changes in bodily functions at different ages, seasons and climate. The holistic doctrine of the Galenic 'six non-natural things' – air, food and drink, sleep and wakefulness, exercise, bodily evacuations and emotions – was peculiarly suited to the social realities of the eighteenth-century Enlightenment.[20] Although this classical framework was a component of traditional humoralism, Cullen sought to adapt it to his own vitalistic scheme of nerves and sensibility, creating a simple set of 'common sense' rules for prudent living that could appeal to all his clients. Besides expressing scepticism about compliance, Cullen was also keenly aware of the paradox involved in his task: the creation of a society of potential 'hypochondriacs' ever more dependent on medical attention.

In Chapter 5, the focus shifts to disease and the problem of 'ague' that afflicted inhabitants of Scotland's lowlands during the latter third of the eighteenth century. For more than a century, the medical literature had increasingly restricted the vague term 'ague' to particular types of fever with distinctive intermittent characteristics. Historians have been attracted to the study of past diseases and more recently resorted to adopt ecological models to understand their movements and fluctuations.[21] The idea that each society and age reveals a unique blend of circumstances and social responses to illness demands that these phenomena be examined within specific geographical, political, economic, and cultural contexts. Moreover, a paleoecology of health and disease needs to use current scientific information to solve its puzzles. The study of 'ague' in Britain suggests that this condition referred to what is currently understood under the term malaria.[22] The analysis is based on a number of contemporary sources. They include the collection of parish reports, institutional records from the Kelso Dispensary and the Edinburgh Infirmary, medical student notebooks, and the writings of prominent Scottish physicians who managed patients afflicted by this disease. Following a careful review of the evidence, the paper concludes that ague in Scotland was mostly an import, a disease continuously brought in from England, the Continent, and tropical British colonies. Its eventual disappearance in the late-eighteenth century was not linked to any medical insights or practices. Instead, it was intimately connected with the country's unique geography and climate, as well as the agricultural and industrial revolutions that took place on its soil.

A study of mining and its health hazards in eighteenth-century Scotland follows. Traditionally, miners were frequently ill and lived short lives. This essay describes in detail the rudimentary extraction and refinement techniques employed in the 'lead hillies' of Lanarkshire, linking them to a somewhat elusive occupational and medical condition: lead poisoning.[23] To understand its protean manifestations, the inquiry reviews successive efforts designed to connect this disease to a number of activities and environments since Antiquity. As the extraction of this metal became more profitable, their health became a greater concern, prompting a number of medical studies to determine the causes of their sickness as well as to design therapies to reverse its manifestations. This study primarily seeks to understand the social construction of Scottish 'mill reek' based on a number of contemporary medical writings and clinical cases admitted to the Edinburgh Infirmary under the traditional rubric *colica pictonum*—colic of the Pictons. Promoted by a number of academic physicians with interests in chemistry, this condition became an attractive subject for a series of clinical and experimental studies. These inquiries created further impetus for studies concerning the toxic action of lead.[24] Paradoxically, the therapeutic successes in reversing some of the gastrointestinal and neurological symptoms were based on the traditional depleting practices opposed by many physicians and gradually falling into disfavour.

Section III features three essays that highlight the deep chasm between eighteenth-century medical theories and practices. While Edinburgh physicians such as William Cullen and James Gregory readily accepted a new view of the human body governed by the nervous system in constant contact with environmental stimuli, their therapeutic efforts remained steeped in traditional humoralism.

Chapter 7 reconstructs the framework of clinical knowledge at the Royal Infirmary of Edinburgh between the years 1770–1800. The study is primarily based on a particular literary genre: student casebooks and lecture notes. As discussed elsewhere, clinical cases are among the most important documents for understanding the organisation, representation, and transmission of health-related knowledge.[25] They furnish valuable empirical information and are essential in reconstructing the actual therapeutic management of individual patients. Often, they depict unique stories of suffering based on narratives of the sick and their interpretations by professionals. Carefully analysed, clinical cases reveal much about the mechanisms of clinical decision-making and conditions governing the medical marketplace, thus exposing issues of professional rhetoric and authority, as well as patient power. With the advent of hospitals during the eighteenth century and their capacity to manage large numbers of patients, the popularity of casebooks soared. Hospital cases became a new form of medical discourse constructed within particular institutional 'ecologies' and shaped by social and professional needs.

This study is restricted to an analysis of selected teaching cases dealing with 'pulmonary consumption', a widespread ailment and probably the most common and deadly disease during the eighteenth century.[26] Persons suffering from this scourge were seldom admitted to hospitals except when there was still hope of recovery. In all instances, the student-copied cases were matched with notes taken from clinical lectures delivered by the professors managing these patients. The intent was to employ a clinically complex disease and follow the words and actions of notable Edinburgh physicians and understand decision-making at the bedside. Not surprisingly, the inquiry detected significant differences in approach and emphasis among medical authorities. The result is an intimate glimpse of the ambiguities of eighteenth-century medical practice in hospitals.

Chapter 8 attempts to contribute to the understanding of eighteenth-century gynaecology by examining a number of 'female complaints' that led to admission and treatment at the Royal Infirmary of Edinburgh during the last quarter of the century. Issues of female fertility and procreation were at the forefront of Britain's national concerns about preserving its population. This story acknowledges the existence of a vast feminine critique on the subject of male-dominated gynaecology in recent times. However, instead of taking sides on this issue, the paper offers a multi-layered historical context for understanding the flow of medical power together with the uncertainties surrounding medicine's ideas and practices. The analysis is based on medical publications, hospital registers, medical students' casebooks and lecture notes, all focusing on the distinctive behaviour and pathology of female bodies, especially menstruation and the role of the womb.[27] Knowledge was shaped by traditional social beliefs in the physical inferiority of women, their relative unhealthiness and natural destiny as procreators and homemakers. In constructing 'female troubles', male physicians created a series of disorders linked to systemic debility and excessive sensibility.

At the same time, this study also tries to understand the social and cultural contexts of clinical encounters between poor urban females and the academic males in charge of the teaching ward. Most disorders of this kind were still considered within the purview of domestic healing while others were judged 'improper' for institutional care. In Britain's competitive marketplace, however, boundaries for dealing with 'female diseases' remained fluid between 'irregulars', midwives, surgeons, male-midwives and gentlemen physicians, all wishing to expand the range of their practice by claiming expertise. Moreover, the growing popularity and professional standing of midwifery threatened gentlemen physicians who were determined to preserve their hold on women's diseases.[28] Eighteenth-century institutional gynaecology exemplified the ambiguities and contradictions surrounding both the explanations and management of female disorders in Edinburgh. It remained a poorly understood area of medicine, a casualty of traditional cultural biases and medical impotence.

Hysteria and hypochondriasis were widely considered fashionable nervous conditions in eighteenth-century Scotland caused by an affluent, civilised existence. Chapter 9 examines the paradoxical assignment of these traditional labels within the new context of charitable hospital practice.[29] After exploring the shifting constructions of rising vapours, relaxed fibres, fragile nerves, and an irritable uterus, the inquiry returns to archival information obtained from Edinburgh Infirmary patient registers, as well as medical student notebooks and lecture notes. These sources reveal that, faced with a new hospital clientele composed of poor people, physicians reconstructed and redefined the boundaries of these traditional diseases. A number of famished lower-class women were subjected to institutional 'hysterisation' despite Foucault's statement to the contrary, while lethargic and introspective men with gastric complaints received the hypochondriasis label.[30] Despite clinical ambiguities and flexible nosological labels, both disorders were primarily managed as somatic conditions, their causality expanded to include the tribulations and deprivations of the poor. By attempting to expose some of the puzzles surrounding the eighteenth-century construction of prominent neuroses in hospitals, this investigation concludes that both hysteria and hypochondriasis came to represent broad and ambiguous complexes of physical and mental suffering submerged within particular environmental, social and cultural contexts.

While the collected essays mostly extend and contribute to the complexity of a particular medical site in Scotland, namely Edinburgh, the information presented in the various studies should cast further light on the nature of the Enlightenment as a cultural phenomenon. In spite of all its paradoxes and contradictions, Scotland's medical institutions delivered what healing schemes since the dawn of history accomplished. They recognised and legitimised disability and suffering, made sense of the abnormal sensations and appearances through descriptions, labelling and explanations, provided reassurance and thus lessened anxiety, and furnished remedies to lessen pain and other troubling symptoms. Beyond such functions, Scottish contributions guided medicine towards a truly modern outlook regarding notions of health prevention, clinical scepticism and experimentation, and the pedagogical advantages of managing patients in hospitals.

Notes

1. For an overview, R.L. Emerson, 'Scotland', in A.C. Kors (ed.), *Encyclopedia of the Enlightenment*, 4 vols (Oxford: Oxford University Press, 2003), Vol. 4, 47–52; see also by the same author 'The Contexts of the Scottish Enlightenment', in A. Brodie (ed.), *The Cambridge Companion to the Scottish Enlightenment* (Cambridge: Cambridge University Press, 2003), 9–30.
2. Consult the contributions in T.M. Devine and J.R. Young (eds), *Eighteenth-Century Scotland: New Perspectives* (East Linton: Tuckwell Press, 1999).
3. P. Wood and C.W.J. Withers, 'Introduction: Science, Medicine and the Scottish Enlightenment: An Historiographical Overview', in C.W.J. Withers and P. Wood (eds), *Science and Medicine in the Enlightenment* (East Linton: Tuckwell Press, 2002), 1–16; P. Wood, 'Science in the Scottish Enlightenment', in Brodie, *op. cit.* (note 1), 94–116.
4. See, for example, J.R.R. Christie, 'The Origins and Development of the Scottish Scientific Community', in *History of Science*, 12 (1974), 122–41; J. B. Morell, 'Reflections on the History of Scottish Science', *ibid.*, 81–94; A.C. Chitnis, 'Universities: Medicine and Science', in *The Scottish Enlightenment* (London: Croom Helm, 1976), 124–94.
5. R.L. Emerson, 'Science and the Origins and Concerns of the Scottish Enlightenment', *History of Science*, 26 (1988), 333–66; T.L. Hankins, *Science and the Enlightenment* (Cambridge: Cambridge University Press, 1985); C. Lawrence, 'The Nervous System and Society in the Scottish Enlightenment', in B. Barnes and S. Shapin (eds), *Natural Order: Historical Studies of Scientific Culture* (Beverly Hills, Calif.: Sage Publications, 1979), 19–40.
6. See R.B. Sher, 'Science and Medicine in the Scottish Enlightenment: The Lessons of Book History', in P. Wood (ed.), *The Scottish Enlightenment: Essays in Reinterpretation* (Rochester, NY: Rochester University Press, 2000), 99–112.
7. For details, J.V. Pickstone, *Ways of Knowing: A New History of Science, Technology and Medicine* (Chicago: University of Chicago Press, 2001).
8. A. Ophir and S. Shapin, 'The Place of Knowledge: A Methodological Survey', *Science in Context*, 4 (1991), 3–17.
9. See J. Habermas, *Structural Transformation of the Public Sphere: An Inquiry into a Category of Bourgeois Society*, trans. T. Burger and F. Lawrence (Cambridge, Mass.: Harvard University Press, 1989).
10. T. Broman, 'The Habermasian Public Sphere and "Science in the Enlightenment"', *History of Science*, 26 (1998), 123–49; see also S. Sturdy, 'Introduction: Medicine, Health and the Public Sphere', in S. Sturdy (ed.), *Medicine, Health and the Public Sphere in Britain, 1600–2000* (London: Routledge, 2002), 1–24.

11. P. Wood, 'Science, the Universities, and the Public Sphere in Eighteenth-Century Scotland', *History of Universities,* 13 (1994), 99–135.
12. C.W.J. Withers, 'Towards a History and Geography in the Public Sphere', *History of Science,* 37 (1999), 45–78.
13. A.J. Kidd, 'Philanthropy and the Social History Paradigm', *Social History,* 21 (1996), 180–92.
14. A.L. Turner, *Story of a Great Hospital: The Royal Infirmary of Edinburgh 1729–1929* (Edinburgh: Oliver & Boyd, 1937), 39–67.
15. G.B. Risse, *Hospital Life in Enlightenment Scotland: Care and Teaching at the Royal Infirmary of Edinburgh* (New York: Cambridge University Press, 1986).
16. L. Rosner, 'The Royal Medical Society', in *Medical Education in The Age of Improvement* (Edinburgh: Edinburgh University Press, 1991).
17. Dissertations Read to the Royal Medical Society, 95 vols (Edinburgh: 1751–1833), MSS Collection, Edinburgh University Library.
18. G.B. Risse, 'The Brownian System of Medicine: Its Theoretical and Practical Implications', *Clio Medica,* 5 (1970), 45–51.
19. A. Wear, 'The History of Personal Hygiene', in W.F. Bynum and R. Porter (eds), *Companion Encyclopedia of the History of Medicine,* 2 vols (London: Routledge, 1993), Vol. 2, 1283–1308.
20. See R. Porter, 'Flesh and Form', in *Flesh in the Age of Reason* (New York: W.W. Norton, 2003), 227–43; W. Coleman, 'Health and Hygiene in the Encyclopédie: A Medical Doctrine for the Bourgeoisie', *Journal of the History of Medicine,* 29 (1974), 399–421.
21. W. Balée, 'Historical Ecology: Premises and Postulates', in W. Balée (ed.), *Advances in Historical Ecology* (New York: Columbia University Press, 1998), 13–29.
22. M.J. Dobson, 'Marshlands, Mosquitoes and Malaria', in *Contours of Death and Disease in Early Modern England* (Cambridge: Cambridge University Press, 1997), 306–27.
23. T.C. Smout, 'Lead Mining in Scotland, 1650–1850', in P.L. Payne (ed.), *Studies in Scottish Business History* (London: Cass, 1967), 103–35.
24. A.C. Aufderheide, 'Lead Poisoning', in K.F. Kiple (ed.), *The Cambridge World History of Human Disease* (New York: Cambridge University Press, 1993), 820–7.
25. G.B. Risse and J.H. Warner, 'Reconstructing Clinical Activities: Patient Records in Medical History,' *Social History of Medicine,* 5 (1992), 1–23.
26. C. Lawlor and A. Suzuki, 'The Disease of the Self: Representing Consumption, 1700–1830', *Bulletin of the History of Medicine,* 74 (2000), 458–94.
27. A. Lord, '"The Great Arcana of the Deity": Menstruation and Menstrual Disorders in Eighteenth-Century British Medical Thought', *Bulletin of the*

History of Medicine, 73 (1999), 38–63.

28. A. Wilson, *The Making of Man-Midwifery: Childbirth in England, 1660–1770* (Cambridge, Mass.: Harvard University Press, 1995).
29. For hysteria, see G.B. Risse, 'Hysteria at the Edinburgh Infirmary: The Construction of a Disease, 1770–1800', *Medical History,* 32, 1 (1988), 1–22; M.S. Micale, *Approaching Hysteria: Disease and Its Interpretations* (Princeton, NJ: Princeton University Press, 1995), 33–107.
30. J. Mullan, 'Hypochondria and Hysteria: Sensibility and the Physician', *The Eighteenth Century: Theory and Interpretation,* 25 (1984), 141–74.

PART I:
MEDICAL INSTITUTIONS

1

For God and Country: Duties and Rewards of Charity at the Edinburgh Infirmary

Within a 'public sphere' framework, this essay discusses the meaning and rewards of charity to specifically establish voluntary hospitals during the eighteenth century. The creation and management of the Edinburgh Infirmary serves as a convenient case study to revisit the perceived motives and actions of donors as well as the expectations and duties of the recipients – the 'deserving' poor allowed to enter the institution. Linked to this gift relationship were medicine's professional interests, especially the acquisition of clinical skills and therapeutic knowledge that created tensions between charitable and scientific objectives. Hospital-based relationships with colleagues and patients prompted new educational guidelines and ethical standards.

Introduction

> The present age has given examples of Charity which may be very properly recommended to imitation.... Among those actions is that of having contributed to an hospital for the sick.... No man can question whether wounds and sickness are not really painful; whether it be not worthy of a good man's care to restore those to ease and usefulness.
>
> Samuel Johnson (1758)[1]

In 1818, during a series of interviews with hospital managers, physicians and surgeons, a special committee appointed by the General Court of Contributors sought to probe a number of problems and deficiencies in the operation of the Royal Infirmary of Edinburgh. The performance of the institution's overseers, especially their efforts to obtain charitable contributions was cited. In the course of the interviews, it was learned that the current administration had successfully raised funds 'independently of the general anxiety to obtain donations'. Indeed, four years earlier, managers secured permission from the General Assembly of the Church of Scotland to conduct a general collection at churches over the entire 'kingdom'. In addition, they had made 'domiciliary visits' throughout the city of Edinburgh for a similar purpose. 'I have reason to know', said one respondent, 'that the Managers have at all times during my acquaintance with the hospital been zealous and active to increase the funds of the charity by every means in their power.'[2]

Hospitals became one of the most visible outlets for private philanthropy. Enthusiasts have judged the voluntary hospital movement in eighteenth-century Britain as one of the most noteworthy achievements of a century characterised as the 'Age of Charity'.[3] As explained by the surgeon, John Aikin (1747–1822),

> Providence has planted in our natures a benevolent principle which without waiting for duty to incite or reason to approve, inclines us by an involuntary emotion to relieve the distress of our fellow creatures to counterbalance the various evils and miseries of life.[4]

In supporting hospitals for 'every species of calamity entailed on human nature' the nation displayed a benevolence and humanity greater than that of other contemporary European states.[5] Modern historians, for their part, came to characterise this enterprise as a convenient stepping-stone in the quest for medical power. Sceptics charged that infirmaries were sinister laboratories for medical experimentation and true gateways to death. 'The chief indictment of hospital work at this period', wrote Thomas McKeown, 'is not that it did no good, but that it positively did harm.'[6] Such a profound divergence of opinion about the role and value of eighteenth-century hospitals deserves re-examination.

Recent scholarship on the role of 'associated philanthropy' in eighteenth-century Britain stresses the complexity surrounding charitable endeavours while examining the distinctive solutions that these voluntary institutions provided.[7] Building upon this historiography, the current analysis is limited to the care of the sick. It probes the interplay of forces responsible for the establishment and operation of a provincial British hospital, the Royal Infirmary of Edinburgh, during the eighteenth century. It seeks to present the charitable enterprise from the perspective of both benefactors and recipients. Donors, managers, caregivers, patients and students, all interact within a complex web of motives and actions. Using a variety of sources, this discussion attempts an examination of the forces involved in the genesis, development, and management of the institution. Broad public appeal, successful fundraising and responsible administration provided the foundations for assisting patients considered worthy of receiving care. Promising shelter and rest, regular meals, and basic nursing along with professional medical advice, hospitals attracted a wide sector of the working poor that lived primarily in urban areas and their immediate surroundings. In turn, the presence of sick individuals in the wards lured medical students to such institutions from around the world, anxious to witness and learn the intricacies of clinical management (Chapter 7).[8]

The meaning and aims of voluntary charity

Philanthropy played a central role in the genesis of voluntary hospitals in Britain. For a millennium and a half, charity had been considered a key Christian virtue.[9] As new relief institutions emerged during the sixteenth and seventeenth centuries, their governance increasingly fell into the hands of laypersons such as merchants, lawyers, and even physicians who replaced royalty, nobles and increasingly discredited clerics. Those imbued with a strong voluntary ethos not only established new criteria and boundaries for charitable relief to the poor; they also set novel standards for institutional management and fiscal accountability. Instead of random alms-giving and posthumous bequests, the new commercial philanthropy sought long-term commitments and focused contributions. During the eighteenth century, such collective benevolent efforts originated from an extensive patchwork of local community groups and societies under the guidance of patrons, officers and subscribers.[10]

Earlier conceptions of the poor as God's chosen people had already shifted from mostly spiritual to economic issues in the sixteenth century, a transformation reflected in the classification of paupers into those deserving and not deserving of charitable assistance. The former – 'the poor of Jesus Christ' – were perceived as having unwittingly fallen into that condition through circumstances beyond their control. This group had been traditionally composed of vulnerable members of society – the very young, old, the infirm, widows, and orphans – but the scope widened to include the working classes of both sexes. By contrast, 'the poor of the Devil', constituted a motley group of able-bodied but wilfully idle individuals which included unruly beggars and potential criminals, chronic drunkards and lunatics endowed with a 'mendicant spirit'. [11]

Such distinctions among the poor combined traditional Christian notions of morality with early modern mercantilist criteria. In seventeenth-century Europe, charity remained organised at the community level. Earlier in England, reformulation of the Poor Laws in 1563 and the Act of 1601 established a tradition of locally financed and administered relief outside the religious frameworks. Based on a mixture of religious and secular motives, British reforms continued into the eighteenth century, leading to the establishment of charity schools, orphanages, workhouses, prisons, and hospitals called 'infirmaries'.[12] The latter term specifically designated institutions of a purely medical nature to be distinguished from many traditional European establishments that functioned as old age residences, shelters, and convalescent homes.[13] Much of this activity was designed to bridge the growing chasm between the rich and the poor, as well as, maintain public order.

From the beginning, modern charitable assistance was closely linked with employment and health. A growing capitalist market economy relied on a healthy labour force. Additionally, if workers were forced to abandon their activities because of illness, they placed their autonomy and the future of their families at risk. Sickness was ubiquitous. However, it was now considered important to confront and ameliorate its effects. For European nations to become both politically and economically powerful, they needed expanding and healthy population capable of furnishing enough manpower for the successful expansion of agriculture, manufacturing, and commerce. Thus modern national ascendancy and economic well-being were closely linked to prosperous societies. It was also important to maintain large standing armies and to create a larger base of tax-paying citizens. Such geopolitical objectives could only be achieved with populations whose numbers and productivity were enhanced through improvements in their material welfare.[14] To be ultimately successful, enactment of social policies that included measures to preserve and mend the health of workers was imperative. As a result, eighteenth-century 'police' assigned greater priority to questions of health and medicine (Chapter 4).[15]

Given their social utility, health-enhancing activities targeted the working poor and were quickly sponsored in many European countries through centralised bureaucratic organisations. Mercantilist efforts to improve health were organised under the rubric of 'medical police', allowing physicians significant contact with the lower sectors of the population for the first time in history.[16] Suddenly, the range of health-related activities widened. Greater emphasis was placed on environmental health, infant and maternal welfare, as well as military and naval medicine. The underlying premise of this medicalisation effort was that human sickness could be adequately prevented, controlled, and even removed by the conscious and deliberate application of enlightened views concerning health and disease.[17]

In Britain, however, efforts to improve the size and health of the population were left to local and private initiatives rather than governmental action. For this purpose, English tradition brought the mobilisation of public opinion for needed reforms through 'political arithmetic', the collection and presentation of statistics illustrating particular problems. Beginning with John Graunt's *Natural and Political Observations Upon the Bills of Mortality* published in 1662 and William Petty's *Essays in Political*

Arithmetic of 1687, Britons diligently gathered the demographic data necessary to persuade potential reformers of the deplorable health conditions among working people in the British Isles.[18] Rapid urbanisation and the problems of early industrialisation played important roles in creating these problems. Unlike other European countries – notably France and the German states – Britain in the early-eighteenth century had retained only five establishments devoted to care of the sick–poor in the entire United Kingdom. In 1545, Henry VIII had abolished all religious institutions in England, including a series of hospitals. As a result, only the municipal authorities in London had founded a few new establishments from bequests of wealthy merchants.[19]

While numerous parishes during the eighteenth century provided relief and assistance to their paupers in almshouses established under the Poor Laws, this rudimentary welfare system left a significant gap for members of the lower-class, working population. In what Foucault perceived as 'functional discrimination', the British welfare system categorised them as 'deserving' poor, a characterisation based on notions of moral discipline and economic productivity, as well as social control.[20] The widely accepted social contract between the classes in Georgian Britain was based on the idea that it was 'as much the duty of the poor to labour when they are able as it is for the rich to help them when they are sick'.[21] 'On the lower classes of our fellow citizens alone', wrote Thomas Bassnett Percival, a chaplain and son of the famous medical ethicist, 'we depend for food, lodging, and all the conveniences and comforts of life.' 'But health is essential to their capacity for labour', he continued, 'and in this labour, I fear, it is too often sacrificed.'[22] Employment, in turn, allowed people to join the burgeoning consumer society and contribute to the prosperity of the nation.

This lopsided relationship between the affluent and labouring classes of Britain paralleled older hierarchical social relations. The responsibility of providing assistance fell on the wealthy classes. Thus, Percival argued, the obligation to provide relief was based on the notion that 'he who at once toils and suffers for our benefit, has a multiplied claim to our support, and to withhold it would be equally chargeable with folly, ingratitude and injustice.'[23] Private benefactors were drawn from particular social groups with established cultural values of piety, generosity and virtue. Their aid included free medical assistance, either at home, or increasingly in institutions such as infirmaries and dispensaries. Young and productive people were the preferred recipients of charitable medical care. The disabilities afflicting heads of family were of particular concern because of the potential destitution of their dependants. In turn, those who received charity had few opportunities to reciprocate the kindness except for offering promises to sustain their 'deserving' behaviour and contribute to the national wealth.[24]

Much has been written about the motivations for charitable assistance.[25] Historians have traditionally stressed the individual piety and altruism of donors,[26] but there is growing consensus that gifting is a complex form of social exchange involving reciprocal relationships. Such a framework, derived from anthropological models, is not meant to solely view charitable acts through the lens of modern cynicism. Rather, it realistically dissects the social and psychological factors involved in the process.[27] Gifts were never entirely disinterested, and individual donors had much to gain in moral reputation and social status. Self-promotion, vanity and a sense of purpose energised philanthropists. Their voluntary participation could be assessed as personal investments for political and cultural influence as well as economic gain. Often spurred by the leadership of a prominent local personality, benefactors clustered into committees and boards sponsoring meetings, elections, reports, and social functions. Admission to such networks contributed to the establishment of urban elites identified by their piety and humanitarianism. In fact, it could be argued that the social contacts were more valuable to affluent donors than the charitable sums provided.[28] Their ultimate reward was the 'esteem of mankind'.[29] Often, this charitable impulse contributed to create visible public improvements that enhanced the image and status of an entire community and country.[30]

During the eighteenth century, Enlightened humanitarianism in Britain came to represent a new sensibility toward the plight of the poor, combining Christian devotion with social utility. A veritable renaissance of urban centres with their prospering early industries created opportunities for its more affluent dwellers to become involved in civic affairs. The purpose was to 'civilise' provincial towns such as Edinburgh through the establishment of clubs and learned societies, libraries, bookstores and printed sources.[31] With the central government unwilling to address social ills, and relief to the poor failing, volunteers took up the challenge at the community level. Charity shifted from individual to institutional forms of giving, creating more social distance between donors and recipients.

Britain's voluntary hospital movement embodied the traditional human gift relationship: a moral commitment to giving and receiving traced to the dawn of time.[32] For donors with strong religious beliefs, the philanthropic impetus to provide temporary shelter for those who were sick and had no one to care for them went back to the very origins of the hospital in early Christianity.[33] Quoting the Scriptures, charity was inseparable from piety, it was considered Christ-like. Donors were quite self-congratulatory, frequently posing as generous and pious souls. These religious dimensions of

charitable giving were not only portrayed as Christian but also Protestant. 'Since the Reformation has banished ignorance and restored Christianity, we have nobly distinguished ourselves by donations of another kind, such as are truly styled charities', read one funding appeal citing the Scriptural recommendations contained in the Gospel of St Matthew as 'an exercise of that most Christian virtue'. A theology based on 'good works' instead of predestination energised the faithful. The celestial hereafter remained the ultimate destination. Nevertheless, the focus had shifted towards the more pragmatic goal of focusing on current needs of particular communities.

Another popular impetus for charity was based on perceptions generated from demographic and economic data. One could demonstrate love for the country by saving the distressed 'lives of multitudes' who had fallen ill and be potentially lost to the community. One typical eighteenth-century representative of the British philanthropic movement was John Bellers, a Quaker merchant, who in 1714 published a work titled *Essay Towards the Improvement of Physick* based on London's mortality statistics. According to Beller's calculations, almost half of the twenty thousand deaths each year in London from an 'army of diseases' could have been prevented or cured. In fact, charged Bellers, Britain lost about one hundred thousand inhabitants each year 'for want of timely advice and suitable medicines'. For Bellers, this represented a significant drain of national resources because each worker was actually worth £200 to the British economy.[34] Bellers suggested that part of the problem could be remedied through the foundation and construction of hospitals or infirmaries. His proposal to protect and restore the productivity of the working poor illuminated the link between charitable efforts and economic development with its demands for a healthy workforce.

Framed in this fashion, hospitals became useful instruments in the war against poverty. According to political arithmeticians such as Bellers, hospitals also contributed indirectly to the nation's power and wealth. By providing medical treatments designed to speed the recovery of gainfully employed individuals, especially breadwinners, families of the sick were also spared from destitution, and the impact on the local economy lessened. Indeed, from a welfare point of view, hospitals were perceived to be an excellent investment of local resources. Philanthropic giving was perceived as a welcome form of taxation for the affluent to avoid higher welfare rates, maintain their class hegemony, and contribute to an active workforce. Thus, from the 1720s onward, the enterprise of erecting several infirmaries in London and the provinces became a source of civic pride and charitable achievement.[35]

Hospital foundations were traditionally created by specific bequests left by persons in their wills. A collective of charitable individuals capable of coordinating a sustained fundraising drive was necessary to avoid the unexpected, unreliable, and precarious reliance on individual bequests. Fundraising focused on specific monetary targets and wise spending on rent or construction of a house for the patients. Each local foundation was, therefore, the creation of a philanthropic group: a 'democracy' of donors or subscribers that included a broad spectrum of upper- and middle-class members, from the landed classes to the clergy, businessmen, professionals, and artisans. From the start, each benefactor – individual, corporate body, parish, or community organisation – pledged to contribute money and promised to continue this support on a long-term basis. Indeed, infirmary patrons throughout the country usually went on to pledge money or stock. Their payments were made quarterly, annually, or even in the form of life memberships. Others made donations in kind, including free labour, building materials, supplies and furnishings. In certain locations, additional funds were collected from special Sunday church collections, benefit concerts and theatrical performances together with the placement of charity boxes at inns.[36] To spark a charitable campaign, the philanthropic association usually relied on the services of a prominent civic leader willing to lend his prestige and social connections. In an attempt to add further momentum, publicity in the form of announcements or declarations of purpose circulated in pamphlets and newspapers. From a financial point of view, benefactors selected the model of a joint stock company from the business world for their financial arrangements. Each donor making a pledge became a subscriber or stockholder in this charitable enterprise. In exchange for their gifts, benefactors were entitled to participate in the annual assemblies and given 'dividends' in the form of printed 'letters' for admission to the hospital to be bestowed to 'deserving' individuals of his or her acquaintance. The right to nominate or recommend for entry a specific number of patients to newly created hospitals was a perk as long as subscription was paid. Moreover, according to their personal expertise or influence, many donors became members of the hospital's board of governors, responsible for guiding and managing the institutions. Not surprisingly, such stewardship had important social advantages. Periodic assemblies of subscribers, meetings of managers, and festivities allowed the ruling elites to come together, share and enjoy their charitable interests and experiences. Subscribers usually attended annual convocations while managers held monthly meetings. In the process, they garnered prestige and created new networks of influence and patronage. Thus, to prospective British donors the enterprise of erecting hospitals seemed to offer excellent opportunities for combining notions of personal piety with social and commercial self-interest.[37]

From its inception, the British drive to establish and operate voluntary hospitals attracted cynics and detractors. Intentions of certain donors became more transparent. Bernard Mandeville's (1670–1733) satiric comment, in 1723, that 'pride and vanity have built more hospitals than all of the virtues together' was part of this physician-turned-social-critic's view of contemporary charity as 'counterfeited' virtue in the new commercial world. Mandeville agreed with the proposition that 'to have sufficient hospitals for sick and wounded' was 'an indispensable duty both in peace and war' but he took issue with the notion that giving money would 'make a full atonement in the next world for the sins committed in this'.[38] Mandeville's efforts to make distinctions between religious and mercantile charitable motives actually led to a further unification of both purposes in a country striving for trade and economic prosperity.[39] With the proliferation of charitable projects, the hunt for suitable benefactors accelerated and some charitable institutions vying for funds began employing professional fund-raisers to beef-up their endowments. 'The open competitions between different hospitals and the animosity with which their patrons oppose one another may prejudice weak minds against them all', was Samuel Johnson's judgement in 1758.[40] As time went on, the sick–poor lodged in hospitals seemed to become a convenient backdrop for eager patrons bent on displaying social conscience and discharging their benevolent obligations in a most public manner. From that point of view, contributions or subscriptions to hospital funds could even be viewed as initiation fees to elite communal brotherhoods focusing on charitable activities to foster social recognition and advancement.

Edinburgh's 'pious and necessary design': the making of an infirmary

Authors have already pointed out the considerable political and economic, albeit humiliating, effects of Scotland's 1707 union with England. In particular, Edinburgh had lost its identity and social prominence previously accorded to the city as seat of Parliament.[41] A crowded town of about twenty-five thousand inhabitants in the early decades of the century, it continued to stagnate within its old medieval walls. Its citizens made efforts to restore some the grandeur. Among them was a program of public works designed to prevent unemployment. Town Council member George Drummond (1687–1766), soon to be Edinburgh's elected Lord Provost, supported the plan.[42] In a related effort, Drummond's friend, the surgeon John Monro (1670–1740), Deacon of the Incorporation of Surgeons, sought to promote the city as a centre of medical and surgical learning. While first ostensibly directed towards the procurement of a professorship for his surgeon son

Alexander, Monro's efforts culminated in the establishment of a chemical laboratory in 1721. With support from powerful local political figures such as Archibald Campbell and the Royal College of Physicians, a number of practitioners were appointed professors at the new Faculty of Medicine in 1726.[43]

A pamphlet issued in 1721 also laid out a rationale for creating a voluntary hospital in the city. The anonymous publication was attributed to Alexander Monro Primus (1697–1767), who had recently been elected the first Professor of Anatomy at the University. The brochure was believed to express views he shared with his father.[44] This document was a typical example of the confluence of religious, humanitarian, economic, and medical considerations involved in such a charitable foundation. The religious justification reiterated the notion that 'as men and Christians we have the strongest inducements and obligations to this sort of Charity, as it is warmly recommended and enjoined in the Gospel as one of the greatest Christian Duties.'[45] Contemporary Scottish Presbyterianism strongly favoured the practice of a selfless public virtue or 'benevolence' for the fulfilment of God's laws and the attainment of human happiness and perfection. Influenced by the philosopher Adam Ferguson (1723–1816) and other moderate ministers from the Church of Scotland, such 'love of mankind' was also an essential part of a program designed to raise the reputation of Scotland. The co-operative 'public spirit' needed to be preserved.[46] Monro's 1721 pamphlet also revealed a secular rationale for building an infirmary congruent with Enlightenment notions of the plight of the sick poor. 'Humanity and Compassion naturally prompt us to relieve our Fellow Creatures when in such deplorable Circumstances', he wrote, 'naked, starving and in the outmost Distress from Pain and Trouble of Body and Anguish of Soul.'[47] In Scotland, humanitarianism was considered the most prominent moral virtue of the times. Compassion was framed within contemporary notions of 'sensibility' and 'sympathy'. Both were important physiological concepts linked to new theories on the functioning of the human nervous system (Chapter 4). Sensibility was not only a vital capacity for perceiving and reacting to outside stimuli but its meaning had been extended to become a desirable moral and social quality – a capacity for feeling – subject to refinement and balance. Later in the century, prominent moral philosophers, such as Glasgow's Francis Hutcheson (1694–1746) and others such as David Hume (1711–76) and Adam Smith (1723–90) encouraged the cultivation of this natural instinct. 'Gentle sensibility' was considered essential for enhanced emotional exchanges, especially for those who wished to bestow charity and benevolence on others.[48] For Scots, 'sympathy' or humanity was another virtuous component of human nature closely linked to sensibility and thus to the nervous system.[49] Based on the work of another Scottish academic, Robert Whytt (1714–66), Cullen wrote that 'the nerves and nervous fibres of the body have all a sympathy and consent with one another' (Chapters 8 and 9.[50] While physicians used the notion of sympathy to explain reciprocal influences between bodily organs and the functional integrity of the human organism, philosophers expanded this notion to social relationships. For Adam Smith, David Hume, and others, sympathy became the capacity to reach out, connect and identify with other persons' sentiments and troubles. It was considered a natural feeling-part of a person's 'language of the heart that makes us feel for the distresses of our fellow creatures'.[51] Sympathy as 'gentle virtue' fuelled benevolence and contributed to morality in an age of narcissism and indifference to others generated by the growth of modern society (Chapter 4).[52]

The commercial impact of charitable actions was duly recognised as another rationale for establishing a hospital in Edinburgh. The 1721 pamphlet explained that 'as the Relief is a Duty, so it is no less Advantage to the Nation, for as many as are recovered in an *Infirmary* are so many working Hands gained to the Country.'[53] In Edinburgh, the plight of 'deserving' urban servants was a particular case in point. Male or female, they worked for low wages in most local households, performing a variety of tasks, from the menial to the intimate. Their frequent turnover generated unemployment and destitution. Illness only exacerbated the problem, as employers often sought to rid themselves of their helpers for fear of contagion and payment of medical bills.[54] Their institutional rehabilitation resonated with the goals of improving the physical and moral condition of the working poor. Finally, Monro's brochure recognised an important role for hospitals in pedagogy: 'that students in Physick and Surgery might hereby have rather a better and easier Opportunity of Experience than they have hitherto had by studying abroad'.[55] Preventing Scots from seeking medical training on the Continent while attracting foreign students to Edinburgh was a key objective with obvious economic implications. Clinical teaching at a local institution could become a critical factor in improving the reputation of medical studies in the city.[56] Like Leyden's teaching hospital, the St. Caecilia Gasthuis, an infirmary in Edinburgh would function as a university-affiliated institution for the promotion and dissemination of clinical knowledge.

In spite of Monro's persuasive arguments, the appeal failed. After a few years, however, another effort was launched by a more powerful and established institution: the Royal College of Physicians. Since 1682 some of its Fellows had volunteered to treat poor patients twice a week in their own hall, providing them with free advice and medicines at cost. By the early 1720s, however, this charitable gesture was thought to be somewhat futile, since many of the needy individuals seeking help sold their medicines for food. In response, the College established a free drug repository and then a dispensary funded by mandatory contributions from the College's Licentiates and Fellows. Yet, a more dependable solution for providing medical treatments was to institutionalise the needy in a hospital. Thus, the College decided to launch another fund-drive for establishing an Infirmary. Coincidentally, Drummond discovered in 1725 that the owners of a fishery company, for which he had been a manager, wanted to dissolve their failing business. Sensing an opportunity, the College and Drummond persuaded the owners of the fishery to transfer their shares to the Bank of Scotland where they would form the basis for a charitable fund 'as to be of Universal Use and Advantage to the Nation'. Among the philanthropic options was a Society for the Propagation of Christian Knowledge, a Linen Manufactory or a Hospital for the Sick and Wounded. In light of the College of Physicians' initiative and with support from surgical circles, the latter alternative seemed most attractive.

Not surprisingly, another anonymous pamphlet – the author was probably again John Monro – strongly supported this choice by arguing once more that the expected influx of students to attend the local Medical School was unlikely to occur 'unless for the opportunity of hospitals to learn the practice in'. In fact, Scottish students would avoid the expenses of travelling abroad for their training.[57] To broaden the appeal, the anonymous author waxed eloquently about the potential of such a hospital to enhance Scotland's, and in particular Edinburgh's, prominence abroad. He went on to make the standard demographic and economic arguments that 'the strength and power' of the community depended on the 'riches and numbers of inhabitants'. 'I imagine it would be no hard matter to demonstrate that a hospital for sick and wounded would increase both in this country', he concluded. Such an institution could also play another useful role: to screen out beggars who claimed to be sick, and to expose those who had made fraudulent claims, treating only those suffering from legitimate sickness. This function would gain substantial support among landowners that were burdened with relief of the poor on their estates, and at a time when the authorities claimed the country was being overrun 'by multitudes of strange beggars'.[58] Support for such 'undeserving' individuals took away funds that could be distributed to the 'real' objects of charity, notably the old and infirm.

As collective efforts to secure funds for the establishment of the Infirmary got under way, the College of Physicians made another pledge in

1727. It promised to send some of their Fellows on a voluntary basis to 'faithfully attend' patients at the proposed facility, a visible gesture of support designed to bolster the fundraising campaign. However, a similar offer from the Incorporation of Surgeons was eventually declined, in part because of a gradual political shift in Edinburgh's Town Council away from supporting craft guilds. Drummond and Monro Primus leaned in favour of academic and professional interests represented by the University and the College of Physicians. In fact the surgeons' leadership was even excluded from playing a role in the future management of the institution. This development prompted locals to characterise the planned establishment as the 'Physicians' Hospital' and a few years later triggered efforts to create a rival surgical institution.[59]

Given these multiple rationales and professional objectives, how did Edinburgh's philanthropic groups actually raise funds?[60] The release of the fisheries stock was followed in 1727 with a subscription campaign. With city approval and support from the Bank of Scotland, Drummond was ultimately successful in rounding up 352 subscribers who collectively pledged the necessary sum of £2,000 to purchase the entire stock before June 1727.[61] The list of contributors constituted a veritable who's who in Scotland. Cited among the aristocratic donors were the Duke of Hamilton and the Earls of Buchan, Findlater, Lauderdale, Leven and Loudon, as well as the Marquis of Lothian and the Countess of Bute and Forfar. Also contributing were members of prestigious families such as the Erskines, Dundas and Drummonds. The list included senators from the College of Justice. Other lawyers, ministers, merchants, writers, physicians and surgeon-apothecaries, even goldsmiths and sea captains were among the first contributors. Additional funds came from collections taken at the more than seventy parish churches on a specific 'Infirmary Sunday'. In addition, the Honourable Ladies of the Assembly of the Church of Scotland organised several 'benefit nights'. At a general meeting of the hospital contributors, held on 13 January 1728, it was announced that the entire sum had been subscribed. Armed with income from these securities, a small house near the College on Robertson' Close was leased and outfitted to become the first Infirmary. The institution – soon dubbed the 'Little House' – opened its doors on 6 August 1729 under the supervision of a housekeeper and with an initial capacity of six beds.

Rules for management of the Infirmary had already been formally approved. From the start, a court of twenty managers was elected. Four to six were to be replaced annually. These men represented distinct constituencies beginning with the Lord Provost of Edinburgh or his deputy, the Dean of the Guild. Other members were the Deacon Convenor of

Crafts, and the President of the College of Physicians together with four additional Fellows. Two of the physicians had to be university professors. There was also the Professor of Anatomy and two members from the Corporation of Surgeons, one senator from the College of Justice, another member from the Faculty of Advocates and a Clerk to the Signet, a Minister of the Gospel, and six contributors residing in or near Edinburgh. In turn, the Court of Managers selected twelve 'ordinary' individuals from their ranks 'whose residence and business will best allow them to look after the affairs of the hospital'. Two of these men were designated 'visitors', charged with touring the Infirmary at least once a month, by turns, closely inspecting 'the treatment and diet of the patients, the conduct of the housekeeper or mistress, the behaviour of servants and patients and the whole economy of the house'.[62]

To ensure the propriety of the Infirmary's financial affairs, the managers hired a full-time treasurer to be in charge of receiving donations, rents and other income as well as disbursing funds 'for the ordinary economy of the house'. He was assisted by an accountant who abstracted all transactions and inserted them into books with the help of a 'clerk of corporation', a person who wrote all 'extracts, orders, memorials and other such papers' necessary to document the management of the Infirmary. Two annual meetings, in January and again in July, brought together all twenty Edinburgh managers for the election of a treasurer, hospital clerk, and housekeeper, as well as to set salaries for the hospital personnel. Local newspapers published in advance the dates for these gatherings. Before the general assembly, the twelve 'ordinary' managers closest to the actual administration of the establishment were required to 'lay upon the table' the records of their administration. These records included lists of patients admitted to the house. The 'ordinary' managers, in turn, demanded that the treasurer, physicians, clerks, apothecary, and housekeeper presented their reports at least four times per year in the months of February, May, August, and November. Given the amount of business that required their attention, managers actually met once every month. After examining the records, the ordinary managers made decisions about personnel matters, purchases, and repairs. Careful minutes were kept regarding what was said and decided at all these meetings.[63]

Such arrangements offered an unusual degree of transparency to the proceedings and financial management while fostering co-operation among members of Edinburgh's elite citizenry in this charitable enterprise. Open voting and majority rule reflected a degree of egalitarianism not found in corporate and parliamentary proceedings among the ruling classes. As a result, the democratic government and financial management of the Edinburgh Infirmary served to weld together leading sectors of the city. It provided civic cohesion and upward social mobility to numerous donors.[64]

Even prospective patients became aware of the importance of this enterprise, often seeking repeated admissions to the hospital as if it were an 'entitlement' of their 'deserving' status. In its first year of operation, however, the 'Little House' could only admit a total of thirty-five patients. A few additional individuals were seen in the consulting room on an outpatient basis. Compared with the 350 original donors, including the twenty managers, the ratio was overwhelmingly in favour of those dispensing, rather than receiving, charity. Nevertheless, the enterprise was considered a success. As a result, in 1736, King George II incorporated the hospital as the Royal Infirmary of Edinburgh through a royal charter.

In addition to displaying the monarchy's political authority, royal patronage was meant to spur further acts of benevolence.[65] By this time, Edinburgh surgeons had set up their own hospital financed by several practitioners willing to attend patients. Founders uttered similar charitable rationales for its establishment, namely that it would prove profitable for Scotland since rehabilitated workers were the 'riches of a trading nation'. Surgeons would no longer be forced to complete their training in Leyden and Paris. The hospital featured a surgical theatre that could accommodate more than fifty students. Indeed, this institution was purposely designed for the benefit of surgical students and apprentices who were willing to pay for the privilege of visiting the patients. Plans for creating a school of midwifery were also contemplated (Chapter 8).[66]

In spite of careful screening of admissions, the 'Little House' rapidly became inadequate for the needs of the sick poor seeking care. Overcrowding also hampered clinical rounds and the performance of operations. Clinical teaching languished. In 1738, the managers readily admitted that the 'reputation of the house will rise in proportion as the number of patients cured increases'.[67] Questions of efficiency and pedagogy prompted a call to erect a much larger building for housing more patients available for study. This decision probably owed a great deal to the success of the surgical teaching facility, which was also planning its own expansion. After negotiations between the Infirmary managers and the Incorporation of Surgeons, the two institutions were merged in 1738. Surgeon-apothecaries, who provided the bulk of medical care in Edinburgh, won access and educational opportunities for their apprentices in a future facility.[68]

Planning a new hospital building, based on designs by the famous architect Robert Adam (1728–92), followed that same year. Two fundraising pamphlets – the first penned by 'Philanthropus' in 1738, and the other by 'Philasthenes' ('friend of the weak') a year later – laid out some of the rationales for engaging in this project. Both documents mirror some of the arguments already presented in the 1721 article attributed to Alexander

Monro Primus. 'Philanthropus' was emphatic about attracting large numbers of students from outside Scotland. A self-proclaimed, unabashed 'lover of this country', the author was determined to foster the city's prosperity.[69] Instead of going to Oxford and Cambridge or abroad for their medical studies, the hope was that Dissenters and Catholics from England and Ireland, as well as the Scots themselves, would matriculate in Edinburgh. The economic advantages for Edinburgh in hosting students would appeal to the commercial and scientific interests of the city and generate broad support. Guesthouses and innkeepers, merchants and shopkeepers, taverns and other entertainment establishments, even book dealers would all become recipients of the students' largesse, not to mention university professors, extramural teachers and tutors who lectured by charging fees. In fact, following the example of surgical apprentices who paid to attend their hospital, the new Infirmary would receive a sizeable income from selling admission tickets. According to 'Philasthenes', the costly construction project needed to be developed in several stages because of a paucity of available funds.[70]

While financial and pedagogical motives seemed to drive this new charitable effort, religion was never excluded. For many, charity remained a key Christian virtue conferring blessings on benefactors as well as morally recharging the recipients. Healing the sick remained a central aspect of Christian good works, exemplified by the published sermon of a Scottish minister, Ninian Niving, raising funds for the Infirmary. 'Jesus Christ descends from his throne on his Father's right side, lays aside his robes of light, and clothing himself with rags, assumes the various diseases incident to humankind', he preached. Niving asserted that 'the Lord begs to build him a house to reside in while some of his faithful servants, eminent for their skill in physick, minister to his cure.'[71] He also reassured his audience that 'persons to be received into the hospital want that which makes poverty tolerable.' Implicit in his rhetoric was that patients' recovery hastened their return to their labour and industry, lessening further burdens on the public.[72] An anonymous letter directed to prospective patients stressed that the key objective for donors was to help ameliorate the link between disease and destitution, 'to find the honest labourer whose family has long pined with hunger' because of his indisposition, restore the breadwinner to health and save his family.[73] By contrast, sick inmates from the local jail were not admitted. Oddly, this prohibition was couched in hygienic terms; denying admittance prevented the spread of 'gaol fever' among hospital inmates. This was a somewhat disingenuous position, however, since Infirmary physicians routinely accepted other contagious cases, including patients suffering from smallpox and venereal disease.[74]

Support for the new Infirmary building came from a cross-section of Scottish merchants, professionals, and prominent landowners.[75] The local citizenry – rich and poor – was inspired to mount a truly collaborative effort supported by the Town Council, the Scottish Masonic brotherhood, as well as workers such as plumbers, slaters and glaziers, who freely contributed part of their materials and labour. Merchants made gifts of timber and stone; farmers and carters supplied carriages. Bedding, furnishings, dishes and other supplies were also donated. Built of stone on a two-acre parcel of land, the foundation was laid in 1738. This 'noble piece of masonry' resembled a large Palladian townhouse with numerous and ample windows to facilitate ventilation.[76] The first patients were admitted to the partially completed building in December 1741. While still under construction, the Infirmary managers continued to seek further funding. A donation from the Earl of Hopetoun in 1742 created enough income to outfit a five-bed ward for housing patients that were considered incurable. The outfitting of twelve cells on the ground floor to house affluent 'mad' people led to additional income. In 1748, a special agent, Adam Anderson, was hired in London to raise more funds among the wealthy. To entice his fickle prospects, Anderson followed the fashionable trend to make advertising attractive. He displayed a set of prints depicting the Adam-designed building in its full splendour. Additional prints went to Ireland and the British colonies. A number of bequests followed. Scotsmen living abroad became involved in the fundraising drive, while the sister of George Drummond sought assistance from Quaker communities in England. Names of all contributors were recorded and a copy displayed at the Infirmary for public viewing.

Financial considerations also prompted the creation of a twenty-four-bed soldiers' ward during the 1745 Scottish rebellion. The costs of hospitalisation were borne by the soldiers themselves, with the stipulated daily charges deducted from their pay by the army's paymaster and turned over to the Infirmary's treasurer. Army commanders freely supplied the institution with guards and provisions. Subsequent arrangements between the British Army and the city of Edinburgh led to the assignment of a Royal Invalid Fund to the Infirmary, an endowment that provided steady income for expenses related to the care of sick and invalid members of the armed forces.[77] Upon its final completion in 1748 with a capacity of about 150 beds, the Infirmary quickly became a source of civic pride. Benevolence had created a veritable city landmark; 'undoubtedly the most noble of the institutions in Edinburgh reared by the hand of charity.'[78] The building set new standards of hospital construction and its floor plan became a blueprint for similar institutions at home and abroad. Following the organisation of clinical lectures at the Infirmary by John Rutherford (1695–1779), Professor of the Practice of Physic, receipts from student tickets soared, prompting managers to authorise the creation of a medical teaching ward. The additional expense to outfit this ward was easily met by this growing source of revenue.[79] In the late 1750s, the Infirmary also participated in a decentralised system of care organised by the Royal Navy for its sick seamen. This created an additional ward especially devoted for the care of sick mariners. This equally financially rewarding commitment increased markedly during the war with France, as fears of a possible invasion of Britain in the mid-1790s prompted a squadron from the British North Sea Fleet to be stationed in the Firth of Forth.[80]

This policy of leasing available hospital space not devoted to charitable patients sometimes took some odds turns. First, several rooms were provided to a local apothecary. In 1750, an entire third floor ward was rented to the Hamilton Company and converted into a print shop and warehouse.[81] In that same year, the managers were informed that a Scottish physician, Archibald Kerr, had bequeathed upon his death a 420-acre Jamaican plantation to the Infirmary. However, this unexpected gift of land and slaves yielded modest rents – often delayed or unpaid – while creating for nearly half a century a large volume of paperwork with the authorities in Kingston.[82] More reliable income was obtained from properties located near the hospital. These smaller houses were originally acquired in order to prevent further construction of high-rise buildings in the immediate neighbourhood which might threaten proper ventilation of the Infirmary and compromise the salubrity of the site. Finally, the shrewd managers decided on another potentially profitable venture: a public bathhouse with a separate entrance located on the ground floor of the Infirmary and exclusively intended 'for people of the city'. The idea came from Alexander Monro Primus in 1748, following the earlier closure of a similar establishment sponsored by the Incorporation of Surgeons. Well-appointed and staffed by a retinue of servants and 'rubbers', the marbled 'bagnio' was intended to evoke the splendour of its Roman and Renaissance predecessors. The facilities opened on 1 July 1756 with prospective users paying separate fees for admission, bathing, massage, and meals. Wine and milk were available from the Infirmary's stores.[83]

In 1771, Infirmary managers circulated a new request for special funds to support a ward in the Infirmary exclusively devoted to the care of local servants. As early as 1738, the Infirmary managers had planned to set aside twenty-six beds for the care of sick servants engaged by 'well-disposed families in town'. That is, if the employers were willing to pay for the costs of hospitalisation. But the scheme only became a reality in 1755 when negotiations with the Town Council and the Presbytery of Edinburgh established a mechanism for annual charitable collections at all metropolitan churches to be earmarked for this purpose. Following the first collection on 29 December 1756, two separate ten-bed wards for male and female domestics were established.[84] Servants were frequent inmates from the inception of the Infirmary, and were often singled out as particularly vulnerable and deserving of assistance because of their extreme dependency (Chapters 8 and 9). Because they lived in close personal contact with their affluent masters, servants were also emblematic of the potential for charity to be a bridge between the rich and poor. A pamphlet argued that 'such is the poverty and too often the inattention of some families in this city, that when their servants are taken ill of fevers, or other acute distempers, many of them are left to shift for themselves, without money and without friends.' The petition went on to stress that 'many are so straitened or ill accommodated in their houses' that it was necessary to remove them to rented rooms where they were left alone or in the hands of ignorant individuals, without remedies and food. 'Hereby many useful lives are annually lost to the public', concluded the appeal.[85]

The success of the hospital required the establishment of a General Register of Patients. According to the 1730 regulations, this Register was to enter the names of all incoming patients, with a listing of their residence or parish of birth, together with their age, name of disease, date of admission and dismissal and discharge status.[86] By the early 1740s, the managers added an Admissions and Refusals Book, a Ward Ledger and Prescription Book. Designed to assist the institution's managers in their administrative endeavours, this extensive documentation answered the demands for fiscal accountability from charitable patrons – even though there were periodic recording delay errors and the occasional loss of entire volumes. The registers and journals also came to be of great value to physicians and students attending the Infirmary. Moreover, Edinburgh student-selected case histories and lecture notes based on the management of these patients helped preserve clinical experiences and medical therapies (Chapter 4).

Charity, explained one author, 'is mere ostentation unless proper attention is paid to the application of the sums destined to purposes of public utility.'[87] In 1770, for example, the Infirmary's treasurer's accounts revealed a total income of nearly £2,600. Of this sum, thirty-two percent came from interest earned by the commercial shares and the Scots Invalid Fund.[88] The second most important revenue for the hospital, £412 (16%), derived from the sale of admission tickets to students who wished to make daily rounds with the professors and observe patients. As noted before, the hospital authorities were also authorised to collect for a segregated account used for the care of servants in the Infirmary. In 1770, the Servant Fund brought in about £200, a sum representing eight percent of the total income. Each year, on a pre-arranged Sunday, ministers were urged to make the necessary announcements and collect money at all the church doors of Edinburgh and its suburbs. Placed inside the hospital, a charity box collected £74 (3%) from grateful patients and visitors.[89]

Managing benefactors subscribed to a contemporary 'commercial sense' that demanded brief institutional stays, high cure rates, and quick turnover at a competitive price. Traditional Scottish thrift played an important role in shaping the Infirmary's finances: 'I find that the expense for each occupied bed is far greater in all of the English hospitals that I have examined', boasted John Hope (1725–86), one of the managers. Income, expenditures and admissions were frequently compared – always favourably – with other voluntary hospitals located elsewhere in Britain, notably London. By the end of the eighteenth century, Hope had calculated that Guy's Hospital in London spent £50 per bed, the Manchester Infirmary £60, while Edinburgh during the same period only spent £28, 4 shillings and 4 pence per bed. By the same token, Guy's Hospital mortality rate was 9.3%, London Hospital 13.3%, Glasgow's Infirmary 8%, while the Edinburgh Infirmary's rating was only 6.4%.[90] Although the multiple records were partially created to prevent financial mismanagement and avoid corruption, donors delighted in establishing additional rules, privileges and duties.[91] Endless meetings were conducted to check every minute event in the life of the Infirmary, from temperature in the venereal disease ward to a laundry allowance for medical clerks, whitewashing of walls to the use of the kitchen for chemical experiments. These decisions provided visibility to the managers and gave them an exalted feeling of having carried out good work.

By the 1790s, the war against Napoleonic France began to take its toll on the British economy, and competition for the dwindling philanthropic support increased. The Infirmary experienced its first fiscal deficit in 1790. It was attributed to higher prices for 'housekeeping' goods. Measures were instituted to economise, especially with respect to the consumption of alcoholic beverages for therapeutic purposes. By 1795, an extraordinary meeting of the Infirmary managers seriously considered limiting the number of admissions and closing several wards since current expenditures greatly exceeded revenues. At the same time, the Commander of the Army and the Royal Navy were urged to increase their allowances for housing sick soldiers and sailors. While revenues from the sale of student 'licenses' or tickets now made up about a third of the annual revenues, the Infirmary's charitable base needed to be broadened. Managers hoped that a new 'scheme for the subscription of small sums of money' would attract additional subscribers.[92]

Five years later in making an appeal for additional funds needed to run the Edinburgh Infirmary, James Gregory (1753–1821), professor and manager, agreed to restrict admissions. He reasoned that it was more humane to keep some of the sick–poor out of the hospital than to provide inadequate care and create institutional crowding conducive to the propagation of infections, a notorious condition prevailing in Parisian institutions.[93] Gregory tried to shame prospective donors into contributing by declaring that 'the wealth of Edinburgh and of Scotland in general is greater at present than it ever was. I do not believe [that] the charity of the people is diminishing', he added, 'for their sake I hope it is increasing too, as it will cover a multitude of sins.'[94] Gregory's calls, however, went unheeded. Fissures were developing in Edinburgh's social fabric as the ever more affluent classes moved away from the city's traditional centre. By 1801, the managers of the Infirmary admitted that expenses had 'increased in a degree which the ordinary funds of the Infirmary are unable to bear'. In requesting more subscriptions, they were careful not to blame poor management for their 'difficulties and encumbrances' but denounced the wartime economic slump. In the long run, increased charitable donations were the only salvation.[95]

The 'gift relation': expectations and obligations of charitable patienthood

Charity in Edinburgh, like elsewhere, was selective. Admission to the Infirmary was restricted to individuals marked 'by their work and honest industry' and usefulness 'to the Commonwealth'.[96] 'Deserving' persons 'desirous of accommodation' usually requested subscription letters from donors they either knew personally or from whom they had been referred. They brought these letters to the Admissions Room. According to the Infirmary's statutes, particular attention was given to endorsements from the most generous benefactors. Many sick–poor secured the required letters of recommendation while others were sent directly by their employers. Those without letters were mostly turned away except in emergency situations, including accidents requiring immediate care.[97] Other individuals or groups able to pay for their care, including soldiers and seamen, could be admitted. In the end, however, exceptions to these rules occurred, since the basic premise of this charitable enterprise was to mitigate the suffering of poor labouring people who asked for help.

Printed copies of subscribers' letters were inserted in local newspapers and also mailed to ministers of many parishes in Scotland. The forms contained standard language absolving the hospital of any responsibilities for conveying patients to and from the infirmary. Many referrals came from the countryside for individuals who had no means for returning to their homes after discharge. Thus, the Edinburgh Infirmary informed subscribers that if they issued a letter, they, and not the hospital, would be financially responsible for such return transportation.[98] A deposit for burial expenses was expected in the event relatives did not claim the deceased. Practitioners were appalled that infirmaries demanded such sums for funeral expenses, a not altogether auspicious initiation rite for often-terrified newcomers.[99] Pregnant women and the elderly were seldom admitted. The same was true for children who at times only entered with their mothers, particularly if they both suffered from fevers or venereal diseases.[100] When the beds allocated for charitable cases were already filled, a few individuals called 'supernumerary' could enter upon payment of a security deposit and monthly charges. In 1764, house physicians were given discretionary powers to receive and admit patients who could not pay for their care but were deemed to 'merit compassion'.[101] The reality of confronting poor, often malnourished people with multiple diseases must have been shocking to physicians labouring under romantic notions of a robust and sturdy workforce.

To bolster the reputation of the charity, incoming patients were expected to recover or at least not perish while hospitalised. To avoid the latter outcome, candidates were duly screened in the Infirmary's Admissions Room. Here the sick–poor were often portrayed as coming from an 'unthinking class' who had been led astray by illness. Many experienced difficulties in mastering the formalities of hospital admission.[102] The admitting physicians determined whether their ailments were 'proper' or medically suitable for hospital treatment by listening to their most important source of information: patient narratives. The process of interrogation continued later in the various hospital wards, and patients were responsible for providing 'fair' – truthful – reports. Not unexpectedly, problems in communication were frequent, given the profound differences of status, income, education, and language between the poor and the medical establishment. As new arrivals sought to negotiate their admission, physicians repeatedly complained of inaccurate answers to their questions.[103] Because of such difficulties, patients were often admonished for providing 'dull', 'confused', 'indistinct', 'inconsistent', and even deliberately misleading accounts.[104] In 1769, Francis Home (1719–1813), a frustrated professor attending the Infirmary, declared that 'the vulgar have no talent in describing their situation and add a great many fancies of their own'.[105]

Distortions and deceit were not uncommon. Persons suspected of harbouring a dangerous contagious disease or those who tried to conceal 'any circumstance relating to their diseases' were quickly rejected. Those feigning illness to obtain shelter and food were particularly unwelcome. Veracity and mutual trust were essential ingredients for establishing a satisfactory patient–physician relationship; they often determined the clinical outcome. Deception subverted the social order and very meaning of humanitarian assistance articulated by the benefactors and violated the newly minted compact. Veracity was also critical for medical management and could have significant consequences for the attending physician's reputation. Malingering was especially suspected during the winter months when a warm bed, rest, and three meals a day were attractive enough to overcome concerns about being subjected to potentially harmful medical treatments.[106] Another professor attending the Infirmary, William Cullen (1710–90), had a favourite target: impostors. He frequently employed Infirmary nurses as informers to unmask individuals who, in contemporary medical jargon, suffered from *morbus simulatus* (simulated disease) (Chapters 8 and 9). Pregnancy and chronic, possibly incurable conditions such as established cases of pulmonary consumption were considered 'improper' and promptly dismissed (Chapter 7).[107] Another notable exception was for those patients considered 'mad'; admission was denied and the individuals referred to the City Bedlam.

Placed within distinct wards, 'proper' patients pledged to adhere to institutional rules. They entered into a social contract with their new hosts who took complete control of their lives. Inmates were expected to unconditionally conform to a hierarchical system that demanded deference, obedience, and gratitude. Sickness was providential, requiring patience and stoicism; a stay in the hospital created opportunities for redemption. In return, the managers vowed to protect all inmates under the terms of their 'charitable' mandate. Besides tending to the body, hospitals were also expected to reclaim the soul. To 'mend the morals', patients needed to 'learn what they owe to God and neighbour'. Indeed, medical authors considered hospitals ideal establishments for mounting such an educational effort. Religious services were part of a 'system of comfort and improvement' designed to insure that they returned to the outside world as 'good members of society'.[108] In Edinburgh, inmates attended religious services on Sundays. Services were conducted by the hospital's own chaplain who also led communal prayer meetings twice a week and was otherwise available to meet with individual patients.[109] Closely linked to morality was the issue of patient physical cleanliness. On admission, inmates were examined and often discovered 'infected with vermin'. As one observer admitted, 'it seems impossible to answer for the transit of the louse'.[110]

Despite institutional shortcomings, patients at the Edinburgh Infirmary considered themselves lucky to be in a hospital rather than battling illness by themselves in crowded and unhealthy quarters. Opportunities for bed rest, three daily meals and nursing assistance were usually beyond their reach otherwise. As William Buchan (1729–1805), author of the widely read book *Domestic Medicine*, observed, 'the poor oftener perish in diseases for want of proper nursing than medicine'. Indeed, Infirmary physicians occasionally even asked for night nurses to monitor very sick patients because there was no regular night shift. In spite of their lowly status and pay, Buchan characterised these nursing functions as 'noble' and 'god-like',[111] although there were occasional complaints of neglect or incompetence.[112] In fact, the Infirmary statutes mandated that hospital physicians 'learn the dispositions of the different nurses'. Some of nurses, 'from a natural impatience', hardly tolerated the 'caprices of patients' whose minds and bodies were debilitated by disease. Others were 'too sympathising', disposed to excuse the faults of inmates instead of reporting them.[113]

During daily medical rounds and when apothecaries distributed medicines, inmates were told to remain silent. Physicians were told to take into consideration the 'feelings and emotions' of patients and avoid discussing a case in their presence. According to Thomas Percival (1740–1804), the author of a treatise on medical ethics, the interrogation of patients was to be conducted in a low tone of voice and kept confidential. Females were to be treated 'with the most scrupulous delicacy' (Chapter 8).[114] Compliance with therapeutic measures was critical and integral to the duties of being a charity patient. Refusal to follow doctors' orders constituted a breach of institutional rules and grounds for dismissal. While the emphasis was on regimen – rest and diet – recovery by means of drug therapy or physical methods such as bloodletting, electricity, and massage were generally attempted.

Regardless of whether they prescribed drugs or other therapeutic measures, the very presence and attention of medical professionals could inspire confidence and respect, offering its own therapeutic effect. In one case of jaundice, for example, 'a disease that admits but few remedies', Cullen deliberately prescribed a palliative remedy, explaining, 'it is necessary to give our patient some confidence in us and a good opinion of our attention'.[115] Indeed, in attendance were some of the best known British physicians and consultants to the affluent classes. In the eyes of Scottish society, these men brought to the Infirmary the best knowledge and clinical skills eighteenth-century medicine could offer. But instead of arrogance and pride, the basis for an ethical relationship with suffering patients consisted of 'tender sympathy', an especially desirable trait for gentlemen physicians. As another Edinburgh professor, John Gregory (1724–73), explained, 'sympathy naturally engages the affection and confidence of a patient, which, in many cases, is of the utmost consequence to his recovery'.[116] These attributes were of course essential in private practice where relationships were guided by the rhetoric of sensibility. In hospital practice, the approach to poor inmates was more pragmatic: it was for the benefit of society to return them as soon as possible to their previous roles and duties. Nevertheless, the poor also needed to be treated with 'delicacy'. One contemporary student praised the hospital physicians' 'humanity and fellow feeling' to patients that bestowed 'honour to themselves, to their countries and to the university'.[117]

In 1774, the Edinburgh Infirmary adopted strict new regulations 'for better preservation of good order and harmony'. Patient socialising was restricted to members of the same sex. Card games were forbidden. Among the stipulations were injunctions against talking too loudly or using foul language, quarrelling or smoking tobacco – behaviour common among rowdy soldiers and sailors, as well as unruly servants. Patients were told to restrict their diets to the articles prescribed for them, and to not convey or accept victuals from visitors. Cupboards were to be kept clean and in proper order. Attention was to be paid to all hospital property from bed clothing, pots and bottles, to fire utensils and phials. No one was allowed to leave the ward without permission except for walking on the mound behind the hospital.[118] Posted at the main gate, a porter monitored access to the building. Contempt for or violations of the rules were promptly punished with expulsion 'for irregularities'.

Moreover, ambulatory patients were required to perform a variety of chores. Since regular working habits determined their 'deserving' status, resuming some forms of labour was considered salutary. Inmates could not refuse to assist the nurses and carry out domestic tasks necessary for the running of an institution with a very limited staff. This included helping to feed other bedridden patients and participate in cleaning and laundry activities. In Edinburgh, patients also prepared surgical dressings from old rags; they were involved in cotton spinning when ordered by the physicians and surgeons. The first refusal 'to draw cotton' carried a penalty of no victuals for that day; the second was punished with immediate dismissal.[119]

The paternalistic attitude of the donors and physicians toward their charges sought to bring order into a house of sorrow. Historians have underscored the strict control and depersonalisation of hospital patients together with the brutality of nurses and the callousness of zealous administrators.[120] Housed in crowded wards, inmates were obviously exposed to the detrimental effects of forced intimacy, lack of privacy, and 'accidental noise'.[121] They witnessed at close range disgusting sights, and smells of the suffering and dying. Repeated admonitions to the staff demanding that they respect the patients' feelings and treat them with 'delicacy and kindness', suggests frequent instances of abuse. Like other British voluntary hospitals, the Edinburgh Infirmary allowed patients who 'think themselves aggrieved' the right to officially complain to the managers at their meetings or directly to the physicians during 'daily circuits'.[122] Not surprisingly, few if any dared come forward.[123]

However, positive aspects of life in an eighteenth-century hospital cannot be ignored. Patients were welcomed into a community of sufferers; visitors were allowed and many bribed the nurses to smuggle articles of food and clothing into the premises. Convalescents received permission to leave the institution and could often be found in nearby pubs. Seldom have patients, individually and collectively, been considered important factors in improvement and recovery. Yet, besides rendering assistance with grooming and feeding the bedridden, inmates offered mutual encouragement and generated empathy through gestures and words. 'All hearts are soften by distress', wrote one inmate, 'inured to suffer, they have learned to feel and pity other's sorrows as their own'.[124] Humour – 'harmless jest' – lightened patients' burdens. 'Social chat' and visits with neighbours were considered 'soothing', easing the anxieties of institutionalisation. 'Some tell their dreams and all are struck to find their neighbour's dreams so like their own.'[125] A contemporary witness spoke of his 'dear companions in affliction, joined in one common misery'. He observed that 'grief attracts by stronger bonds than pleasure ever knew'.[126] Many patients 'liked their lodgings' and kept coming up with new complaints to extend their sojourn (Chapter 7).[127] Infirmary records reveal that former inmates also returned for further care 'when again attacked with sickness'. Indeed, Thomas Spens, one of the attending physicians, noted that 'the patients are very glad to come back to it', whether in dire straits or not.[128] Others made it a habit to linger at particular times of the year, as Cullen's remarks suggest: '[Patients] had been long accustomed to lodge in hospitals and expected to meet with good entertainment and pass part of the winter with us'.[129]

Dying patients prompted a redrawing of the hospital's traditional boundaries, displacing older hospice functions that centred mainly on spiritual care. As hospitals became medicalised, the very mission that sought to transform them into houses of recovery drastically changed the cultural meaning of institutionalised death. Attitudes about death were already in flux. Instead of being characterised as the ultimate foe, polite society tended to portray the event as a natural transition, even a gentle friend, with family and friends assuming a central role in the passing. For physicians, death was a natural bodily event reflecting the cessation of vital functions. Instead of withdrawing, physicians were expected to be present at the deathbed and often contribute to the peaceful process with the administration of sedatives so those patients would die 'without a struggle'. Since mortality rates reflected unfavourably on hospital performance and the charitable enterprise, dying patients quickly became institutional liabilities. Thankfully for the managers, many were allowed to leave voluntarily and die at home surrounded by their family and friends. Cullen understood popular cultural practices since he had lived in the centre of Edinburgh before the city expanded and became segregated by class. He explained that 'it is a custom in this country that people must not be allowed to die out of sight of their friends', a practice reminiscent of traditional death vigils.[130] However, the same was no longer acceptable in medicalised eighteenth-century institutions. Assemblies of relatives and friends who tried to express social solidarity during the dying process created additional fears of environmental contamination in hospital wards as well as the potential for disease transmission. These fears were based on the new tenets of public hygiene. When Cullen discovered 'six or seven gossips [friends] in the room and as many candles lighted up' in 1773, the physician acted quickly. 'I had the light carried away, made the persons go out and had the room ventilated'. Cullen's efforts apparently bore fruit: 'Next day I found a difference of symptoms', he claimed.[131]

There were no longer religious obligations following death.[132] One author suggested the 'scene of parting life' be 'veiled as much as possible' to avoid depressing other inmates.[133] With rare exceptions, contact with the dead was minimised due to the dread of contagion. Bodies were promptly removed to special mortuaries before being released for burial elsewhere.[134] Regulations only allowed post-mortem examinations if proper permission was secured from the deceased's next of kin or close friends. This created a formidable hurdle because the general public considered dissections 'violations of the dead'[135] and often expressed 'horror and apprehension' about their performance.[136] In one fatal case of 'typhus fever', Cullen explained that 'I was desirous to have a dissection but the interposition of his friends was violent and prevented us'.[137] In Edinburgh three hospital managers also had to agree to the importance of the examination before a dissection could be authorised. This arrangement was justified as preventing 'the violation of the feelings of those most nearly concerned'. But the managers were equally keen to avoid any negative publicity arising from the practice of cutting corpses, which may have jeopardised the loyalty of institutional subscribers. These rules, together with a carefully orchestrated low institutional mortality, were responsible for the paucity of autopsies at the Edinburgh Infirmary.[138]

Journals, newspapers, and reports boasted of the Infirmary's cure rate. These publications provided statistical proof and bought recognition for the hospital's charitable accomplishments. Even for inmates who failed to respond to treatments, the discharge category 'relieved' implied a positive outcome. As in private practice, hospital practitioners needed to pay attention to the 'prejudices' of patients who reacted with fear and distrust to medical intervention. But reassuring inmates and their next of kin was not enough. Hospital management took place in full view of the public, and those entrusted with the day-to-day operations of the institution were quite aware of the image they needed to project to the community.[139] Beyond them was the city of Edinburgh with its large constituency of influential subscribers, a circle of managers, and the professional colleges of physicians and surgeons. Above all else, maintaining a good opinion of the Infirmary was essential to the success of the charity.

In the end, the Infirmary's 'noble and benevolent provision' entitled donors to its 'best acknowledgements of gratitude and love.'[140] As part of the responsibility to benefactors, patients were told to publicly express their appreciation for the privilege of obtaining free shelter, food, and medical care. Before leaving the Infirmary, inmates were expected to engage in an institutional ritual of personally acknowledging and giving gratitude for what they had received. When asked by a board of inquiry how patients had felt about their hospital confinement, Spens responded that 'patients generally declare great satisfaction with their general treatment in the Hospital'. He added that 'after having quitted the Hospital, [they] have frequently expressed themselves to the same effect'. Andrew Duncan Sr (1744–1828), one of the attending professors to the Edinburgh Infirmary, testified that 'I have a hundred times in the street got the blessing of patients for the care they had met in the Infirmary'.[141] For better or worse, their lives had been changed by an experience they would never forget.

Hospitals and medicine's professional interests

While especially attentive to the needs of Britain's growing economy, Bellers' call for the creation of hospitals also considered the interests of the medical profession. In Britain's competitive medical marketplace, for a physician wishing to 'get himself talked of', the appointment to a local hospital became highly desirable and status-enhancing. It was 'the best method for adding to notoriety and practice'.[142] While such posts were usually voluntary and medical advice given free of charge, the assignments provided valuable public exposure and reputation essential for building a prosperous private practice. Caring for the poor constituted genuine compassion and Christian behaviour; it energised the soul and was compatible with professional dignity.[143] To reassure managers, candidates for hospital work needed certain professional qualifications. Most institutions, including the Edinburgh

Infirmary, only allowed access to practitioners who were Fellows of their respective Royal Colleges. Since competition could be fierce, social connections were key. One contemporary, who sought to lampoon the contested nature of such appointments, counselled, 'prostitute [your] talents or barter virtue'.[144]

Eighteenth-century infirmaries also became indispensable in medical and surgical instruction, and in the acquisition of knowledge and experience. William Blizard (1743–1835), a prominent London surgeon, called hospitals 'the principal pillars of a rational system of instruction in the healing art'.[145] Bellers envisioned hospitals as 'great nurseries' and called for the construction of university-affiliated institutions at Oxford and Cambridge endowed 'with different wards for each distemper'.[146] Practitioners, he and others argued, could markedly improve their knowledge and education through the frequent observation of sick people congregated in hospital wards (Chapters 2 and 7). Clinical instruction in hospitals already claimed a long tradition reaching back to the sixteenth century at the University of Padua. What was new from the 1750s onward was the proposed scope of such instruction. The entire population of an infirmary was viewed as potential educational material and proponents of clinical instruction expected that such institutional arrangements would supply the needed corpses for anatomical dissection and the study of pathology.[147]

In the opinion of many observers, new voluntary institutions could become veritable storehouses of clinical experience. Instead of shuttling daily between a handful of private cases and being completely dependent on patients for return visits, practitioners would dramatically increase their case load more than ten- or even twenty-fold without having to spend days and nights in their carriages, travelling from one customer to another. 'These hospitals', wrote Bellers, 'will breed up some of the best physicians and surgeons because they may see as much there in one year as in seven anywhere else'.[148] It is therefore not difficult to understand why prominent physicians and surgeons joined the ranks of the local fundraising committees and societies to establish infirmaries.

But the hospital not only provided enhanced opportunities for the observation of diverse diseases and trauma. The issue of clinical continuity through serial bedside observations and supervised therapy was equally critical. Instead of sporadic and brief private visits during the course of an illness, hospital physicians had regular access to the bedside. Thus, they could truly observe the course of any given condition from admission to discharge. In their own quest for empirical evidence, surgical apprentices were particularly keen on gaining practical experience and operating skills.

Among the new criteria increasingly employed in diagnosis were anatomical findings made at the time of an autopsy. Surgeons were particularly eager to ascertain the effects of their handiwork, and post-mortem examinations became the hallmark of progressive hospital surgeons who diligently sought such feedback to improve their operating strategies and postoperative management.[149] The availability of unclaimed cadavers in hospitals also provided surgeons of opportunities to perfect surgical speed and dexterity. A nearly quantum leap in diagnostic and prognostic acumen ensued.[150] But there were also potential drawbacks associated with such exposures to corpses. Physicians attempting to preserve the traits of gentility and sensibility worried about the dehumanising effects of dissections on the medical student. They feared it might render 'his heart hard and his deportment unfeeling'.[151]

In the domestic household arrangement adopted by the Infirmary, relations between managers, practitioners, apothecary, staff and patients were carefully structured along formal hierarchical lines. All activities were closely monitored and regulated through detailed accounting systems that furnished order and thrift. Communications among professionals were usually made in writing and officially presented at monthly meetings held by the managers. In turn, the 'internal economy of the family' came under the direction of a housekeeper or matron in charge of clerical personnel, cooks, porters, and servant-nurses responsible for hygiene, records, furnishings, supplies, and meals.[152] Given the powers awarded to governors, managers, and matrons, attending physicians strived to exercise control over patients. At the Edinburgh Infirmary they were able to decide the admission and dismissal of patients, assisted by two hired and resident medical clerks. The clerks were also on hand during official rounds, writing down the clinical information and therapeutic orders in ward journals. They were also entrusted with keeping the patient registers up-to-date. In spite of language barriers, all these men attempted to sharpen their interviewing skills and revise the criteria used in the definition and diagnosis of particular diseases. At the Infirmary, Cullen's *Nosology* prevailed although its author insisted that it should be periodically amended on the basis of further knowledge derived from hospital practice. By 'walking the wards' and making bodily inspections, physicians, surgeons, and their clerks had new opportunities to detect the physical signs of disease (Chapters 7 and 8).

Because they commanded exclusive access to inmates and were the only ones prescribing drugs and other therapeutic methods, Infirmary physicians were able to ascertain ever more clearly the effects of their therapies.[153] Practitioners began to test certain drugs in hospital wards, army barracks, and naval vessels, believing that is was their professional and moral duty to discover new treatments. Some of the medicines were new; others were already well known but compounded in novel ways or administered in different dosages.[154] 'Hospital patients are on several accounts the most proper subjects for an experimental course', declared Aikin. They were 'accustomed to obey orders' and strictly confined to the wards. In private practice, physicians carried out a 'timid and narrow' practice, but free of restraints in hospitals they could 'exert their genius'. Aikin concluded that 'the improvement of medical knowledge is greatly indebted to hospitals for the opportunities they afford of experimental practice.'[155] Not surprisingly, complaints about human experimentation in hospitals became more frequent. Because of the strict control of the charity, managers, professors, apothecaries, and even house physicians carefully monitored treatments. In Edinburgh, Infirmary physicians were restricted in prescribing medicines; they were told to limit their orders to items from the hospital's own list of drugs. Still, some testing took place. Home insisted that conclusions from trials conducted at the Infirmary's teaching ward were quite useful. In his opinion, they were deemed more credible than results derived from private practice 'as they are performed before so many spectators, reviewed in clinical lectures and preserved in the private books of each gentleman present'.[156] Moreover, hospital patients would be the first 'to reap the benefits from new Knowledge'.[157] Home also conceded that 'it is of great use in medicine to show that what we trust [in] does not deserve our confidence'.[158] James Gregory's remark about physicians 'playing with the human hide – *corio humano ludere* – reflected his uneasiness, shared by other practitioners, about the morally dubious character of medical testing.[159] 'The hospital was instituted and the managers of it appointed for the relief of the sick–poor, not for the general interests of science', he wrote later.[160] Gradually, therapeutic scepticism emerged as a result of using traditional and new remedies hitherto insufficiently tested in private practice.[161]

While elite Edinburgh physicians and their students benefited the most from their involvement with the Infirmary, the attending surgeons and their apprentices struggled. From its inception, the politics of the Infirmary's associated philanthropy had favoured local physicians. The original sponsor, the Royal College of Physicians, continued to use this charitable enterprise as an instrument to advance the professional interests of medicine. Britain's armed forces, however, required a growing cadre of military and naval surgeons; therefore hospitals such as the Royal Infirmary of Edinburgh also became key training grounds for fledgling apprentices under the auspices of local surgical corporations.[162] The arrangement for a monthly rotation of surgeons visiting the hospital was rapidly becoming unwieldy as the number of Fellows of the Royal College of Surgeons nearly doubled. Irregularities in attendance caused delays in surgery and continuity of patient care. Some of those placing their names on the list were newly qualified, lacking the experience and maturity of their peers. A paucity of autopsies created by the Infirmary's burdensome rules prevented valuable feedback and a lack of clinical surgical lectures created unfavourable conditions for the education of surgeons.[163] According to the 1792 university guide, the condition of patients seen in the surgical ward was not as adequately documented as that of inmates in the medical unit, and a majority of the managing surgeons failed to produce daily progress notes. 'This great abuse should be corrected by the managers of the Infirmary', the document concluded.[164]

By the early 1790s, a new generation of hospital-trained Edinburgh surgeons tried to press the Infirmary managers to improve conditions for their patients and students. In June 1792, the Royal College of Surgeons requested the establishment of a separate ward to house postoperative patients. The request was based on the notion that the 'impure' air in the regular ward often proved fatal or retarded their recovery, especially during the summer months.[165] The Infirmary managers responded by vacating a small fever ward in the upper story of the new wing. Because surgeons were somewhat tainted from grave-robbing practices and commerce with anatomical specimens which generated public disgust, managers were concerned about institutional 'irregularities in the dissection of dead bodies'. In 1794, they highlighted a particular incident in which the attending surgeon, John Bell (1762–1820), carried off a number of body parts for his collection of pathological samples. A special hospital committee quickly condemned this violation of the rules and expelled Bell, stating that 'any indecorums of that nature if rumoured abroad might be of essential prejudice to the hospital'.[166] That same year, the College of Surgeons was also told to select more senior members to attend the hospital. At the end of the century, its president, James Lew, agreed that two senior ordinary surgeons selected by the College were needed to make rounds in the surgical wards filled with a 'degree of bustle and confusion'. This arrangement would protect the interests of patients and the growing number of students who could not 'get near enough neither to see the patient or hear the opinion of the attending surgeon'. However, the Infirmary managers were determined to make such personnel selections themselves and rejected the proposal.[167]

The increasingly bitter controversy continued with a pamphlet war between James Gregory, the prestigious academic and hospital manager, and John Bell, also an extramural lecturer. Each asserted differing visions of professional life. The conflict revealed the critical importance of access to the now famous Infirmary for the fortunes of Edinburgh medicine and surgery – the former basking in worldwide recognition, the latter still mired in mediocrity but strenuously aiming to improve its image and scope of practice.[168] Gregory insisted that only the most senior and established surgeons ought to be part of the attending rotation; Bell defended the access of better, scientifically educated, junior surgeons with proven skills. The ultimate aim of the Edinburgh managers in curtailing the role of surgery was clear. By insisting on the seniority system represented by older, less well-trained surgeons, the managers sought to buttress the profile of elite medicine in the city against surgeon–apothecaries who were increasingly expanding the scope of their practices as a prelude to becoming general medical practitioners (Chapter 8).[169] Moreover, medicine attempted to expand its own base of practice by infiltrating the field of surgery. The Edinburgh guide for prospective students recommended that 'although many students mean to dedicate themselves entirely to the practice of medicine, they should all attend the surgical ward for one season because every physician ought to be acquainted with the general principles of surgery'.[170]

Additional insights into the complexity of clinical and surgical events were obtained by placing 'political arithmetic' in the service of medicine. Vital statistics provided knowledge concerning the dynamics and frequency of urban disease.[171] Clinical data compiled from hospital experiences also helped understand some of the complexities surrounding the behaviour of several diseases as well as methods to deal with them. It seemed clear that extending the practitioner's opportunities to visit with the sick would eventually revolutionise medicine.[172] Surgery would benefit even more from access to hospitals, expanding its legitimate access to human dissections, improving indications for interventions, perfecting techniques and decreasing postoperative mortality. To gauge progress, surgical statistics became equally important benchmarks for individual operators and institutions. In the end, donors and sponsors, patients and visitors, all contributed to create the perception that hospital-affiliated practitioners possessed superior knowledge and perhaps more effective remedies.

Conclusion

In the absence of governmental responsibility, those with power and wealth in British society organised private and often expensive charitable associations to build hospitals. This philanthropic investment promised rich dividends in personal salvation, moral development, social recognition, civic pride, economic growth, and even national enhancement. Referring to donors of a newly established public dispensary, Andrew Duncan Sr wrote in 1778 that 'I am convinced that it will add somewhat to the respectable character which they hold as citizens of Edinburgh'.[173] To achieve these social agendas, the eighteenth-century voluntary hospital movement became a unique focus for such charitable efforts. A confluence of interests, religious and commercial, influenced patient admissions. The politics of fundraising together with the charitable impulse of benefactors became aligned with the managers' demand for financial balance and the physicians' ambitions for fame and status. Those who were allowed admission to the hospital were mostly young adults who had been in reasonable good health just prior to their present illness. They usually suffered from ordinary acute or subacute conditions.

High cure rates confirmed the skills and superiority of hospital physicians, who used the growing reputations to bolster their private practices. Given the average hospitalisation period of less than three weeks in Edinburgh, patient turnover was timely, allowing for increases in the total number of individuals treated, a statistic that suggested the Infirmary was a dynamic, efficient, and productive charity worthy of additional bequests. Hospital practice also formulated a new medical ethos. The rules created a physician–patient relationship influenced by the pragmatic goals of functional recovery, experimentalism, and pedagogy forged across social classes. This renegotiated moral and social contract sought to retain the physician's earlier ideals of gentility and scholarship. It also brought the physician into closer collaboration with other groups of practitioners. To play their roles, poor patients, for their part, demanded dignity and civility.[174]

At the end of the eighteenth century, the Royal Infirmary of Edinburgh was selected as a premier example of that country's dramatic improvement. Fulfilling its duties to 'sick and helpless fellow creatures' avoided poverty among the 'deserving' poor and represented nothing less than 'civilisation'.[175] Hospital management and medical activities involved all sectors of Edinburgh society, fostering channels of communication and interaction in an atmosphere of politeness and charity. For more than half a century, hundreds of students from around the world had walked the Infirmary wards before embarking on their careers. Most of them, in private practice or employed in Britain's armed forces continued to recognise the hospital's contribution to the nation's medical reputation and manpower. The Annual Report for the year 1802 put it most succinctly: 'The Royal Infirmary of Edinburgh has been established above seventy years; and during that period, it has uniformly maintained its claim to the public favour. By this Institution, the Poor under the pressure of disease, are provided with everything which can tend to their comfort and relief; and many lives are annually saved to Society through the attention and abilities of the Medical Gentlemen to whom the care of the Patients is committed.'[176]

Notes

1. S. Johnson, Essay 4, Saturday, 6 May 1758, in *The Idler*, 5th edn, 2 vols. (London: J. Rivington, 1790), Vol. I, 16–18.
2. Royal Infirmary of Edinburgh, *Report of a Committee on the State of the Hospital* (Edinburgh, 1818), 58.
3. For reference R. Bremner, *Giving: Charity and Philanthropy in History* (New Brunswick, N.J.: Transaction Publishers, 1994); S.N. Katz and E.L Queen (eds), *Philanthropy in the World's Traditions* (Bloomington: Indiana University Press, 1998).
4. J. Aikin, *Thoughts on Hospitals* (London: J. Johnson, 1771), 5.
5. W. Nolan, *An Essay on Humanity: Or a View of Abuses in Hospitals With a Plan for Correcting Them* (London: J. Murray, 1786), 9.
6. T. McKeown and R.G. Brown, 'Medical Evidence Related to English Population Changes in the Eighteenth Century', *Population Studies* 9 (1955–6), 125. This judgement has been uncritically repeated in numerous subsequent publications. McKeown's assumption was that if nineteenth-century hospitals were overcrowded and lethal, then earlier institutions must have been even more deadly.
7. K. Wilson, 'Urban Culture and Political Activism in Hanoverian England: The Example of Voluntary Hospitals', in E. Hellmuth (ed.), *The Transformation of Political Culture: England and Germany in the Late Eighteenth Century* (New York: Oxford University Press, 1990), 164–84.
8. For details see G.B. Risse, *Hospital Life in Enlightenment Scotland, Care and Teaching at the Royal Infirmary of Edinburgh* (New York: Cambridge University Press, 1986), 279–95.
9. C. Jones, 'Some Recent Trends in the History of Charity', in M. Daunton (ed.), *Charity, Selfinterest and Welfare in the English Past* (London: Palgrave Macmillan, 1996), 51–63. For historians, charity has become a somewhat controversial topic of study. See K. Waddington, *Charity and the London Hospitals, 1850–1898* (London: Royal Historical Society, 2000), 21–57.
10. Two traditional works are W.K. Jordan, *Philanthropy in England* (London: G. Allen & Unwin, 1959); D. Owen, *English Philanthropy, 1660–1960* (Cambridge, Mass.: Belknap Press, 1965), 36–61.
11. M. Mollat, *The Poor in the Middle Ages: An Essay in Social History*, trans. A. Goldhammer (New Haven: Yale University Press, 1986); T. Riis, 'Poverty and Urban Development in Early Modern Europe (15th–18th/19th Centuries: A General View', in T. Riis (ed.), *Aspects of Poverty in Early Modern Europe* (Florence: Le Monnier, 1981), 1–28; see also R. Jütte, *Poverty and Deviance in Early Modern Europe* (Cambridge: Cambridge University Press, 1994).

12. A.L. Beier, *The Problem of the Poor in Tudor and Early Stuart England* (London: Methuen, 1982); L.H. Lees, *The Solidarities of Strangers: The English Poor Laws and the People, 1700–1948* (Cambridge: Cambridge University Press, 1998); for a brief overview, consult I. Loudon, 'Poor Relief Under the 'Old' Poor Law', in *Medical Care and the General Practitioner, 1750–1850* (Oxford: Clarendon Press, 1986), 231–4.
13. For literature on continental hospitals, see C. Jones and M. Sonenscher, 'The Social Functions of the Hospital in Eighteenth-Century France: The Case of the Hotel-Dieu of Nimes', *French Historical Studies,* 13 (1983), 172–214; A.E. Imhof, 'The Hospital in the 18th Century: For Whom?', in P. Branca (ed.), *The Medicine Show* (New York: Science History Publications, 1977), 141–63. For Italian hospitals S. Cavallo, 'Charity, Power, and Patronage in Eighteenth-Century Italian Hospitals: The Case of Turin', in L. Granshaw and R. Porter (eds), *The Hospital in History* (London: Routledge, 1989), 93–122.
14. See for example, A.W. Coats, 'The Relief of Poverty, Attitudes to Labour and Economic Change in England, 1660–1782', *International Review of Social History,* 21 (1976), 98–115.
15. The topic has been more extensively explored in recent years. See D.T. Andrew, *Philanthropy and Police: London Charity in the Eighteenth Century* (Princeton, N.J.: Princeton University Press, 1989); H. Cunningham and J. Innes (eds), *Charity, Philanthropy and Reform: From the 1690s to 1850* (New York: St. Martin's Press, 1998).
16. G. Rosen, *From Medical Police to Social Medicine, Essays on the History of Medical Care* (New York: Science History Publications, 1974).
17. For a comprehensive synthesis of medicine during the Enlightenment see G.B. Risse, 'Medicine in the Age of Enlightenment', in A. Wear (ed.), *Medicine in Society: Historical Essays* (Cambridge: Cambridge University Press, 1992), 149–95. Other useful secondary sources are P. Gay, 'Enlightenment: Medicine and Cure', in *The Enlightenment,* 2 vols (New York: Knopf, 1966–9), Vol. 2, 12–23; E. Lesky, 'Johann Peter Frank and Social Medicine', *Annales Cisalpines d'Histoire Sociale,* 4 (1973), 137–44.
18. J.H. Cassedy, 'Medicine and the Rise of Statistics', in A.G. Debus (ed.), *Medicine in Seventeenth-Century England* (Berkeley: University of California Press, 1974), 283–312; see also T. Frängsmyr, J.L. Heilbron and R. Rider (eds), *The Quantifying Spirit in the Eighteenth Century* (Berkeley: University of California Press, 1990).
19. B.G. Gale, 'The Dissolution and the Revolution in London Hospital Facilities', *Medical History* 11, 1 (1967), 91–6. For more details, L. Granshaw, 'The Rise of the Modern Hospital in Britain', in Wear, *op. cit.* (note 17), 197–218.

20. M. Foucault, 'The Politics of Health in the Eighteenth Century', in C. Gordon (ed.), *Power/Knowledge, Selected Interviews and Other Writings 1972–1977* (New York: Pantheon, 1980), 169.
21. J. Bellers, *Essay Towards the Improvement of Medicine* (London: Sowle, 1714), 6. On Bellers, see G. Clarke (ed.), *John Bellers, His Life, Times and Writings* (London: Routledge & Kegan Paul, 1987).
22. T.B. Percival, 'A Discourse Addressed to the Gentlemen of the Faculty, the Officers, the Clergy and the Trustees of the Infirmary at Liverpool', in T. Percival, *Medical Ethics* (Manchester: S. Russell, 1803), 119.
23. *Ibid.,* 119.
24. 'The motives must be disinterested because those who receive the munificence cannot so much as acknowledge the obligation' in 'Proposal to Augment the Foundling Hospital Fund', *Gentleman's Magazine,* 17 (1747), 163–4.
25. S. Cavallo, 'The Motivations of Benefactors: An Overview of Approaches to the Study of Charity', in J. Barry and C. Jones (eds), *Medicine and Charity Before the Welfare State* (London: Routledge, 1991), 46–62.
26. See F.K. Prochaska, *The Voluntary Impulse: Philanthropy in Modern Britain* (London: Faber, 1988).
27. According to D.T. Andrew, the waters of motivation are treacherous and murky. See Andrew, *op. cit.* (note 15), 12; see also M.E. Fissell, 'The "Sick and Drooping Poor" in Eighteenth Century Bristol and its Region', *Social History of Medicine,* 2 (1989), 35–58.
28. For details, R. Porter, 'The Gift Relation: Philanthropy and Provincial Hospitals in Eighteenth-Century England', in Granshaw and Porter, *op. cit.* (note 13), 149–78.
29. Andrew, *op. cit.* (note 15), 21.
30. Quite useful here is A.J. Kidd, 'Philanthropy and the Social History Paradigm', *Social History,* 21 (1996), 180–92.
31. For details, P. Borsay, *The English Urban Renaissance: Culture and Society in the Provincial Town, 1660–1770* (Oxford: Clarendon Press, 1989), 296–300. Another insightful case study is A. Wilson, 'The Birmingham General Hospital and its Public, 1765–79', in S. Sturdy (ed.), *Medicine, Health and the Public Sphere in Britain, 1600–2000* (London: Routledge, 2002), 85–106.
32. M. Maus, *The Gift*, trans, W.D. Halls (New York: Norton, 1990).
33. For details, G.B. Risse, *Mending Bodies, Saving Souls: A History of Hospitals* (New York: Oxford University Press, 1999), 69–116.
34. Bellers, *op. cit.* (note 21), 1–3.
35. For an incisive analysis of the politics behind charitable hospital projects, see A. Wilson, 'Conflict, Consensus and Charity: Politics and the Provincial

Voluntary Hospitals in the Eighteenth Century', *English Historical Review,* 111 (1996), 599–619. For a view of institutions devoted to paupers see F.A. Macdonald, 'The Infirmary of the Glasgow Town's Hospital: Patient Care, 1733–1800', in P. Wood (ed.), *The Scottish Enlightenment: Essays in Reinterpretation* (Rochester, NY: Rochester University Press, 2000), 199–238.

36. K. Wilson, *The Sense of the People: Politics, Culture and Imperialism in England, 1715–1785* (New York: Cambridge University Press, 1995), 76.
37. According the R.A. Houston, the donations served both the internal and external aims of polite culture. See his *Social Change in the Age of Enlightenment: Edinburgh, 1660-1760* (Oxford: Clarendon Press, 1994), 234–89; also J.H. Jamieson, 'Social Assemblies of the Eighteenth-Century', *Book of the Old Edinburgh Club,* 19 (1933), 31–91.
38. E.J. Hundert (ed.), B. Mandeville, *The Fable of the Bees: And Other Writings* (1723) (Indianapolis: Hackett Pub., 1997), 114-5. For details, E.J. Hundert, *The Enlightenment's Fable: Bernard Mandeville and the Discovery of Society* (Cambridge: Cambridge University Press, 1994).
39. Andrew, *op. cit.* (note 15), 30-41.
40. Johnson, *op. cit.* (note 1), Vol. I, 19.
41. See J.S. Shaw, *The Management of Scottish Society, 1707–1764: Power, Nobles, Lawyers, Edinburgh Agents and English Influences* (Edinburgh: J. Donald, 1983); and T.C. Smout, 'The Anglo-Scottish Union of 1707: The Economic Background', *Economic Historical Review,* 16 (1963–4), 455–67.
42. See A.C. Chitnis, 'Provost Drummond and the Origins of Edinburgh Medicine', in R.H. Campbell and A.S. Skinner (eds), *The Origins and Nature of the Scottish Enlightenment* (Edinburgh: J. Donald, 1982), 86–114; M. Barfoot, *Lord Provost George Drummond, 1687–1766* (Edinburgh: Scotland's Cultural Heritage, 1987).
43. J.B. Morell, 'The Edinburgh Town Council and its University, 1717–1776', in R.G.W. Anderson and A.D.C. Simpson (eds), *The Early Years of the Edinburgh Medical School* (Edinburgh: Royal Scottish Museum, Edinburgh, 1976), 46–65. For a recent revisionist account, R.L. Emerson, 'The Founding of the Edinburgh Medical School', *Journal of the History of Medicine,* 59 (2004), 183–218.
44. For autobiographical information on Monro, H.D. Erlham, 'Alexander Monro, primus', *University of Edinburgh Journal,* 17 (1953–5), 77–105; and more recently R.E. Wright–St. Clair, *Doctors Monro: A Medical Saga* (London: Wellcome History of Medicine Library, 1964), 27–37.
45. Edinburgh Infirmary, *An Account of the Rise and Establishment of the Infirmary or Hospital for Sick Poor, Erected at Edinburgh* (Edinburgh, *ca.* 1730), 2.

46. A. Ferguson, *An Essay on the History of Civil Society* (1767), ed. D. Forbes, (Edinburgh: Edinburgh University Press, 1966). For details about the role of the Scottish Church, consult A.L. Drummond and J. Bulloch, *The Scottish Church, 1688–1843: The Age of Moderates* (Edinburgh: St Andrew's Press, 1973); and more recently R.B. Sher, *Church and University in the Scottish Enlightenment* (Edinburgh: Edinburgh University Press, 1985), 187–212.
47. Edinburgh Infirmary, *op. cit.* (note 45), 2. Portions of the pamphlet and a detailed account of the developments in Edinburgh can be found in A.L. Turner, *Story of a Great Hospital: The Royal Infirmary of Edinburgh 1729–1929* (Edinburgh: Oliver & Boyd, 1937), 39–67.
48. J. Dwyer, 'Enlightenment Spectators and Classical Moralists: Sympathetic Relations in Eighteenth-Century Scotland', in J. Dwyer and R.B. Sher (eds), *Sociability and Society in Eighteenth-Century Scotland* (Edinburgh: Mercat Press, 1993), 115; see also J. Mullan, *Sentiment and Sociability: The Language of Feeling in the Eighteenth Century* (Oxford: Oxford University Press, 1988).
49. For Enlightenment views of human nature, J.B. Schneewind, *The Invention of Autonomy: A History of Modern Moral Philosophy* (Cambridge: Cambridge University Press, 1998).
50. W. Cullen, 'An Essay on the Hypochondriac Disease' (in a Letter), Cullen Papers, MSS Collection, Glasgow University Library, 20.
51. John Gregory, *Lectures on the Duties and Qualifications of a Physician* (London: W. Strahan and T. Cadell, 1772), 19.
52. J.A. Dwyer, *Virtuous Discourse: Sensibility and Community in Late Eighteenth-Century Scotland* (Edinburgh: J. Donald, 1987), 95–116. For an overview C.J. Berry, *Social Theory of the Scottish Enlightenment* (Edinburgh: Edinburgh University Press, 1997).
53. Edinburgh Infirmary, *op. cit.* (note 45), 2.
54. Houston, *op. cit.* (note 37), 87–101.
55. Edinburgh Infirmary, *op. cit.* (note 45), 2; see also P.M. Eaves Walton, 'The Early Years in the Infirmary', in Anderson and Simpson, *op. cit.* (note 43), 71–80.
56. For a comparative view in another Scottish city, F.A. MacDonald, 'The Infirmary of the Glasgow Town's Hospital, 1733–1800: A Case for Voluntarism?', *Bulletin of the History of Medicine,* 73 (1999), 64–105. For Bristol see M.E. Fissell, 'Charity Universal?', in *Patients, Power and the Poor in Eighteenth-Century Bristol* (New York: Cambridge University Press, 1991), 74–93; Fissel's PhD dissertation on this topic is 'The Physic of Charity: Health and Welfare in the West Country, 1690–1834', University of Pennsylvania, 1988.
57. 'A Letter from a Gentleman in the Country to his Friend in Edinburgh' (Edinburgh, 1725), 9. This publication is quoted in R.M. Stott, 'The

Incorporation of Surgeons and Medical Education and Practice in Edinburgh, 1696–1755', PhD dissertation, University of Edinburgh, 1984, 113.

58. This quote from the Haddington Justices of the Peace in 1724 is quoted in Stott's dissertation, *ibid.*, 143.
59. A more detailed account of the personalities and politics involved can be found in C.J. Lawrence, 'Medicine as Culture: Edinburgh and the Scottish Enlightenment', PhD dissertation, University College London, 1984, 103–9.
60. A. Borsay, 'Cash and Conscience: Financing the General Hospital at Bath, ca. 1738–1750', *Social History of Medicine,* 4 (1991), 207–29.
61. W. Maitland, 'Infirmary', in *The History of Edinburgh From its Foundation to the Present Time,* IX Books (Edinburgh: Hamilton, Balfour and Neil, 1753), Book VI, 450–1.
62. Edinburgh Infirmary, 'List of the Original Subscribers and Other Donors to the Infirmary or Hospital for Sick Poor, Erected at Edinburgh', in *op. cit.* (note 45), 6–9. More details concerning administrative arrangements in hospitals can be found in W.B. Howie, 'The Administration of an Eighteenth-Century Provincial Hospital: The Royal Salop Infirmary, 1747–1830', *Medical History* 5, 1 (1961), 34–55.
63. Several volumes of the 'Minutes of Managers' from the Royal Infirmary of Edinburgh have survived and offer a wealth of information regarding the activities and decisions of the hospital managers. They are: vol 1, February 1728 to December 1741; Vol. 2, January 1742 to January 1749; Vol. 3, from February 1749 to December 1760; Vol. 4, from January 1761 to December 1775; and Vol. 6, January 1789 to December 1800, MSS Collection, Edinburgh University Library.
64. Wilson, *op. cit.* (note 36), 73–82.
65. For this topic, see F.K. Prochaska, *Royal Bounty: The Making of a Welfare Monarchy* (New Haven: Yale University Press, 1995), 1–13.
66. Pamphlet titled *Memorial Concerning the Surgeon's Hospital* (Edinburgh: 18 February 1737), 7; see also Stott, *The Incorporation of Surgeons, op. cit.* (note 57), 159–62.
67. R.I.E., *op. cit.* (note 63), Vol. 1, 20 April 1738, 147. This statement contradicts notions that the benefactors tried to accept individuals on the basis of need in opposition to medical notions of potential curability.
68. I am indebted to information contained in an unpublished paper written by Michael Barfoot: 'Pedagogy, Practice and Politics: The Gregory–Bell Dispute and the Nature of Early 19th Century Edinburgh Medicine'.
69. Philanthropus, *A Letter From a Gentleman in Town to His Friend in the Country Relating to the Royal Infirmary of Edinburgh* (Edinburgh, 1738), 6 and 9.

70. Philasthenes, *A Letter From a Gentleman in Town to His Friend in the Country Relating to the Royal Infirmary of Edinburgh* (Edinburgh, 1739), 4–5. Given the similarity in title and content, scholars have assumed that both pamphlets came from the same author.
71. N. Niving, *Jesus Christ in the Poor, or the Royal Infirmary of Edinburgh Recommended to the Charity of Well-Disposed Christians* (Edinburgh: Sands, Brymer, Murray & Cochran, 1739), 3.
72. *Ibid.*, 17–18; see also R. Goldberg, 'Charity Sermons and the Poor: A Rhetoric of Compassion', *The Age of Johnson,* 4 (1991), 171–216.
73. Anonymous, *Letters to the Patients in the Royal Infirmary of Edinburgh* (Edinburgh: J. Reid, 1772), 5. This pamphlet was apparently written by a medical student.
74. R.I.E., *op. cit.* (note 63), Vol. 6, 2 November 1789, 21.
75. Edinburgh Infirmary, 'List of the Original Subscribers and Other Donors to the Infirmary or Hospital for Sick Poor, Erected at Edinburgh', *op. cit.* (note 45), 19–30
76. See C. Stevenson, 'The Charitable Construction of the Edinburgh Royal Infirmary', in *Medicine and Magnificence, British Hospital and Asylum Architecture, 1660–1815* (New Haven: Yale University Press, 2000), 111-21.
77. Risse, *op. cit.* (note 8), 92–7.
78. H. Arnot, *The History of Edinburgh* (Edinburgh: W. Creech, 1779), 546.
79. R.I.E., *op. cit.* (note 63). Vol. 3, 1 January 1750, 38.
80. For the care of sailors. see G.B. Risse, 'Britannia Rules the Seas: The Health of Seamen, Edinburgh, 1791–1800', *Journal of the History of Medicine,* 43 (1988), 1–22.
81. R.I.E., *op. cit.* (note 63), Vol. 3, 7 March 1750, 48.
82. *Ibid.*, Vol. 3, 7 January 1751, 78.
83. *Ibid.*, Vol. 3, 5 April 1756, 141.
84. Risse, *op. cit.* (note 8), 98–101.
85. *Appeal for Funds Made in Behalf of Lord Provost, Magistrates and Council, for Funding of the Special Servants Ward at the Infirmary* (Edinburgh, 31 January 1771), 1. Printed for public distribution, this pamphlet is available in the Edinburgh Room of the Edinburgh City Library.
86. Further information about the singularly complex system of medical records established at the Edinburgh Infirmary in Risse, *op. cit.* (note 8), 43–56.
87. G. Foster, *An Essay on Hospitals* (Dublin: W.G. Jones, 1768), 40.
88. This information was extracted from the Treasurer's Account Book, one of the few surviving administrative records from the eighteenth century. MSS Collection, Edinburgh University. For more details about financial matters in British infirmaries consult W.B. Howie, 'Finance and Supply in an

Eighteenth-Century Hospital, 1747–1830', *Medical History*, 7, 2 (1963), 126–46.

89. 'Petition from the Managers of the Infirmary for Collection in the Churches to Maintain a Ward for Admitting Sick Servants Ordered to be Observed Sunday, 8 August 1773', in 'Minutes of Town Council', Vol. 90, meeting of 16 July 1773; see also Risse, *op. cit.* (note 8), 34–43.
90. R.I.E., *op. cit.* (note 2), 90.
91. A. Borsay, 'Persons of Honor and Reputation: The Voluntary Hospital in an Age of Corruption', *Medical History*, 35, 3 (1991), 281–94.
92. R.I.E., *op. cit.* (note 63), Vol. 6, 15 June 1795, 228. For conditions in England, see A. Berry, 'Community Sponsorship and the Hospital Patient in Late Eighteenth-Century England', in P. Horden and R. Smith (eds), *Locus of Care: Communities, Institutions and the Provision of Welfare Since Antiquity* (London: Routledge, 1998), 126–49.
93. 'Everybody who knows anything about hospitals will acknowledge that it would be much better to admit only 150 patients all of whom may be comfortably accommodated and properly taken care of, than to receive into the hospital all that desired to be admitted as used to be done in the Hotel Dieu at Paris', in James Gregory, *Memorial to the Managers of the Royal Infirmary* (Edinburgh: Murray and Cochrane, 1800), 182.
94. *Ibid.*, 180.
95. Royal Infirmary of Edinburgh, *Annual Report for the Year 1801* (Edinburgh: J. Hay, 1802), 2.
96. This qualification was spelled out in the 'Rules for Admitting and Dismissing Patients' approved by the Edinburgh Infirmary managers on 2 November 1730.
97. [J. Stedman], 'A Power is Lodged with the Physicians and Surgeons, and Even with the Clerks, to Admit Patients in Case of Sudden Accidents, as Fractures, Dangerous Wounds, Contusions, or Where Lives are in Immediate Danger', in Anonymous, *The History and Statutes of the Royal Infirmary of Edinburgh* (Edinburgh: Balfour & Smellie, 1778), 76.
98. *Ibid.*, 10. See also R.I.E., *op. cit.* (note 63), Vol. 4, meeting of 14 March 1774, 308–9. For more details about the transportation of the sick see H.W. Hart, 'The Conveyance of Patients To and From Hospital, 1720–1850', *Medical History*, 22, 4 (1978), 397–407.
99. 'I have taken occasion to censure that spirit of penurious economy which makes charity so unlike itself and often defeats its benevolent intentions', in Aikin, *op. cit.* (note 4), 55.
100. See cases of Christian S. and Janet W. in James Gregory, Clinical Notes and Lectures (Edinburgh, 1779–80), MSS Collection, Royal College of Physicians, Edinburgh.

101. R.I.E., *op. cit.* (note 63), Vol. 4, 7 May 1764, 77.
102. Details in Turner, *op. cit.* (note 47), 91–115.
103. See case of Saunders B., in D. Rutherford, Clinical Lectures by Dr Daniel Rutherford MD (Edinburgh, 1799), MSS Collection, Royal College of Physicians, Edinburgh.
104. Risse, *op. cit.* (note 8), 108–12. For details, see S. Shapin, *A Social History of Truth: Civility and Science in Seventeenth-Century England* (Chicago: University of Chicago Press, 1994), 8–17.
105. F. Home, Clinical Lectures Delivered in the Year 1769, taken by John Goodsir (Edinburgh, 1769), MSS Collection, Royal College of Physicians, Edinburgh, 2. Some of the patients were characterised as 'extremely given to complain'. See case of Margaret Mc Cullock, in Rutherford, Clinical Lectures, *op. cit.* (note 103).
106. 'We know that falsehood prevails among men', William Cullen told his students, exhorting them to routinely challenge the testimony of incoming patients if the accounts appeared odd or inconsistent. See W. Cullen, Clinical Lectures (Edinburgh, 1772–3), MSS Collection, Royal College of Physicians, Edinburgh, 651.
107. Risse, *op. cit.* (note 8), 235–7.
108. W. Blizard, *Suggestions for the Improvement of Hospitals and Other Charitable Institutions* (London: H.L. Galabin, 1796), 81.
109. [Stedman], *op. cit.* (note 97), 23.
110. R.I.E., *op. cit.* (note 2), 5.
111. Buchan, *Domestic Medicine* (New York: R. Scott, 1812), XV.
112. Cullen, *op. cit.* (note 106), 504.
113. [Stedman], *op. cit.* (note 97), 89.
114. C.D. Leake (ed.), *Percival's Medical Ethics* (Baltimore: Williams & Wilkins, 1927), 72–3.
115. Cullen, *op. cit.* (note 106), 145.
116. John Gregory, *op. cit.* (note 51), 21; see L. Haakonssen, *Medicine and Morals in the Enlightenment: John Gregory, Thomas Percival and Benjamin Rush* (Amsterdam: Rodopi, 1997), 46-93.
117. Anon., *op. cit.* (note 73), 5.
118. R.I.E., *op. cit.* (note 63), Vol. 4, 2 July 1774, 315-6.
119. *Ibid.*, Vol. 3, 5 February 1750, 39.
120. An interesting circumstance is described by William Cullen in his clinical lectures dealing with a young boy who apparently suffered from epilepsy: 'I think the boy has got a tonic remedy of a more powerful kind than any we can employ. His ordinary home is forty miles from any practitioner of physic and his father is unable to keep him in the hands of physicians and apothecaries... where he would most trust to their attentions, so he has put

him in here. But the boy is of a condition above the vulgar and has been bred a little better, he has more delicacy, attention, and care and was not a little shocked at being put in here, and was struck with a considerable dread and awe. When he was left alone, he did not dare to look out from the chamber; it was proposed that he might go out to the back court for the sake of the air, but he found a soldier, a strange sort of animal to him, whereupon he immediately shrunk back into his cell with a good deal of fear. In short, this boy has been under a considerable dread ever since he came in', Cullen, *op. cit.* (note 106), 125–6.

121. See cases of Elizabeth S. and Margaret B. in W. Cullen, Clinical Cases and Reports, taken by Richard W. Hall (Edinburgh, 1772–3), MSS Collection, National Library of Medicine, Bethesda, Maryland, USA.
122. R.I.E., *op. cit.* (note 63), Vol. 4, 2 July 1774, 316.
123. W.B. Howie, 'Complaints and Complaint Procedures in the Eighteenth- and Early Nineteenth-Century Provincial Hospitals in England', *Medical History* 25, 4 (1981), 345–62.
124. J. Wilde, *The Hospital, A Poem in Three Books Written in the Devon and Exeter Hospital, 1809* (Norwich: Stevenson, Matchett, and Stevenson, 1810), 27. I am indebted to Dr William B. Howie for pointing out this unique and invaluable source. See his essay 'Consumer Reaction: A Patient's View of Hospital Life in 1809', *British Medical Journal,* 3 (1973), 534–6.
125. *Ibid.*, 32. Dr Howie was of the opinion that given the standard of education in late eighteenth-century Britain, few hospital inmates would have been capable of writing such an account.
126. *Ibid.*, 61.
127. Instead of attempting to cut short their hospital stay, Thomas Spens later testified that 'great difficulty is experienced in prevailing on the patients to quit the hospital after they are no longer proper subjects for the Infirmary' R.I.E., *op. cit.* (note 2), 8.
128. *Ibid.*, 9.
129. Cullen, *op. cit.* (note 106), 60.
130. *Ibid.*, 186–7.
131. *Ibid.*
132. Case of Adam C. in James Gregory, Cases of Patients Under the Care of James Gregory MD (Edinburgh, 1781–2), MSS Collection, Royal College of Physicians, Edinburgh.
133. Blizard, *op. cit.* (note 108), 70.
134. E.M. Sigsworth, 'Gateways to Death? Medicine, Hospitals and Mortality, 1700–1850', in P. Mathias (ed.), *Science and Society, 1600–1900* (Cambridge: Cambridge University Press, 1972), 97–110.
135. Aikin, *op. cit.* (note 4), 56.

136. Blizard, *op. cit.* (note 108), 72.
137. Cullen, *op. cit.* (note 106), 578; see also G.B. Risse, 'Typhus Fever in Eighteenth-Century Hospitals: New Approaches to Medical Treatment', *Bulletin of the History of Medicine,* 59 (1985), 176–95.
138. Risse, *op. cit.* (note 8), 261–6; see also Sigsworth, *op. cit.* (note 134), 97–110.
139. James Gregory, *Additional Memorial to the Managers of the Royal Infirmary* (Edinburgh: Murray & Cochrane, 1803), 382–3.
140. Anon., *op. cit.* (note 73), 5.
141. R.I.E., *op. cit.* (note 2), 68.
142. P. Mac Flogg'em (pseud.), *Aesculapian Secrets Revealed* (London: C. Chapple, 1813), 42.
143. Leake, *op. cit.* (note 114), 125.
144. Mac Flogg'em, *op. cit.* (note 142), 43.
145. Blizard, *op. cit.* (note 108), 34.
146. Bellers, *op. cit.* (note 21), 14.
147. G.B. Risse, 'Clinical Instruction in Hospitals: The Boerhaavian Tradition in Leyden, Edinburgh, Vienna, and Pavia', *Clio Medica* 21 (1987/88), 1–19.
148. Bellers, *op. cit.* (note 21), 10–11.
149. For Edinburgh, see Risse, *op. cit.* (note 8), 261–6; for England see S.C. Lawrence, *Charitable Knowledge: Hospital Pupils and Practitioners in Eighteenth-Century London* (Cambridge: Cambridge University Press, 1996); for France, see T. Gelfand, *Professionalizing Modern Medicine* (Westport, Conn.: Greenwood Press, 1980), 178–86.
150. G.B. Risse, 'A Shift in Medical Epistemology: Clinical Diagnosis 1770–1828', in Y. Kawakita (ed.), *History of Diagnostics,* Proceedings of the 9th International Symposium on the Comparative History of Medicine – East and West (Osaka: Tanaguchi Foundation, 1987), 115–47.
151. Such were the comments of Thomas Gisborne, a friend of Thomas Percival. See R. Porter, 'Thomas Gisborne: Physicians, Christians and Gentlemen', in A. Wear, J. Geyer-Kordesch and R. French (eds), *Doctors and Ethics: The Earlier Historical Setting of Professional Ethics* (Amsterdam: Rodopi, 1993), 252–73.
152. For more details, Risse, *op. cit.* (note 8), 34–56.
153. A.H. Maehle, *Drugs on Trial: Experimental Pharmacology and Therapeutic Innovation in the Eighteenth Century* (Amsterdam: Rodopi, 1999).
154. J.W. Estes, 'Drug Usage at the Infirmary: The Example of Dr Andrew Duncan, Sr', in Risse, *op. cit.* (note 8), 351–84.
155. Aikin, *op. cit.* (note 4), 79–81.
156. F. Home, *Clinical Experiments, Histories, and Dissections* (London: Murray, 1782), IX; see J.F. Enders, 'Francis Home and His Experimental Approach

to Medicine', *Bulletin of the History of Medicine,* 38 (1964), 101–12.
157. Aikin, *op. cit.* (note 4), 81.
158. Home, *op. cit.* (note 156), 58. For details, Risse, *op. cit.* (note 8), 177–228.
159. Gregory, *op. cit.* (note 93), 143.
160. Gregory, *op. cit.* (note 139), 507.
161. E.H. Ackerknecht, 'Therapeutics', in *Medicine at the Paris Hospital, 1794–1848* (Baltimore: Johns Hopkins University Press, 1967), 129–38.
162. C.H. Creswell, 'The Early Association of the Incorporation of Surgeons with the Royal Infirmary', in *Royal College of Surgeons of Edinburgh* (Edinburgh: Oliver & Boyd, 1926), 208–33.
163. Barfoot, *op. cit.* (note 68); see also J. Woodward, *To Do The Sick No Harm: A Study of the British Voluntary Hospital System to 1875* (London: Routledge & Kegan Paul, 1974).
164. [J. Johnson], *A Guide for Gentlemen Studying Medicine at the University of Edinburgh* (London: Robison, 1792), 46.
165. R.I.E., *op. cit.* (note 63), Vol. 6, 4 June 1792, 137.
166. *Ibid.*, Vol. 6, 5 May 1794, 200.
167. *Ibid.*, Vol. 6, 7 November 1800, 379 and 1 December 1800, 394.
168. Barfoot, *op. cit.* (note 68). See also J. Bell, *Answer for the Junior Members of the Royal College of Surgeons of Edinburgh to the Memorial of James Gregory* (Edinburgh: P. Hill, 1800). For developments in London, see W.F. Bynum, 'Physicians, Hospitals, and Career Structures in Eighteenth-Century London', in W.F. Bynum and R. Porter (eds), *William Hunter and the Eighteenth-Century Medical World* (Cambridge: Cambridge University Press, 1985), 105–28.
169. See O. Temkin,'The Role of Surgery in the Rise of Modern Medical Thought', *Bulletin of the History of Medicine,* 25 (1951), 248–59; Barfoot also makes this point in his 'Pedagogy, Practice and Politics', *op. cit.* (note 68); see also I. Loudon, 'Medical Practitioners, 1750-1850 and the Period of Medical Reform in Britain', in Wear, *op. cit.* (note 17), 219–47.
170. [Johnson], *op. cit.* (note 164), 47; see also B. Bell, 'Observations on the Modes of Attendance of Surgeons of Edinburgh on the Royal Infirmary, in a Letter addressed to the Royal College of Surgeons' (Edinburgh, 1800).
171. W. Black, *An Arithmetical and Medical Analysis of the Diseases and Mortality of the Human Species,* 2nd edn (London: Crowder, 1789); see U. Tröhler, '"To Improve the Evidence of Medicine": Arithmetic Observations in Clinical Medicine in the 18th and Early 19th Centuries', *History and Philosophy of the Life Sciences,* 10 (1988), suppl. 31–40; A. Borsay, 'An Example of Political Arithmetic: The Evaluations of Spa Therapy at the Georgian Bath Infirmary, 1742–1830', *Medical History,* 44, 2 (2000), 149–72.

172. Aikin, *op. cit.* (note 4), 76–81.
173. A. Duncan Sr, *Medical Cases Selected from the Records of the Public Dispensary of Edinburgh* (Edinburgh: C. Elliot, 1778), IX.
174. Wrote Percival: 'Hospital physicians and surgeons… should in their deportment to unite *tenderness* with *steadiness*, and *condescension* with *authority*, as to inspire the minds of their patients with gratitude, respect and confidence', in Leake, *op. cit.* (note 114), 71.
175. An engraving of the Infirmary can be found in Anonymous, *A New Guide to the City of Edinburgh*, 3rd edn (Edinburgh: T. Brown, 1797), 80–1; see also A.H. Stirling, *A Sketch of Scottish Industrial and Social History in the Eighteenth and Nineteenth Centuries* (London: Blackie & Son, 1906), 72.
176. R.I.E., *op. cit.* (note 95), 1.

2

Debates and Experiments: The Royal Medical Society of Edinburgh

Like other Scottish clubs and societies, this student-run organisation was a public forum where medical students could present their own papers and hone rhetorical skills. This essay is a first attempt to present and analyse the broad range of dissertations composed and presented during the last two decades of the eighteenth century. The documents offer a valuable window into contemporary Scottish medical science. Behind a façade of didactic exercises, the Society gradually shifted from an elite debating club into an institution adopting new epistemological foundations for the acquisition of medical knowledge that included the design and execution of human and animal experiments.

Introduction

> It is the inevitable tendency of the Scot mind to follow out every line to its terminus... In humble cottages as well as in University societies, the Scot is disputing in every spare moment of his time, from morning till night.
>
> John Watson (1907)[1]

On Saturday, 31 October 1778, a group of Edinburgh medical students belonging to the Royal Medical Society assembled for the season's inaugural meeting. The forty-second session came to order under the direction of senior president Andrew Wardrop, who a few months earlier had signed a petition to King George III requesting a royal charter for this student-led organisation. Another academic year was about to begin at the University, and the atmosphere in the Medical Hall, which opened two years earlier, was festive and expectant. Among the scheduled speakers were two junior presidents, Edward Stevens and John Ford. Stevens was experimenting on the nature of gastric juice. Ford had joined the Society in December 1776 and planned to graduate the following year. Both were friends of another student, John Brown (1735–88), a former president of the Society who was becoming a vociferous critic of the medical theories held by William Cullen (1710–90), the doyen of Edinburgh academic medicine. Stevens' presentation narrowly examined the behaviour of metals during the process of calcination. Ford's essay was about the search for the best method of studying medicine and its branches. Apologising for his inadequacies, including the necessary rhetorical skills, Ford vowed to discharge his duty by addressing the paper to men of his own rank who hoped to conduct themselves as gentlement and pursue their studies with determination. Custom and rules allowed for subsequent discussion of these papers with final copies handed to the session president. Bound in yearly folios, these dissertations constitute a unique collection of documents essential for a full understanding of Scottish medicine during its period of highest accomplishments.

Background and organisation

Several prominent medical students attending the University first established the Medical Society of Edinburgh in 1734. They included John Fothergill (1712–80), later a fashionable London practitioner, and George Cleghorn (1716–89), subsequently appointed professor of anatomy in Dublin. Formally constituted in 1737, the Society was the oldest Scottish medical organisation exclusively run by, and devoted to, medical students. The stated objective of this fraternity was 'the improvement of medical knowledge', considered essential to bolster the scientific and professional authority of practitioners. To implement the program, the fledgling physicians pledged to meet regularly and present their own learned papers and clinical cases obtained from the local Infirmary. The idea was to engage the entire membership in wide-ranging scholarship and promote freewheeling discussions. Like other social functions in Edinburgh, these youthful gatherings initially took place in the convivial atmosphere of a tavern. After holding regular meetings in a room placed at their disposal in the Edinburgh Infirmary, the students moved into their own building in 1776 and received a royal charter from George III on 14 December 1778.[2]

A product of a new urban culture and morality, the Society became one of several voluntary organisations in eighteenth-century Edinburgh that, in an era of growing commercial complexity, played an important role in Scotland's development. The organisation was a tangible expression of the Scottish Enlightenment, a new cultural movement responsible for gradually transforming Scotland from a backward, poor country into a prosperous British province.[3] In Edinburgh, this ideology of self-improvement brought together leading aristocrats, clergymen, philosophers, literati, lawyers, and medical men, turning the abandoned seat of royalty into a cultural hub known as the 'Athens of the North'.[4] Other learned associations, among them the Philosophical Society and the Royal Physical Society, also shared Enlightenment values and interest in scientific matters. Their elite memberships included most of the intellectual luminaries residing in Edinburgh.[5] Early leaders of the Royal Medical Society supported freedom of expression, polite learning, humanitarianism and personal virtue. They were keen on fostering a scholarly and professional image for young men who had committed themselves to the study of medicine. At the beginning, the institution was closely linked to the Edinburgh Society for the Improvement of Medical Knowledge, a professional group of local physicians, surgeons, and university professors founded in 1731.[6] Later, the Aesculapian Club (1773) and Harveian Society (1782) – both founded by Andrew Duncan, Sr. (1744–1828) – also became sites for convivial medical meetings.[7]

Much has been written about Scotland's ideological background favouring what one recent author has coined a 'system of voluntary face-to-face relationships between independently minded individuals' within a 'society'.[8] Supported by traditional elites and a growing, prosperous middle-class clubs and societies created networks for social, intellectual and professional exchanges. According to Adam Smith (1723–90), associations between men from the middling ranks were the products of 'sensibility' and 'sympathy'. Such qualities of social responsibility and reciprocal fellowship provided a sense of moral autonomy and personal identity for those people who pledged to work for the reputation and dignity of the profession (Chapter 7).[9]

In the 1760s, when the University of Edinburgh achieved an international reputation as one of the best places for medical learning in Europe, natives as well as foreigners eagerly flocked to the city for the purpose of attending lectures and obtaining doctoral degrees.[10] University education was considered extremely important for establishing a successful medical practice. One satirical observer recommended that any 18-year-old with a smattering of Greek and Latin who wished to become a physician should 'enter himself as student in Edinburgh', lingering there for some three years before obtaining a degree. Equipped with a diploma, many newly minted doctors headed for London where they could 'astonish the natives'.[11] Scottish university studies had abandoned the tutorial system and replaced it with a scheme based on lectures and demonstrations given for a fee by several intramural professors and extramural lecturers. This permissive and somewhat unstructured arrangement drew a growing crowd of independent-minded students to Edinburgh; welcomed consumers ready to boost the local economy. These young men were free to select their classes, hire tutors and repeat courses at whim. They 'shopped' and paid for lecture courses given by popular teachers, listening to their presentations and taking extensive notes. Between class attendance, students filled local rooming houses and crowded alehouses with what the American student Samuel Bard (1742–1821) – later president of the College of Physicians and Surgeons in New York – called 'schemes of dissipation'.[12]

Amid the multiple urban distractions, the Royal Medical Society provided a welcome oasis of structure and propriety. The Society offered opportunities for professional fellowship as well as individual involvement and peer-controlled dialogue. Its sponsorship of polite discussions in an atmosphere of moderation and reasonableness stood in sharp contrast to the official fragmented, depersonalised and laissez-faire academic program. It was the ideal complement to medical studies at Edinburgh University. As Fothergill remarked, the Royal Medical Society came to develop a growing reputation as an active local community, a 'seminary of physic'.[13] With the help of a Library Committee, publications were obtained through direct purchase, exchanges with other learned societies in Britain and the Continent, and gifts from former members. Natural history specimens were also gathered for study.[14] Later, in 1751, the Society decided to collect all papers prepared and delivered by students, preserving them in folios for the perusal of its members.[15]

The Society began as a forum with opportunities 'for display of eloquence and for saying plausible and ingenious things' among well-born gentlemen who could uphold the dignity of the profession because of their social status.[16] By the 1770s, however, its original character experienced significant changes as medicine expanded its professional horizons to include employment in the armed forces, hospitals and dispensaries. Thus, Society members were increasingly drawn from a pool of students representing diverse social backgrounds and religious affiliations. A new ethos of sincerity, motivation, and the search for knowledge, based on Baconian and Newtonian principles, came to dominate the meetings. This discussion, therefore, focuses on a broad survey of surviving papers for the years 1778–92. It attempts to describe the nature, scope, content, and methodology employed in the preparation of these papers, and reach a number of conclusions. The choice of years is not arbitrary. This period coincided with a very active and sometimes contentious era in the life of the Society as it became increasingly polarised under the impact of certain highly publicised debates and controversies (Chapter 3). Following receipt of the prestigious Royal Charter, membership multiplied rapidly. Between the 1782–3 and 1787–8 sessions alone, the Society grew by nearly a third, counting 257 members – by far the highest number for the eighteenth century – only to decline during the 1790s by about fifty percent.[17]

Students needed to be enrolled in university courses for at least six months before applying for membership in the Society. Candidates required a letter of recommendation signed by at least six current members. The petition for a seat in the Society had to be formally presented at one of the sessions by another associate before being subjected to a ballot. The Society's laws demanded at least a two-thirds majority vote in favour of admission. No candidate receiving insufficient votes could be presented more than three times during the entire academic year. Once their request was accepted, new members were invited to officially subscribe to the laws and regulations of the organisation, including faithful attendance of the meetings, presentation of papers, and payment of various and expensive fees. A special Program Committee was elected each February. It assigned topics and dates for the delivery of student essays six months in advance of the scheduled presentations. With the Committee's approval, however, new students could write on subjects of their own choosing. Authors needed to provide three copies to the Society's officers well in advance of the scheduled delivery for perusal and study by the membership at large.

Governance of the Society was distributed among four presidents elected for each academic session, These men were ranked by seniority and charged with chairing the meetings, which included conducting roll calls at the beginning and end of the private and public business segments. They also accepted written versions of student papers, dealt with visitors, monitored presentations, and tried to moderate the ensuing discussion. All meetings of the Society were held in Edinburgh every Friday or Saturday evening during the academic year, from early November until April at 7pm. On average, the leadership scheduled twenty-four sessions each year, including a few extraordinary meetings on Saturdays to consider urgent administrative matters. There was no fixed deadline for adjournment, only a limit on the transaction of private Society business before the presentations and debates. As long as an ordinary member resided in Edinburgh, he was expected to participate in the discussions. Those who graduated and moved elsewhere became extraordinary members excused from compulsory attendance. Students who failed to comply with all regulations were subject to substantial fines.[18]

Closely linked to the University of Edinburgh, the Society was an ideal forum for students to rehearse their academic requirements for obtaining a doctoral degree. Considerable emphasis was, therefore, placed on the oratory, literary and debating skills of its elite members. Newcomers were required to engage in rituals deemed preparatory for launching a successful medical career. At the core were three presentations: one based on a clinical case; another, a response to a specific question; and the last, a commentary on well-known medical aphorisms. Information for the clinical case was usually drawn from records of the Edinburgh Infirmary (Chapter 1). Answers to queries proposed by other members included well-argued and researched summaries of contemporary knowledge. Such student papers were increasingly supplemented with additional evidence derived from personal observations. Aphorisms derived from the writings of famous medical authors from the Hippocratic collection to recent times. By the late 1770s, however, the aphorism requirement was often replaced with an additional clinical case presentation, presumably a sign of the increasing importance being accorded to clinical subjects within the Edinburgh Medical School curriculum. If the multiple presentations of a candidate were deemed satisfactory, the student was officially incorporated into the Society and became eligible for elected office, especially that of junior or senior president. Such positions constituted valuable stepping stones for a future academic career, particularly as extramural lecturer in Edinburgh.[19]

New arrivals were quickly assimilated, adopting the values and social manners of genteel professionals within a rigid, hierarchical organisation ruled by seniority. Many viewed their membership as a vehicle for achieving status and identity, even 'honourable fame'.[20] Custom suggested that freshmen members show deference to their elder peers and avoid the appearance of presumptuous expertise about the topics they were presenting. In 1780, student Philip Holland, admitted his question should have been put to a professor 'who has great abilities and a very extensive practice' rather than to a student 'who comes to be informed rather than to inform'. But, he conceded, 'we must conform to the rules of this Society and endeavour to give a very short and we fear very superficial answer'.[21] Much has been made about the didactic nature of these literary exercises. Imitating their professors, the students' essays marshalled the existing evidence and seldom expressed a particular point of view.[22] Many students began their presentations by indicating that their subject lacked originality and much had already been said and written about it by others. Most begged forgiveness for their hasty and imperfect productions, hoping that 'the candour of the Society will excuse and the ingenuity of the members will supply its numerous deficiencies'. Others humbly apologised in advance for inadvertent omissions and errors contained in their 'imperfect and undigested notes'[23] or for being longwinded.[24] Pledging to abide by the authority of eminent authors, they expressed indebtedness to those whose opinions coincided with their own. Some members even publicly admitted outright ignorance of the subject they were scheduled to deliver, claiming that it had been impossible to properly prepare a paper in the few months between assignment and delivery dates.[25] A few with brief essays were candid enough to cite additional 'distractions' and 'other avocations' as excuses for their lack of preparation.[26]

In 1771, the current Society president, Andrew Duncan Sr, reassured his fellow students that professors 'know that their opinions are compared without partiality or prejudice. They are not ignorant of the freedom with which objections to the doctrines they teach are here started'. According to Duncan, faculty members indeed 'approve of your endeavours to impugn these doctrines'.[27] Despite such rhetorical encouragement, students remained cautious about expressing views that clearly clashed with the belief and theories of their professors and other recognised medical authorities. They wished, after all, to graduate, and it was much safer to tow the official line. Increasingly, however, in the early 1780s, several Society members started to shed the prescribed cloak of modesty and deference. Discussing the effects of emotion during the 1787–8 session, one student was quite assertive about his conviction that the passions were all stimulants. To soften his bravado, he quickly added that 'we are not magisterial in opinion; nor would we, dictator-like, obtrude our conceptions, but, in the humility of inquiries would propose them to more ocular discerners. And, therefore, opinions are free and open'.[28] Another member somewhat sarcastically pledged that he would not take upon him 'flatly to contradict the assertion of grave physicians clad in the dignity of professorial robes nor the implicit assent which many are inclined sadly to pay to the dictatorial effusions of their pens'.[29] Every 'real lover of science' had an obligation to present original observations and opinions even if they clashed with current beliefs (Chapter 3).[30]

After each student paper was delivered, the floor opened for 'judicious remarks', a formal discussion involving those attending the meeting. In his previously quoted memoirs, Samuel Bard remembered spending nearly four hours debating the issues, using all his knowledge and rhetorical skills to defend his newly formed opinions. Like Scottish men of letters as well as ministers of the Kirk, such native propensity for debate and discussion was considered necessary and fruitful. Exercises in argumentation were considered appropriate pathways to knowledge and truth. Historians have characterised the dynamics of such contested dialogues as being 'corporatist'[31] since they transcended individual opinions and allowed for a collective construction of knowledge.

The assumption was that the Royal Medical Society was composed of committed, polite gentlemen who respected each others beliefs but were ready to engage in critiques and express contrary opinions as a way to improve their own judgement and knowledge. According to Fothergill, 'questions, no doubt, were here disputed and decided which long experience would have declined. But it exercised their faculties, gave them both sides of arguments, taught them to doubt, and habituated them to observation'.[32] To be sure, debates honed rhetorical skills useful in philosophical debates and consultations; but were of dubious value for settling practical medical questions. Yet, balanced reasoning and lucid writing, eloquence and conviction, were all desirable skills for properly-educated gentlemen physicians who needed to acquire sufficient professional authority in their dealings with affluent patients.[33]

Epistemological issues: system-building and the scientific method

One of the key issues periodically presented and discussed in the Society was the perceived lack of progress in medicine. In the face of widely acclaimed contemporary discoveries in physics and chemistry, this judgement was quite troubling to a profession in search of authority and control of the medical marketplace. Given the divergent views about the role of theory, especially the construction of medical systems,[34] such arguments dominated the presentations. They centred on the appropriate methodology used in promoting new medical knowledge. Here, students found themselves in a real quandary. From the Society's inception, members of the local Medical School had strongly promoted a rational and systematic arrangement of medical knowledge, first adhering to the schemes formulated by the Dutch physician Hermann Boerhaave (1668–1739).[35] By the 1770s, however, the ideas of Cullen, professor of the practice of medicine, had come to dominate Edinburgh's medical establishment. Although not an original thinker, Cullen nevertheless managed to construct a coherent system of explanations concerned with bodily behaviour in health and disease by weaving together a number of recent experimental findings in neuromuscular physiology. Students were loath to challenge the status quo and advocate further studies. To do so would run the risk those new facts would strain or challenge their master's doctrine.

To complicate matters, Cullen tried to diffuse the unique nature of his system by considering it just a heuristic tool for organising all medical knowledge.[36] During the 1778–9 session, two students, John Ford and J.P. Harris, tried to wrestle with this issue. Ford advocated a combination of reasoning (philosophy) and observation (induction) to elucidate the truth or error of current scientific knowledge. Personal judgement rather than dependence on school opinions were supposedly the key. While acknowledging the need for a comprehensive medical theory, Ford also attempted to stress that theory was not a proper guide for clinical activities at the bedside.[37] In fact, Ford went on to praise Sydenham's empirical approach. He declared that it would be better to rely on the intuitive conduct of an old nurse rather than a physician who 'mechanically' followed rational doctrine. Harris, for his part, justified his conclusions by simply labelling them inductive; in his words, a 'recapitulation of effects established upon experience and the result of actual observations not being drawn from the intuitive reasoning of theories nor the fallacious conclusions of analogies'.[38] He believed that science had been impeded in its progress by ignorance regarding the functioning of the human mind. Other students chimed in, insisting in their papers that a veneration of previous medical authorities and their hypothetical reasoning still held excessive ground. Instead, they proposed a union of 'theory with experiment and observation'. In 1780, John Howell sought to relieve the art of medicine from its present state of uncertainty and error by encouraging 'men of independent fortunes' in the mould of the scientist–gentleman to study medicine 'as an interesting branch of natural physiology'.[39]

In subsequent years, however, the tone of many presentations at the Society became increasingly hostile and critical of what was perceived and labelled as the 'Cullenian' system (Chapter 3). The conclusion, expressed by another student, was self-evident: 'every attempt, hitherto, to establish a safe and reasonable practice under the direction of an adequate or unquestionable theory of science failed miserably'.[40] When it came to drug treatments, theoretical considerations were not helpful. Individual narratives of health-related experiences, including the action of drugs, were valuable testimonials and guides for therapy. Speaking about the effects of opium and alcohol, student Edward Harrison followed an increasingly fashionable empiricism by arguing that 'almost every individual in the civilised world' knew first-hand about the effects of these two popular stimulants. Students experimenting on themselves or using animals as subjects could also make important contributions. Everybody, in fact, was in a position to advance scientific knowledge and the Society's aims of professional improvement. 'My business', announced Harrison, 'is to collect facts; let others reason on them'.[41] Another student, Henry Ainslie, suggested that members first plan a trip to the library and then, informed by good medical authors, consult nature and acquire experience with 'Providence your guide'.[42] No longer should the delivery of 'a view of the subject different from the commonly received' be stigmatising, observed his fellow student, John Lawson, since it was 'the duty of every member to lay before the Society every improvement that may be in his power'.[43] Many of these student pronouncements, of course, were just rhetorical. Yet, one can sense a new and liberating strain within the rather didactic and passive framework of Edinburgh medical education: the student not merely as collector, abstractor, and presenter but active contributor to medical knowledge. This notion created a new impetus among many members of the Society to communicate their own clinical and experimental findings – 'the real fountain' – for new ideas.

The World at large: studying 'natural philosophy'

From modest beginnings in the late 1770s, the Royal Medical Society increasingly engaged in discussions of general scientific topics, a practice that reached its peak in the late 1780s and early 1790s. After years of bitter confrontations related to epistemological and physiological issues, members evidently sought to broaden their horizons. Indeed, in each of the 1790–1 and 1792–3 sessions, students presented a number of papers on a variety of subjects. In 1783, John Duncan had already admitted in his essay that 'the science of medicine has gained considerable advantages from other sciences.... The medical world is certainly much indebted to those ingenious authors who have investigated the laws of mechanics or explored the secrets of chemistry'.[44] These presentations focused on the physical and human environment as key factors in health and disease. This view provided an additional role for physicians in managing both individual and public health (Chapter 4).[45] Thus, a series of student presentations focused on basic issues such as the nature and phenomena of life, theories of generation, sensibility of plants and economy of vegetation.[46] A frequent topic for discussion involved the similarities and differences between the animal and vegetable kingdoms.[47] Questions about the cause of animal heat and preservation of temperature led to a discussion of Lavoisier's work and the role of oxygen.[48] Students queried whether animals acted instinctively, or what the differences were between animals and the intellectual powers of humans.[49]

Additionally, chemical questions abounded. Students followed the interests of their chemistry professors, William Cullen, and later Joseph Black (1728–9),[50] in discussing the composition of air and water, the nature of phlogiston, crystallisation and its causes, and spontaneous evaporation.[51] During several sessions, various members spoke about the nature and causes of heat, combustion and fermentation.[52] Others collected information on the calcination of metals as well as the formation and uses of nitre and vitriolic acid.[53] Another presentation focused on pneumatic chemistry and new theories of respiration. In one instance, contemporary chemistry itself came under attack, as one member, Charles Throckmorton, argued that analysis could not be relied upon because once the substances subjected to examination had been exposed to fire, their nature changed irreversibly and all results would be 'confusing'.[54] During the 1783–4 session, David Skeene favourably reviewed a critical issue: the usefulness of chemistry in discovering the pharmacological action of certain drugs.[55] Here Black's experiments with calcium oxide and other alkaline substances in his quest for finding a compound to dissolve kidney stones played a role in inspiring the students' interests in applied chemistry.

The earthly environment also came under considerable scrutiny. Besides conferring on cause and effect in physics, members presented information on the earth's stratified crust, causes of earthquakes, atmospheric electricity, gravitation and the phenomena of tides, origin of winds, and theory of water spouts.[56] In 1785, R. Miller turned to anthropological themes, discussing possible relationships between the physical environment and the formation of human races.[57] Miller sought the explanation for the various complexions observed among different races.[58] Three years later, the American student, Benjamin Smith Barton, commented on the natural history of North American Indians,[59] and, during the 1791–2 season, natural healing methods of the Indians were highlighted.[60] Richard Pearson, senior student president of the Society's 1785–6 session, expanded on the anodyne virtues of hope by launching into an extensive account of the Orinoco Indians and their new chief's painful initiation rites that included repeated floggings.[61]

Health and disease: physiological and pathological questions

Speaking about the milder clinical manifestations of inoculated smallpox during the 1785–6 session of the Society, one of the students aptly pointed out the key contemporary dilemma when he stated that 'the discussion of medical questions is a business of the most difficult and uncertain nature'. Given the complex structure of the body and the 'hidden nature of the powers which operate upon it' ignorance prevailed. Even 'after the most elaborate investigations', medicine remained 'in great obscurity'.[62] In spite of the perplexities, Society members wrote quite frequently about topics dealing with health preservation. Some of the so-called 'non-naturals', including climate, weather and the seasons received considerable attention (Chapter 4).[63] One of Cullen's followers repeated his teacher's notions about debility and exposure to disease caused by the relaxation of solids.[64] Some essays related to the preservation of health and susceptibility to diseases in various stages of life.[65] Citing experiments made by Lavoisier, Boyle and Priestley, other Society members discoursed on the effects of atmospheric conditions in health and disease such as high pressure and the problems of vitiated air as well as the means for restoring its purity.[66] The influence of climate and life-style on constitution, temperament and complexion, as well as disease in various countries was also explored.[67] Students wondered if there could be advantages for keeping meteorological registers.[68] Finally, the Society heard essays devoted to sleep – an accumulation of excitability – together with effects of exercise.[69] Mental factors were not neglected, with papers on the mechanisms and stimulation of the passions,[70] as well as the impact of grief and fear.[71] There were also presentations on hearing and the role of the tympanic membrane, the physiology of vision, including the perception of distance and probable cause of strabismus.[72]

On the topic of human growth and development, students examined contemporary theories of generation, the nature of hereditary diseases,[73] and the question of sterility. Differences in physical structure between the fetus and adults also prompted discussions on the placenta's role as a pulmonary organ. Growth and nourishment of the fetus, especially during the last months of pregnancy [74] were reviewed, together with obstruction of umbilical circulation and infant death. Ailments prevailing during infancy, the process of ossification in childhood and puberty, and bone formation following fractures were also studied. [75] Some presentations focused on bodily changes taking place at puberty, including an analysis of the structure and functions of glands and causes of menstruation (Chapter 8).[76] Others probed the action of minerals in the body.[77] Due to frequency of bladder stones, several students discussed their formation and composition.[78]

Society members demonstrated great interest in the physiopathology of muscular contraction; the laws of muscle fibres, sentient powers and moving solids, all framed within a vitalistic context. The linkage to nerves and nature of volition sparked repeated presentations and discussions including a paper on the effects of animal magnetism on the human body.[79] Many of the conclusions were based on recent animal experimentation in which the heart was used to study muscular excitement and circulation. In addition to this focus on motions of the heart, students made several presentations on arterial circulation and irritability. Quoting Cullen and Hoffmann's writings, one student discussed arterial atony and its relation to fever.[80] There were also papers on the abolition of animal functions in apoplexy, excessive blood circulation or plethora, and the circumstances retarding the healing of ulcers. Both the nature and properties of blood and its tendency towards putrefaction generated interest, as were haemorrhages and pus formation.[81] Moreover, students dealt with the causes of the blood's inflammatory crust and the notion of blood as the principle of life.[82] Not surprisingly, the nature of inflammation and fever drew centre stage. Members discussed the origin of different fevers, specifically the nature of hectic and typhus fever (Chapter 7).[83] Great concern was expressed about the effects of heat and cold on the human body: some members insisted that cold possessed a sedative quality while others actually considered cold a stimulant.[84] Students were also interested in the nature and action of contagion,[85] often understood as a localised stimulus. Using old humoral theories, contagion was believed to irritate the surface of the body, causing a stagnation of matter and perspiration under the skin that was responsible for the eruptions accompanying several conditions such as smallpox and measles.[86]

Another subject popular with Edinburgh students was the process of food digestion. Members of the Society specifically targeted the nature of saliva, gastric juice and bile for study. Several presented theories of intestinal absorption and discussed the role of the lymphatic system.[87] Bile had already been the topic of a 1757 thesis by Society member Robert Ramsay – later Professor of Natural History at the University. Other students were curious about the effects of biliary secretion and liver function including the appearance of jaundice. Since the seventeenth century, authors had written about 'fermentation' in the digestive tract, while others conceived digestion was a form of mechanical fragmentation, achieved through muscular action. Several Society students examined the nutrient principles in food,[88] and the uses of fat in the animal economy as a possible cause of obesity. In two papers published in 1752, the French naturalist René A.F. de Reaumur (1683-1757) reported on his isolation of gastric juice in birds. He had experimented on his pet buzzard, previously trained to ingest small sponges. Reamur's chemical studies and technique led Benjamin Rush, an American medical student and Society member, to take up this subject for his doctoral dissertation. Rush had arrived in Edinburgh to complete his studies, attending lectures in anatomy, the practice of physic, and chemistry. He was being groomed to assume a new chair of chemistry at the Medical School of the College of Philadelphia.[89] Following Cullen's suggestions, Rush and another student, William Penny, initiated a series of auto-experiments to ascertain the acidic nature of gastric digestion. Both ingested small portions of food, which they subsequently recovered for analysis with the help of emetics. Rush's 1768 thesis concluded that the first stage of digestion took place in the stomach under the influence of gastric acid.[90] In subsequent years, Edinburgh medical students continued to pursue the subject. Among them was Edward Stevens (1755?–1834), who actually became president of the Society following his graduation for the 1778–9 and 1779–80 academic years. Stevens hired a man 'of weak understanding' who had been making a living swallowing and regurgitating stones for public amusement. Using a hollow silver sphere with several compartments resembling a tea strainer, this student was able to study the digestion of several types of meat.[91] Later in Italy, Lazzaro Spallanzani (1729–9) carried out similar trials by regurgitating a sponge tied to a piece of string, confirming the chemical qualities of saliva and gastric secretions to dissolve meat. Stevens and Spallanzani's findings were published in 1780.[92]

Clinical subjects: cases and treatments

From its inception, the Society paid great attention to clinical issues. As early as 1747, members set up a Clinical Board charged with creating opportunities for students to obtain their own practical experiences by providing free medical attention to Edinburgh's sick–poor. Both senior and junior members dispensed this care and also provided destitute patients with supplies of needed drugs.[93] The Society's requirement to present cases closely followed the model instituted by John Rutherford (1695–1779), professor of the practice of medicine. Delivering his hospital lectures after 1748, Rutherford pledged to 'give you the history of the disease, inquire into the cause of it, give you my opinion as to how it will terminate, [and] lay down instructions of cure which will arise' (Chapter 7).[94] Such a systematic approach was widely supported by most medical authors, including William Cullen in his *First Lines of the Practice of Physic.* Students wrote their 'cases' in a similar fashion, merely citing the bare details about particular patients – presumably drawn from the Infirmary – as a convenient way to introduce the discussion of certain diseases.

A case of rabies, presented by P. James during the 1786–7 session, exemplified this approach. 'E.T.' – students only used patient initials – being for some days melancholy and languid, showed signs of horror at the sight of water which was brought into the room. On attempting to swallow a dish of tea, he was affected by violent and painful convulsions of the throat. His breathing laborious and a wild stare appeared in his countenance'. A few weeks before these symptoms presented, a mad dog had bitten him. Following such brief particulars, the presenters made some general comments. In this case, James stressed the absolute certainty of the diagnosis and prognosis of a disease that was always fatal. He also indicated how frustrating and mortifying it was for the physician to realise the limitations of his art except for dispensing 'miserable palliation'. Although 'canine madness' was not infrequent, James indicated 'the disease is still involved in much obscurity'. He felt that physicians needed to be better acquainted with it in order to make an early diagnosis that could prove perhaps to be life saving. 'I presume that the Society is satisfied respecting this case which makes the subject of this dissertation', he concluded, 'and shall therefore proceed'.[95]

The first aspect to be discussed was a brief history of the disease or *historia morbi.* Members usually attempted to trace the featured ailment back to Antiquity and quote to a number of important authors who had written on it. James, for example, mentioned Dioscorides, Galen, and Caelius Aurelianus, but quickly observed that 'a discussion on that head would tend to no useful purpose'. For this student and others, the historical effort was usually thought to be irrelevant – a ritual display of scholarship. The historical analysis was followed by a presentation of the most salient symptoms and physical findings typically associated with the disease. James chose to describe the sequence of events that occurred in a rabid dog before turning to the manifestations of rabies in humans. According to contemporary authors, the incubation time after the fateful bite ranged widely from days to weeks, even years. Indicating that he preferred not 'to trouble the Society with a narrative of the different periods', James settled on a norm of 30–40 days. He then pointed out the characteristics of the dog bite and the subsequent lassitude, and sore throat of the victim. In other cases, students discussed the importance of pulses and their use in medicine,[96] often describing pathognomonic signs. In rabies, James talked about the patients' inability to swallow their own saliva, a phenomenon that made them characteristically foam from the mouth. As more fluid seeped into the larynx, and generalised convulsions ensued, sufferers were noted to emit gurgling, drowning, even howling sounds that simulated dog barks, eerily suggesting the transformation of rabid humans into the animals that had bitten them. Finally, students spoke a great deal about the signs of death.[97]

Although unnecessary in James' dramatic disease, Society members usually went on to discuss additional diagnostic methods.[98] Seeking a differential diagnosis was critical in many ailments, including distinctions between active and passive inflammation, *scarlatina* and *cynanche maligna*, herpes and other skin diseases, bodily discharges in gonorrhoea and syphilis.[99] In the end, the diagnostic label based on symptoms and physical signs needed to be placed within a classification of disease. As James admitted, 'it is customary in papers of this kind to give the definition of the disease from Cullen or some other nosologist (Chapters 7, 8 and 9).[100] In his case, however, he felt that defining and positioning 'hydrophobia' or rabies in a particular category was inadequate. In fact, the usefulness of classifying diseases generated a host of student papers, especially during the 1780s and early 1790s – with opponents of Cullen's nomenclature insisting that to do so was artificial, complex, and unnecessary.[101]

Subsequently, a case presentation before the Society involved an explanation of causality and location, the *sedes morbi* or sites of pathology. Members waxed eloquently about causes, including predisposing causes such as age, sex, habit, non-naturals, and constitution; as well as remote, proximate, and occasional causes.[102] These were hypothetical attempts to make sense of the phenomena, or rationales for explaining the symptoms, signs, and presumed physiopathology of the sickness. They were essential components for a *theoria morbi*, the theory of a disease.[103] James cited the link between the wound produced by a mad animal and the other manifestations of rabies. He also presented a number of pathological findings obtained at post-mortem dissection. Challenging the traditional causality, James tried to convince his audience that hydrophobia was not always present in rabid dogs and that the various symptoms could also be observed in other diseases. One thing was certain: the saliva from the infected animal transmitted the contagion of rabies during a bite but it could also indirectly infect other individuals if the matter was simply deposited on the intact skin or on clothing. Based on the proposed diagnosis and causality, students then went on to formulate a *prognosis morbi* or prognosis of the disease, an easy task for James dealing with a typical and always fatal case of rabies. The final step in the presentation was a discussion of the disease's prophylaxis and method of cure or *curatio morbi.*

Little was known about the specific prevention of infectious conditions, but several Society members engaged in discussions about the advisability of inoculation for smallpox. In their essays, these students attempted to explain the milder symptoms of inoculated, versus naturally acquired, disease.[104] There were also frequent debates regarding the existence of bodily forces capable of achieving a spontaneous recovery, the so-called *vis medicatrix naturae*, or the healing power of nature.[105] Traditionalists also discussed the doctrine of 'critical days'; examples of 'happy crises' of vomiting, diarrhoea and perspiration that signalled a favourable turn in the evolution of a disease. They were seen as 'undeniable instances' of a natural form of mending. Both concepts were survivors of classical humoralism, and increasingly controversial.[106]

With regard to therapeutics, students discussed various arrangements of the materia medica.[107] One student insisted the diversity of medicinal effects did not depend on the nature of individual drugs since their mode of action was always stimulating.[108] Frequently employed remedies were fair topics for student presentations. Some Society members explored the action of purgatives and remedies to check biliary secretion, a mainstay of the traditional depleting practices that were still in vogue.[109] Others inquired into the action and usefulness of opium and sedatives, a fashionable subject in Edinburgh, particularly in the 1780s.[110] Expectorants, especially the use of gum resin in a variety of chest ailments, were discussed.[111] Tonics such as Peruvian bark and camphor,[112] astringents,[113] diuretics,[114] diaphoretics,[115] and emetics – especially antimony preparations[116] – all came up for discussion. Moreover, attention was paid to the effects of bloodletting, including complications such as accidental nerve punctures.[117] Finally, there were papers on useful mercurial preparations for treatment of venereal disease,[118] indications for the administration of arsenic,[119] employment of blisters,[120] and benefits from the use of electricity. Like other presentations before the Society, one can also categorise the clinical essays as traditionally organised literary products that were designed to summarise and convey contemporary knowledge. Systematically arranged, these 'cases' were necessary drills for professional communication between future consulting physicians. They were also rehearsals for those who wished to engage in writing and teaching careers. Beyond the traditional and didactic, however, some students managed to insert unique personal observations and ideas for further discussion and debate.

Twelve Most Frequently Presented Diseases	
Pneumonia	9
Cynanche trachealis (maligna, gangrenosa)	8
Dysentery	8
Phthisis pulmonaris	7
Gonorrhea virulenta	7
Typhus fever	7
Catarrh	6
Dyspepsia	6
Diabetes	6
Scurvy	6
Tetanus	6
Smallpox	6

Among those less common, but intriguing ailments scrutinised by students were intermittent fevers, *colica pictonum*, rickets, and puerperal fever.

Experiments

As in other societies with scientific interests, Society members increasingly included experimental results into their physiological and clinical presentations before the Society. In some instances, they replicated human and especially animal trials already carried out by British and foreign medical authorities for more than a century.[121] On other occasions, the students simply sought to prove the theoretical premises promoted by local medical personalities, regarding bodily excitability and the action of certain drugs. In 1775, for example, during his presidency of the Society, Gilbert Blane (1749–1834) conducted some trials about the effects of antiseptics 'to determine some of the ambiguous points by experiment'.[122] Even several Edinburgh faculty members such as the anatomist Alexander Monro Secundus (1733–1817), chemist Joseph Black (1728–99) and bedside physician Francis Home (1719–1813) had carried out multiple experiments. However, the lack of facilities and equipment continued to hamper their successful execution.[123] Self-experimentation among students was very common and did not require expensive apparatus. Many papers presented to the Society or doctoral dissertation contained results obtained from trials in which the essayist and perhaps some of his close friends subjected themselves to a series of tests. Repeatedly exposed to experimental scrutiny was the action of opium on the human organism. In a paper delivered during the 1783–4 session, the senior president, Edward Harrison,[124] followed in the footsteps of the American student, Samuel Bard, who had carried out on himself and other persons a series of pulse measurements after ingesting certain amounts of opium powder.[125] During the next year, another president, Thomas Skeete, conducted similar tests. With the co-operation of Thomas A. Emmet, William Hayle, and Skeete's landlady, each of the experimenters swallowed a grain of opium and had their pulses continuously monitored for approximately three hours. Confirming Bard's earlier findings, all these human guinea pigs experienced a considerable drop in pulse frequency and strength. Other physiological effects, such as flushed faces, lack of appetite, diminished bodily secretions, and restless sleep convinced Emmet that opium could never be considered a stimulant like wine and distilled spirits which the students also tested extensively to arrive at their conclusions.[126]

Black's studies in the early 1780s helped create a short-lived student-organised Chemical Society. However, one of the Society's experimenters cautioned that isolated trials could sometimes lead to erroneous conclusions, making it 'very improper to establish or repudiate a general doctrine by a single experiment'.[127] Nevertheless, in 1785, the Society decided to appoint an Experimental Committee charged with supervising the creation of a small laboratory and to purchase different 'philosophical instruments', particularly an electrical machine, thermometers, and other equipment. The Committee approved funds to defray expenses for certain projects. Several rooms in the building were set aside for all students to conduct investigations and dissections at their own expense. As gentlemen, of course, most students eschewed a hands-on approach, hiring a dissector–demonstrator to actually carry out many of the gruesome vivisections. While lacking in sophistication, these student efforts reflected the growing belief that information obtained from experiments could be valuable in shaping and settling important theoretical questions.

Most Society-sponsored trials used living animals, already a Galenic practice later revived during the Renaissance and considered of considerable medical utility by the eighteenth century. Nevertheless, a number of authors had begun raising concerns about the cruelty inherent in such practices. In 1751, the Scottish philosopher, David Hume (1711–76), pleaded in his *Essay Concerning the Principles of Morals* for the 'gentle usage' of experimental animals.[128] Even the physician Thomas Percival (1740–1804) spoke in 1775 of the need to carefully define the purposes of animal trials and avoid unnecessary repetitions.[129] Given such early antivivisectionist views, one Society member felt it necessary to justify the practice in a 1794 essay. He insisted that even though animals were 'our humble partners in creation', they nevertheless remained indispensable for the advancement of science even 'when the physiologist puts them on the rack, sacrifices their ease and perhaps his own feelings'. Indeed, animal abuse and torture were absolutely necessary for 'the good of mankind'. Concluded the student: 'I cannot consider hardships imposed on them, in any way, greater than those we are ourselves willing to undergo in proportion to our strength.'[130]

Among the earliest experiments, in March 1785, were several designed to test the action of cold on bodily excitability, an issue prominently involved in the therapeutic debates between the adherents of Cullen and his student John Brown (Chapter 9). Following a presentation by a follower of Brown, William Spooner claimed cold to be a stimulant. He and a number of unnamed students decided to study this effect experimentally with a series of crude trials.[131] They gradually submerged white rabbits in glass bowls filled with a mixture of snow and salt. At first, the animals jumped violently until their feet became frozen to the glass. Following what appeared to be death by exposure to temperatures below thirty degrees Fahrenheit, their chests were opened, disclosing still spontaneously beating hearts. As more time passed and the bodies cooled further, the students continued to subject the organ to needle pricks, checking its dwindling contractions and irritability. Similar attempts were made to observe the effects of heat by pouring boiling water into the bowls. The experimenting students eventually concluded that young animals were more resistant to the effects of cold than adult ones, a phenomenon reversed with exposure to heat. These findings were interpreted to mean that animals displayed a greater capacity to receive stimuli as it achieved maturity, a notion contrary to the accepted laws of vitality articulated by the Italian investigator Lazzaro Spallanzani (1729–99).[132] To extend this opinion to other parts of the natural world, another Society member used maggots, adult wasps, caterpillars and butterflies as subjects. The insects were subjected to varying degrees of heat to confirm their resistance to strong stimuli. The experimenters then turned to vegetables, specifically beans and their seeds, exposing them to changing amounts of air and light in an attempt to link the vital phenomena of the animal and vegetable kingdoms.[133] In the end, this student pronounced his results as corroborating 'the doctrine promulgated by Dr. Brown', exhorting fellow members of their duty to inform the organisation that Brown's notions needed to 'receive every possible support which experiments could give to it' (Chapter 3).[134]

Carried out in May 1785, other experiments used dogs and calves to study the effects of tartar emetic on the stomach. A month later, another Society member went to study the action of blood transfusions. Others conducted chemical tests of bodily fluids.[135] Trials in November 1785 on fowl and rabbits consisted of the placement of a tracheal tube into the airwaves of these animals. The purpose was to determine whether the fatal consequences of breathing 'fixed air' were actually due to effects in the nose and throat or the 'internal surface of the lungs'.[136] Finally, using frogs, an unnamed student sought to investigate the action of tobacco on living animals. After exposing the thorax, the experimenter injected drops of a watery solution into the auricles of the heart, triggering its immediate stoppage and spasms in the lower extremities. Similar symptoms occurred when the solution was infused into the animal's stomach and intestines. In as possibly early as 1786, a set of fifty-one separate experiments attempted to determine whether lead acetate, considered a popular astringent, anti-inflammatory and sedative, actually behaved as a stimulant (Chapter 3). Accordingly, three students and future presidents of the Society, Henry Bowles, John Jachmann, and William Alexander, volunteered to be co-investigators. First, the white powder was given orally, rectally and subcutaneously to a number of young dogs in different dosages and intervals. After a brief period of excitement and higher pulse rates, the animals vomited and became very drowsy and sleepy, their pulses sinking rapidly. However, when the students began injecting a solution of the compound in the jugular vein of other dogs, they nearly instantly perished; on dissection, their organs and muscles showed no signs of irritability when tested by mechanical and electrical means. Further trials using frogs seemed to confirm the hypothesis that lead preparations acted like stimulants which would quickly exhaust the body's excitability.[137]

From this time period, another series of experiments, designed by Edmund Goodwyn (1756–1829), sought to ascertain the nature and possible means for reviving nearly drowned persons. This senior Society president (during the 1786–7 session) criticised earlier authorities, including Albrecht von Haller (1708–77) and Robert Whytt (1714–66) by accusing them of blending 'hypotheses with fact' and sometimes grasping 'at more than the mind can attain'.[138] Goodwyn questioned the usage of the popular but vague notion of 'sympathy' between organs, without seeking an experimental confirmation of its actions (Chapter 4). Together with another student, William Alexander, they designed a number of tests carried out on cats, dogs and rabbits to ascertain the link between respiration and heart action. The animals were submerged and purposely drowned in a container full of ink-coloured water, then had their lungs dissected to detect and measure the presence of fluids and air. After numerous animal experiments, Goodwyn – who had measured his own volume of inspired air – concluded that a chemical element of the blood passing through the lungs – oxygen – was necessary for the maintenance of heart action and to sustain the vitality of the entire organism.[139] His trials reflected a gradual maturing of the student experimentalists. Goodwyn was emphatic in recommending that trials be performed and repeated numerous times with great care and attention in the presence of 'judicious' friends who would act as valuable witnesses and critics. For Goodwyn, the impressions of the experimenter's senses were not always sufficient or correct; it was necessary for others to repeat the trials and confirm his experimental findings. For his part, he pledged to retract his own conclusions if subsequent studies and results proved more credible.

In that same year, William Alexander read a paper about the effects of opium upon healthy and diseased animals. The presentation was based on a series of animal experiments in which he successively injected opium extracts and ether into the subclavian and jugular veins of rabbits. After their prompt demise, their chests were opened to probe for residual cardiac irritability. In another trial, Alexander had frog hearts submerged into aqueous solutions of opium – controls were placed in plain water – to measure their lingering capacity to contract. His conclusion: opium stimulates the body's excitability.[140] Investigations carried out by the Experimental Committee continued to focus on the problem of muscular irritability as well as the physiology of sleep. One member of the Committee, Murray Grant, carried out some trials that lead him to conclude that sleep represented an exhaustion of the body's excitability. This issue became the pivotal interest of the Society's 1790–1 session.[141] Two students conducted studies on plant irritability, which were presented to the Natural History Society of Edinburgh.[142] Another member, Josiah Clerk, revealed that the Experimental Committee had repeated and expanded the original experiments of another Italian investigator, Felice Fontana (1730–1803), which had led to the formulation of laws governing muscular irritability.[143]

Finally, following his stint as president of the 1792–3 session, Alexander Philip Wilson presented to the Society the results of his own three-year study based on animal experiments concerned with the physiological action of opium. In spite of numerous trials carried out by prominent medical authorities such as Robert Whytt and Samuel Crumpe, the subject was still 'involved in the utmost obscurity'.[144] Wilson sought to debunk the notion, supported by other researchers, that opium was a muscular stimulant because of its particular 'sympathy among the nerves'. Trials with frogs that had their aorta completely ligated, however, failed to produce any muscular contractions when a solution of opium was injected into their hearts. Wilson's conclusion was that the drug would only trigger convulsions if it were conveyed by the vascular system to the brain. To prove this path, he simply removed the heart from other frogs, placing his opium solution into the stomach of these animals.[145] The promotion of the experimental method received further impetus with the creation of an Apparatus Committee in 1796 and the establishment of yearly prizes for the best research projects. Sceptical students continued to single out a number of important physiological and therapeutical issues for experimental scrutiny. Their main motivation was to debunk sweeping but vague theoretical claims and to derail the practices of system-building as an ideal path towards medical certainty. However, unsupervised by more seasoned experimentalists, most trials lacked focus and sophistication. They remained subordinated to the didactic approach that characterised most of the Society's activities. Nevertheless, these experimental efforts reveal a growing student desire to participate in, and contribute to, the contemporary construction of scientific knowledge.[146]

Clinical education

In 1785, the Society also became involved in issues surrounding students' access to the Edinburgh Infirmary (Chapter 1). Under the leadership of Thomas Beddoes (1760–1808), one of the presidents during the 1785–6 session, students formed a group called the 'Associated Students'. It included James Mackintosh (1765–1832), later a famous politician, and John Haslam (1764–1844), discoverer of the mental condition termed 'general paralysis'. The group's goal was to protest against recent hospital regulations ratified by the Infirmary's managers that sought to restrict student access to the institution. Claiming that 'much abuse and disorder has been introduced into the House by their presence at all hours of the day in the wards,' the hospital authorities now strictly prohibited students from talking directly with patients. All questions had to be directed to the medical personnel. Access was to be restricted to rounds and clinical lectures. Copying of ward journals and ledgers was permitted during two hours a day before noon and supper and confined to the waiting room (Chapter 7).[147] In their complaint dated 25 June 1785, the Society's members considered the regulations 'injurious and unjust' since they assailed the students' status and reputation as gentlemen. Moreover, the prohibition of having direct contact with patients was deemed very harmful: 'the great object of a student's attendance at an infirmary is to examine the phenomena of diseases by himself and to see the method of treating the sick'.[148] Limited only to observation at certain hours deprived students from witnessing the admission and management of emergency cases and autopsies, two experiences considered critical for the development of future physicians. Edinburgh's didactic model was unsuited for the new demands for improved clinical experience. Besides Beddoes, the ninety-three signatories of the complaint included other Society leaders, among them the other three presidents of the session: Richard Pearson, Samuel Hinds and Casper Wistar.

The Infirmary managers responded to the Society's grievance by pointing out that all surgical interventions and post-mortem examinations were traditionally performed in the amphitheatre, subject to a posted notice, and that students who had purchased admission tickets were certainly always welcome to attend these events.[149] However, the official response deliberately ignored the central issue of direct access to patients – the 'indispensable requisite' raised earlier. Angered students now threatened to withhold the purchase of further hospital tickets. They also vowed to advertise their protest to all medical students and the public via two thousand pamphlets with personal accounts to be published in British, Irish and American newspapers. The hospital authorities were given a 6 September deadline to restore all previous student privileges. Fully aware that the income from student tickets constituted a significant and necessary source of income for the Infirmary, this tactic was a clever attempt on the part of the students to flex their economic muscles.[150] Thus, by 18 August, the Managers were forced to make a few concessions. They expanded the evening visits by an hour and guaranteed access to emergency cases. The copying of clinical cases was restored to four hours per day in a specially designated room.[151] However, these measures still fell short of the original demands and the Society's 'Associated Students' now aimed their complaints directly toward the University's medical faculty. Still at stake was the 'liberty of examining by themselves patients at all times of the day between rounds by the physicians'. Students demanded attendance at the Edinburgh Infirmary be removed from the graduation requirements if the hospital managers failed to allow access. They also threatened to warn potential new students about the restrictions to their clinical studies.[152]

Two weeks later, on behalf of the faculty, James Gregory (1753–1821) responded to Beddoes and his group. Gregory was keenly aware of the potential damage to the School's reputation and enrolments if the confrontation between members of the Society and the Infirmary managers lingered. Indeed, the whole economy of the city could be affected; especially its lodging houses and taverns (Chapter 1). Therefore, Gregory, who was also an Infirmary manager, proposed to restore the students' direct contact with patients, allowing them four hours daily to freely roam the wards. A further concession was to give students all day to consult the ward journals except during rounds when clerks and physicians were making entries into these books. There was, however, a caveat: the professors could only propose such changes, but it was up to the duly-appointed hospital managers to make the final decision. 'The students must consider too that none can have any right or ought to have any privilege about the Infirmary that is inconsistent with the good of the patients', warned Gregory. Indeed, the 'immediate interests of humanity' overrode all educational goals, and the reality of larger numbers of students in the wards would have an injurious effect on the patients. As to the suggestion to drop the student attendance of the Infirmary as a graduation requirement, the professors held firm. Clinical instruction, Gregory insisted, 'has been fully confirmed by many years experience in this University and the truth of it is now universally acknowledged'.[153]

Beddoes and the 'Associated Students' reluctantly accepted Gregory's compromise solution by early September and authorised the faculty to officially present the plan to the hospital managers. However, Beddoes continued to characterise the Infirmary's restrictions as an 'injury and insult' to his fellow students. He warned that they would not tolerate further abuse or withdraw from their studies, leaving 'their old and respected masters'. 'If your laws render submission to indignities necessary to graduation', Beddoes wrote, 'what must be the consequence!' 'Let us not, by reflection, anticipate evils', he concluded.[154] On 5 September 1785, Gregory announced the Infirmary managers had accepted the faculty's compromise proposal. The new regulations went into effect, at least until 1792 when further restrictions were again put in place.[155] Student reaction to the Infirmary's decision went unregistered. The episode, however, disclosed growing student dissatisfaction with their rather passive role in clinical education. Witnessing medical rounds with attending Infirmary physicians, listening to lectures given by rotating clinical professors, and copying selected clinical cases were no longer deemed sufficient. These exercises could not substitute for practical experience through individual bedside contact with patients.

Conclusion

The goal of the Royal Medical Society was to produce gentlemen–physicians who would be prepared to practice medicine in polite society. Their professional training was originally based on the acquisition of gentrified manners, social and debating skills, rhetorical and literary abilities, as well as independence of opinion. Student members delivered papers based on contemporary theoretical claims and classical medical aphorisms, with leaders encouraging discussion and commentary. By the 1770s, however, the genteel physician model began to shift. Traditional codes of honour and etiquette lost favour. Professional reputation rested on the adherence to

Baconian principles in the acquisition of scientific knowledge. Students sought to ascertain the validity of all propositions by subjecting them to empirical scrutiny, instead of merely grounding their ideas in the authority of previous authors. The students showed a fair amount of determination and ingenuity in designing and carrying out their own clinical and experimental studies. While the often-confusing experimental results were highly idiosyncratic, the critical issue was that members of the Society began to believe that many fashionable concepts needed scrutiny. They went on to conduct trials 'with greatest pleasure' even though their results often merely confirmed their own theoretical biases.

This collective enthusiasm for science changed the Royal Medical Society from an essentially philosophical debating club to an organisation that encouraged the acquisition of new knowledge by providing library and laboratory facilities, as well as supporting hospital-based bedside education. Presentations tended to reflect personal opinions, clinical experiences and experimental discoveries. Although hampered by modest resources and often lacking proper guidance and appropriate skills, Society members nevertheless attempted to transcend the prevailing pedagogical models adopted by the University of Edinburgh. These experiences helped shape a new approach to medical knowledge for future physicians studying there. The change of epistemology is epitomised in the words of one of the student experimenters, Alexander P. Wilson. Presenting his investigations on the action of opium in living animals, Wilson declared that 'all that is necessary here is merely to lay before the Society those facts which were ascertained by experiment and which have been confirmed or at least reported by succeeding observations'.[156]

Notes

1. J. Watson, *The Scot of the Eighteenth Century: His Religion and his Life* (London: Hodder & Stoughton, 1907), 24.
2. See announcement 'King Granted Charter Erecting Medical Society Into a Body Politic', in *Scots Magazine,* 41 (February 1779), 106; J.D. Holmes, 'Early Years of the Medical Society', *University of Edinburgh Journal,* (Autumn 1968), 333–40. A four-page pamphlet describes the arrangements for the new building: Medical Society of Edinburgh, *An Account of the Scheme for Building a Hall for the Medical Society at Edinburgh* (Edinburgh, 1771); see also D.C. Macarthur, 'The First Forty Years of the Royal Medical Society and the Part William Cullen Played in it', in A. Doig *et al.* (eds), *William Cullen and the Eighteenth-Century Medical World* (Edinburgh: Edinburgh University Press, 1993), 247–51.

3. The literature on this subject is extensive. Among the most informative works see R. Emerson, 'The Enlightenment and Social Structures', in P. Fritz and D. Williams (eds), *City and Society in the Eighteenth Century* (Toronto: Hakkert, 1973), 99–124; J. Brewer, 'The Most Polite Age and the Most Vicious: Attitudes Towards Culture as a Commodity, 1660–1800', in A. Bermingham and J. Brewer (eds), *The Consumption of Culture, 1660–1800* (London: Routledge, 1995), 341–61.
4. S. Shapin, 'The Audience for Science in Eighteenth-Century Edinburgh', *History of Science*, 12 (1974), 95–121; R.L. Emerson, 'The Philosophical Society of Edinburgh, 1737–1747', *British Journal for the History of Science*, 12 (1979), 154–91.
5. S. Shapin, 'Property, Patronage and the Politics of Science: The Founding of the Royal Society of Edinburgh', *British Journal for the History of Science*, 7 (1974), 1–41; R.L. Emerson, 'The Scottish Enlightenment and the End of the Philosophical Society of Edinburgh', *ibid.*, 21 (1988), 33–66.
6. See J. Jenkinson, *Scottish Medical Societies, 1731–1939, Their History and Records* (Edinburgh: Edinburgh University Press, 1993); D.D. McElroy, *Scotland's Age of Improvement: A Survey of Eighteenth-Century Literary Clubs and Societies* (Pullman, Wash.: Washington State University Press, 1969).
7. For information, consult The Aesculapian Club, *Minutebooks 1773–1934*, MSS Collection, Royal College of Physicians, Edinburgh.
8. N. Phillipson, 'Adam Smith as Civic Moralist', in I. Hont and M. Ignatieff (eds), *Wealth and Virtue: The Shaping of Political Economy in the Scottish Enlightenment* (Cambridge: Cambridge University Press, 1983), 198; K. Tribe, 'Adam Smith: Cultural Critic?', *Journal of Economic Literature*, 37 (1999), 609–32.
9. For details, see A. Smith, *The Theory of Moral Sentiments* (6th edn 1790) (Cambridge: Cambridge University Press, 2002).
10. R. Emerson, 'Scottish Universities in the Eighteenth Century, 1690–1800', *Studies on Voltaire and the Eighteenth Century*, 114 (1977), 453–74; and J.B. Morell, 'The University of Edinburgh in the Late Eighteenth Century: Its Scientific Eminence and Academic Structure', *Isis*, 62 (1971), 158–71.
11. P. Mac Flogg'em (psued.), *Aesculapian Secrets Revealed* (London: C. Chapple, 1813), 10.
12. J. McVickar, *A Domestic Narrative of the Life of Samuel Bard* (New York: A. Paul, 1822), 14.
13. J. Fothergill, *An Essay on the Character of the Late Alexander Russell* (London, 1770), 6; see also C. Camic, *Experience and Enlightenment: Socialization for Cultural Change in Eighteenth-Century Scotland* (Chicago: University of Chicago Press, 1983), 141–233.
14. See Royal Medical Society of Edinburgh, *Laws of the Medical Society of*

Edinburgh Instituted in 1737, Incorporated by Royal Charter in 1778 (Edinburgh: 1775). For an overview, J.R. Christie, 'The Origins and Development of the Scottish Scientific Community, 1680-1760', *History of Science,* 12 (1974), 122–41.

15. *Dissertations Read to the Royal Medical Society (Diss. RMS),* 95 vols (Edinburgh, 1751–1833), MSS Collection, Edinburgh University Library. The student papers are also available in 115 reels of microfilm from Microfilm Academic Publishers, Wakefield, England.
16. This background dominated contemporary medical ethics. See John Gregory, *Lectures on the Duties and Qualifications of a Physician* (London: W. Strahan and T. Cadell, 1772), 2–6.
17. The information is contained in a table attached to the first historical account of the Society: [W. Stroude], 'History of the Medical Society of Edinburgh', in *List of Members, Laws, and Library Catalogue of the Medical Society of Edinburgh* (Edinburgh: W. Aitken, 1820).
18. A more recent source is J. Gray, *History of the Royal Medical Society 1737–1937* (Edinburgh: Edinburgh University Press, 1952).
19. D. Guthrie, *Extramural Medical Education in Edinburgh and the School of Medicine* (Edinburgh: Livingstone, 1965). Many students also attended the meetings of a Speculative Society founded in 1764 'for the improvement of literary composition and public speaking'.
20. [Stroude], *op. cit.* (note 17), XII. The rhetoric of 'honour' often served to disguise the commercial aspect of medical practice. See D. Harley, 'Honour and Property: The Structure of Professional Disputes in Eighteenth-Century English Medicine', in A. Cunningham and R. French (eds), *The Medical Enlightenment of the Eighteenth Century* (Cambridge: Cambridge University Press, 1990), 138–60.
21. P. Holland, 'What are the Peculiarities of Climate and Mode of Living Which Give Use to the Particular Diseases if Different Countries?', *Diss. RMS,* Vol. 12 (1780–1), 189.
22. L. Rosner, 'Eighteenth-Century Medical Education and the Didactic Model of Experiment', in P. Dear (ed.), *The Literary Structure of Scientific Knowledge: Historical Studies* (Philadelphia: University of Pennsylvania Press, 1991), 182–94.
23. J. Adair, 'What Advantages Result From the Use, What Inconveniences From the Abuse of Analysis and Analogy in Medicine?', *Diss. RMS,* Vol. 23 (1788–9), 122.
24. James Currie admitted that 'a full discussion would extend the paper far beyond the limits prescribed by the custom of the Society'. See his essay 'What are the Effects of Cold on the Living Body?', *ibid.,* Vol. 11 (1778), 288–300.

25. T. White, 'What are the Qualities of Bile and What are the Best Remedies for Checking Morbid Secretions of it', *ibid.*, Vol. 17 (1783–5), 473.
26. This formulaic modesty was best expressed by James Carver : 'I have nothing further to add but to beg for the Society's pardon for having given them such an unfinished paper, and to assure them that nothing but want of time and abilities could have made me treat the subject of some importance in such a cursory manner'. See his essay 'What are the Most Probable Causes of Menstruation in the Human Species?', *Diss. RMS*, Vol. 14 (1782–3), 318.
27. A. Duncan, Sr, 'Introductory Address to the Medical Society of Students in Edinburgh', read 2 November 1771 (Edinburgh, 1772), 8.
28. F. Sayers, 'What are the Effects of the Passions on the Body?', *Diss. RMS*, Vol. 21 (1786–8), 258.
29 . W. Alexander discussing a case of colic, during the 1785–6 session, *Diss. RMS*, Vol. 18 (1785–7), 414.
30 . Comments made by S. Alvey in his clinical presentation on erysipelas, *Diss. RMS*, Vol. 20 (1786–7), 279.
31. See abstract of J.J. Christie, 'Edinburgh Medicine in the Eighteenth Century: The View From the Students', *Society for the Social History of Medicine Bulletin,* 19 (1976), 13–15.
32. Fothergill, *op. cit.* (note 13), 7.
33. The issue of medicine as a literary activity is made by L. Rosner, 'The Royal Medical Society', in *Medical Education in The Age of Improvement* (Edinburgh: Edinburgh University Press, 1991), 119–34.
34. For a discussion of medical systems, G.B. Risse, 'Medicine in the Age of Enlightenment', in A. Wear (ed.), *Medicine in Society: Historical Essays* (Cambridge: Cambridge University Press, 1992), 155–67.
35. A. Cunningham, 'Medicine to Calm the Mind: Boerhaave's Medical System and Why it was Adopted in Edinburgh', in R. Porter (ed.), *The Medical Enlightenment of the Eighteenth Century* (Amsterdam: Rodopi, 1995), 64–112.
36. M. Barfoot, 'Philosophy and the Method of Cullen's Medical Teaching', in Doig, *op. cit.* (note 2), 110–32.
37. 'He [physician] must therefore, without prejudice to any peculiar system or received opinion whatsoever, act according to the state of the case before him'. See J. Ford, *Diss. RMS*, Vol. 11 (1778), 152–9.
38. J.P. Harris, 'What is the Modus Operandi of Opium and in what States May it be Admitted as Useful?', *Diss. RMS*, Vol. 11 (1778), 221–6.
39. J. Howell, 'What are the Likeliest Means of Rescuing or at Least Relieving the Art of Medicine From its Present State of Uncertainty and Error?', *Diss. RMS*, Vol. 12 (1780–1), 59–64.
40. R.G. Munro, 'What are the Circumstances that Have Principally

Contributed to Promote or Retard the Progress of Medicine as Science and as Art?', *Diss. RMS*, Vol. 17 (1783–5), 417–46.

41. E. Harrison, 'What are the Agreements and Differences in the Effects of Opium and Alcohol on the Human Body in Health and Disease?', *Diss. RMS*, Vol. 14 (1782–3), 188–211.
42. H. Ainslie, 'How Shall We Best Preserve Health and Cure Disease?', *Diss. RMS*, Vol. 14 (1782–3), 274–94.
43. J. Lawson, 'What are the Effects of Peruvian Bark?', *Diss. RMS*, Vol. 14 (1782–3), 368–83.
44. J. Duncan, 'What Advantages Have Been Derived, or Are to be Expected From Meteorological Registers?', *Diss. RMS*, Vol. 14 (1782–3), 220.
45. See C. Lawrence, 'Ornate Physicians and Learned Artisans', in W.F. Bynum and R. Porter (eds), *William Hunter and the Eighteenth-Century Medical World* (Cambridge: Cambridge University Press, 1985), 153–76.
46. J. Gibney, 'What is the Most Probable Theory of Generation?', *Diss. RMS*, Vol. 23 (1788-9), 301–11; E. Bourne, 'Upon What Principles are We to Account for the Sensibility of Certain Plants?', *Diss. RMS*, Vol. 31 (1793–5), 161–96; T. Garnett, 'What does Life Consist of? How are Those Variations from Health Called Diseases Produced?', *Diss. RMS*, Vol. 21 (1786-8), 365–87.
47. See for example, J. Astbury, 'What Analogy and Connection is there Between the Animal and Vegetable Kingdom?', *Diss. RMS*, Vol. 12 (1780-1), 141; H. Ainslie, 'Is There any Difference Between the Animal and Vegetable Kingdoms?', *Ibid.*, Vol. 14 (1782–3), 1–6.
48. C.F. Brown, 'What is the Probable Theory of Animal Heat?', *Diss. RMS*, Vol. 31 (1793–5), 304–16; W. Marsh, 'What is the Cause of Animal Heat?', *Ibid.*, Vol. 17 (1783–5), 322–41; and J. McLenan, 'In What Manner do Certain Animals Preserve their Temperature Nearly Uniform?', *Diss. RMS*, Vol. 27 (1791–2), 211–241.
49. P. Erskine, 'In What Way are We to Proceed in Order to Ascertain the Nature of the Thinking Principle in Man?', *Diss. RMS*, Vol. 31 (1793–5), 214–27.
50. A.L. Donovan, 'Medicine and Natural Philosophy in Edinburgh', in his *Philosophical Chemistry in the Scottish Enlightenment: The Doctrines of William Cullen and Joseph Black* (Edinburgh: Edinburgh University Press, 1975), 34–48.
51. R. Gray, 'What are the Chemical Effects of Pure Air?', *Diss. RMS*, Vol. 23 (1788–9), 199–224. One published medical dissertation on this subject is J. Stokes, *De Aere Dephlogisticato* (Edinburgh: Balfour & Smellie, 1782). For phlogiston, W. Reid, 'Whether or not There is in Bodies Such a Thing as Phlogiston, the Principle of Fire?', *Diss. RMS*, Vol. 31 (1793–5), 73–117;

E. Ash, 'What is the Nature of the Chemical Process of Crystallization?', *Diss. RMS*, Vol. 23 (1788–9), 158–76; J. Paterson, 'Is Evaporation Performed by Heat Alone?', *Diss. RMS*, Vol. 14 (1782–3), 13–20; W. Russell, 'What is the Cause of Evaporation', *Diss. RMS*, Vol. 26 (1790–1), 1–15; and G. Hunter, 'What is the Cause of Spontaneous Evaporation?', *Diss. RMS*, Vol. 29 (1792–4), 198–207.

52. M. Davy, 'What is the Change Produced in a Dead Animal or Vegetable Substance by Fermentation?', *Diss. RMS*, Vol. 17 (1783–5), 342–53; and R. Drake, 'What is the Nature of Fermentation?', *Diss. RMS*, Vol. 23 (1788–9), 333–61.
53. E. Stevens, 'What is the Cause of the Increase in Weight Which Metals Require During their Calcination?', *Diss. RMS*, Vol.11 (1778), 179; A.P. Anderson, 'What is the Nature and Composition of Vitriolic Acid?', *Diss. RMS*, Vol. 26 (1790–1), 78–97.
54. C. Throckmorton, 'What are the Changes the Blood Undergoes in Diseases?', *Diss. RMS*, Vol. 17 (1783–5), 31–40.
55. D. Skeene, 'Is the Chemical Analysis of Substances of Any Use Towards Discovering their Medical Virtues?', *Diss. RMS*, Vol. 14 (1782–3), 354–67.
56. J. Bradley, 'On the Principal Phenomena of Atmospheric Electricity', *Diss. RMS*, Vol. 26 (1790–1), 433–67; J. Babington, 'What is the Origin of Winds?', *Diss. RMS*, Vol. 31 (1793–5), 13–28.
57. R. Miller, 'How Far Can the Varieties of the Human Species that are Observable in Different Countries be Accounted for From Physical Causes?', *Diss. RMS*, Vol. 19 (1785–6), 144–76; see also J. Bradley, 'Whence the Varieties of Human Species?', *Diss. RMS*, Vol. 27 (1791–2), 95–128.
58. E. Holme, 'To the Operation of What Causes are We to Ascribe the Variety of Complexion in the Human Species?', *Diss. RMS*, Vol. 29 (1792–4), 366–81; similarly R.E. Taylor, 'What are the Causes of the Varieties of Complexion in the Human Species?', *Diss. RMS*, Vol. 31 (1793–5), 274–88.
59. B.S. Barton, 'An Essay Towards the Natural History of the North American Indians', *Diss. RMS*, Vol. 23 (1788–9), 1–17.
60. J.W. Wallace, 'An Inquiry Into the Natural State of Medicine Among the Indians of North America', *Diss. RMS*, Vol. 27 (1791–2), 316–31.
61. R. Pearson, 'What are the Effects of the Different Passions of the Mind on the Body and How are these Effects Produced?', *Diss. RMS*, Vol. 17 (1783–5), 483–97.
62. J. Forsythe, 'What are the Cause or Causes of the Mildness of Inoculated Smallpox?', *Diss. RMS*, Vol. 17 (1783–5), 408.
63. R. Wood, 'Is There a Difference in Diseases as Occurring in Different Climates? How Far is a Change in Climate Adopted for their Cure?', *Diss. RMS*, Vol. 23 (1788–9), 482–7.

64. C. Stanger, 'What are the Most Likely Means of Preserving Health?', *Diss. RMS*, Vol. 14 (1782–3), 89–100.
65. H. Ainslie, 'How Shall we Best Preserve Health and Cure Disease?', *Diss. RMS*, Vol. 14 (1782–3), 274–94; S. Cave, 'To What Particular Diseases do the Four Principal Stages of life, Infancy, Youth, Manhood, and Old Age Fix Upon?', *Diss. RMS*, Vol. 11 (1778), 253–62.
66. T.A. Emmet, 'What are the Circumstances Which Vitiate the Atmosphere and What are the Means Provided by Nature for the Restoration of its Parity?', *Diss. RMS*, Vol. 14 (1782–3), 461–505; W. Younge, 'By What Means is the Purification of Vitiated Atmospheric Air Effected?', *Diss. RMS*, Vol. 17 (1783–5), 71–91.
67. P. Holland, 'What are the Peculiarities of Climate and Mode of Living Which give Use to the Particular Diseases of Different Countries?', *Diss. RMS*, Vol. 12 (1780–1), 189–94.
68. J. Duncan, 'What Advantages have been Derived or are to be Expected From Meteorological Registers?', *Diss. RMS*, Vol. 14 (1782–3), 220–8.
69. G. Bachmetieve, 'What is the Cause of Ordinary Sleep and What is its Use?', *Diss. RMS*, Vol. 17 (1783–5), 306–12; P. Baron, 'What is the Ordinary Sleep and What are the Effects Upon the System?', *Diss. RMS*, Vol. 19 (1785–6), 114–26; R. Cleghorn, 'What is the Nature of Sleep', *Diss. RMS*, Vol. 14 (1782–3), 36–49; T. Spens, 'What are the Effects of Exercise in Preserving Health?', *Diss. RMS*, Vol. 14 (1782–3), 83–6.
70. R. Kentish, Jr, 'How do Passions Operate in Producing and Curing Diseases?', *Diss. RMS*, Vol. 14 (1782–3), 443–60; R. Pearson, 'What are the Effects of the Different Passions of the Mind on the Body?', *Diss. RMS*, Vol. 17 (1783–5), 483–97; and J. Thomson, 'In What Manner Can the Mechanism of the Passions Be Explained?', *Diss. RMS*, Vol. 27 (1791–2), 242–51.
71. J. Bell, 'What are the Effects of Grief and Fear?', *Diss. RMS*, Vol. 31 (1793–5), 151–60; R. Fowler, 'What are the Effects of Grief and Fear?', *Diss. RMS*, Vol. 27 (1791–2), 183–210.
72. W. Yates, 'In What Manner Does the Eye Perceive the Distance of Objects?', *Diss. RMS*, Vol. 29 (1792–4), 332–56; A.P. Wilson, 'Is There Any Hypothesis Hitherto Proposed Capable of Accounting for All the Phenomena of Vision?', *Diss. RMS*, Vol. 31 (1793–5), 41–72.
73. R. Kiernan, 'Do Hereditary Diseases Depend on the State of Fluids or Solids?', *Diss. RMS*, Vol. 14 (1782–3), 7–12.
74. R. Lubbock, 'How is the Increment of the Human Body Effected?', *Diss. RMS*, Vol. 14 (1782–3), 229–55.
75. J. Ruter, 'What are the Diseases Peculiarly Incident to Infancy, their Causes and the Means of Removing Them?', *Diss. RMS*, Vol. 17 (1783–5), 363–77;

T. Wallis, 'What are the Changes Which Take Place in the Human Body at the Age of Puberty?', *Diss. RMS*, Vol. 14 (1782–3), 429–42.

76. A. Knox, 'In What Manner are the Structure and Functions of Glands to be Explained?', *Diss. RMS*, Vol. 29 (1792–4), 208–32; J. Carver, 'What are the Most Probable Causes of Menstruation in the Human Species?', *Diss. RMS*, Vol. 14 (1782-3), 299–318; J. Gahagan, 'Which of the Different Theories of Menstruation Afford the Most Probable View of its Nature and Causes?', *Diss. RMS*, Vol. 23 (1788–9), 293–300.
77. J. Palmer, 'In What Manner do Mineral Poisons Act on Animal Bodies?', *Diss. RMS*, Vol. 31 (1793–5), 138–150.
78. S. Allvey, 'Upon What Does the Formation of Calculi Depend? What is their Chemical Analysis? And, When Formed, What is the Best Method of Dissolving Them?', *Diss. RMS*, Vol. 21 (1786–8), 285–98.
79. R. Cooper, 'On What does the Contraction of Muscular Fibers Depend?', *Diss. RMS*, Vol. 14 (1782–3), 347–54; D. Alexander, 'What is the Analogy Between the Operation of Powers on the Sentient and Moving Solids?', *Diss. RMS*, Vol. 27 (1791-2), 1–14; R. Fowler, 'What are the Effects Which Arise from Unequal Degrees of Excitement in Antagonist Muscles or Fibers of the Same Muscles?', *Diss. RMS*, Vol. 27 (1791–2), 36–73.
80. W. Younge, 'On What Depends the Motion of the Heart and Arteries?', *Diss. RMS*, Vol. 17 (1783–5), 447–58; J. Jones, 'Is an Atony of the Extreme Vessels Part of the Proximate Cause of Fever?', *Diss. RMS*, Vol. 11 (1778), 300–17.
81. J. Law, 'What is the Nature of Plethora and What is its Cure', *Diss. RMS*, Vol. 14 (1782–3), 26–9; J. Wood, 'What is the Cause of the Red Color of the Blood?', *Diss. RMS*, Vol. 27 (1791–2), 15–35; E. Vaisey, 'What is the Nature and Properties of the Blood?', *Diss. RMS*, Vol. 29 (1792–4), 44–56; W. Girod, 'What is the Most Probable Theory of the Formation of Pus, and How is it to be Distinguished Particularly in Diseases of the Heart?', *Diss. RMS*, Vol. 26 (1790–1), 45–53.
82. S. Ferris, 'Can any Degree of Putridity Take Place in the Circulating Blood of the Human Body During Life?', *Diss. RMS*, Vol. 14 (1782–3), 318–34; M. Blake, 'To What Causes May We Attribute the Formation of the Inflammatory Crust of the Blood?', *Diss. RMS*, Vol. 29 (1792–4), 295–365; H. McPherson, 'Is the Blood Possessed of a Principle of Life?', *Diss. RMS*, Vol. 27 (1791–2), 357–83; J. Moultrie, 'Is the Blood Possessed of a Living Principle?', *Diss. RMS*, Vol. 19 (1785–6), 328–43.
83. J. Gahagan, 'What is the Best Theory of Inflammation?', *Diss. RMS*, Vol. 26 (1790–1), 103–20; A. Smith, 'What is the Cause of Fever?', *Diss. RMS*, Vol. 23 (1788–9), 37–47; J.B. Jachmann, 'What is the Proximate Cause of Fever?', *Diss. RMS*, 263–72; W. Alexander, 'To What Cause Can the

Production of Hectic Fever be Mostly Attributed?', *Diss. RMS*, Vol. 17 (1783–5), 261–84; J. Fleming, 'Does the Disease Called Hectic Fever Depend on the Presence of Purulent Matter in the Blood?', *Diss. RMS*, Vol. 23 (1788–9), 26–36; A. Dalzell, 'Is There Any Essential Difference Between Plague and Fevers of the Species of Typhus?', *Diss. RMS*, Vol. 12 (1780–1), 105–12.

84. J. Currie, 'What are the Effects of Cold on the Living Body?', *Diss. RMS*, Vol. 11 (1778), 288–300; A. Coventry, 'What are the Effects of Heat on the Human Body?', *Diss. RMS*, Vol. 14 (1782–3), 101–8; W. Spooner, 'What are the Effects of Cold Upon the Human Body?', *Diss. RMS*, Vol. 17 (1783–5), 234–44; P. Baron, 'What is the Action of Cold on the Living Body?'. *Diss. RMS*, Vol. 19 (1785–6), 193–203.
85. R. Lubbock, 'Are Contagions Producing Idiopathic Disease, Directly or Indirectly Debilitating?', *Diss. RMS*, Vol. 14 (1782–3), 55–69; J. Clothier, 'What is the Most Probable Nature of Contagion and the Best Means of Obviating its Effects Upon the System', *Diss. RMS,* Vol. 17 (1783–5), 198–217; J.H. Gibbons, 'What is the Most Probable Mode of Contagion Operating?', *Diss. RMS,* Vol. 19 (1785–6), 185–90.
86. B. Hird, 'How are Contagious Exanthemata Produced?', *Diss. RMS,* Vol. 17 (1783–5), 354–62. For the issue of insensible perspiration, G. Cayley, 'Is an Obstruction of the Insensible Perspiration of Itself a Sufficient Cause for Disease?', *Diss. RMS,* Vol. 21 (1786–8), 460–84.
87. S. Fitt, 'Are the Proofs Decisive Which are Brought on by Different Authors to Conclude that the Absorption is Only Determined to the Lymphatic System and that the Red Veins do not Absorb at all ?', *Diss. RMS,* Vol. 19 (1785–6) 59–92; and E. Vaisey, 'In What Manner do the Lacteals Perform their Functions?', *Diss. RMS,* Vol. 27 (1791–2), 74–94.
88. B. Kissam, 'How is the Process of Digestion Performed in the Human Stomach?', *Diss. RMS,* Vol. 14 (1782–3), 30–5.
89. W. Miles, 'Benjamin Rush, chemist', *Chymia,* 4 (1953), 37–77.
90. See Benjamin Rush's medical thesis: *De Coctione Cibarum in Ventriculo* ('On the Digestion of Food in the Stomach') (Edinburgh: Balfour, Auld & Smellie, 1768), translated with an introduction by D.F. Musto, *Transactions and Studies of the College of Physicians, Philadelphia,* 32/34 (1964–7), 121–38. See also B. Rush, *The Autobiography of Benjamin Rush* (Princeton, NJ: Princeton University Press, 1948), 434.
91. J.F. Fulton and L.G. Wilson (eds), *Selected Readings in the History of Physiology,* 2nd edn (Springfield, Ill.: C. C. Thomas, 1966), 173–4.
92. Edward Stevens' findings were published in his medical dissertation *De Alimentorum Concoctione* (Edinburgh: Balfour and Smellie, 1777) and translated into English for incorporation into a work of L. Spallanzani,

Dissertations Relative to the Natural History of Animals and Vegetables, 2 vols, trans. T. Beddoes (London: J. Murray, 1784), Vol. I, 303–16. A collection of Edinburgh medical dissertations from 1759 to 1785 can be found in William Smellie, *Thesaurus Medicus Edinburgensis Novus*, 4 vols (Edinburgh: C. Eliot, 1785).

93. Gray, *op. cit.* (note 18), 28; see also a discussion in [Stroude], *op. cit.* (note 17), XXV.
94. Unpublished manuscript of Dr. Rutherford's clinical lectures delivered in 1758. The quotation is from A.L. Turner, *The Story of a Great Hospital: The Royal Infirmary of Edinburgh, 1729-1929* (Edinburgh: Oliver & Boyd, 1937), 131.
95. P. James, 'Rabies', Diss. RMS, Vol.18 (1785–7), 426.
96. M. Darwin, 'What are the Established Varieties of the Pulse, their Causes and Use in Medicine?', *Diss. RMS,* Vol. 11 (1778), no pagination; W. Kent, 'How Far Ought the Physician be Directed in his Prescriptions and Prognosis by the Pulse', *Diss. RMS,* Vol. 26 (1790–1), 54–66.
97. J. Macdonell, 'What are the Symptoms of Death?', *Diss. RMS,* Vol. 14 (1782–3), 517–24.
98. J. Baader, 'By What Means are We to Obtain a Distinct Diagnosis of a Disease?', *Diss. RMS,* Vol. 23 (1788–9), 188–98.
99. E. Long Fox, 'What are the Characteristic Marks which Distinguish Herpes From Other Cutaneous Diseases: What are its Different Species and Most Rational Mode of Treatment?', *Diss. RMS,* Vol. 14 (1782–3), 171–87; H. Black, 'Is the Matter Evacuated in Gonorrhea Different from that in Syphilis?', *Diss. RMS,* Vol. 12 (1780–1), 35–44; H. Owen, 'Do Syphilis and Gonorrhea Depend on the Same Poison?', *Diss. RMS,* Vol. 14 (1782–3), 21–5.
100. James, *op. cit.* (note 95), 426.
101. G. Dunbar, 'How Far Have Nosological Arrangements Been Useful to Medicine?', Diss. RMS, Vol. 21 (1786–8), 485–95; H. Bowles, 'Has Nosology Been Prejudicial or Beneficial to the Interests of Medicine?', *Diss. RMS,* Vol. 23 (1788–9), 282–92.
102. J. Clerk, 'Has the Investigation of Proximate Causes been of Advantage to Practical Medicine?', *Diss. RMS,* Vol. 26 (1790–1), 33–44.
103. This approach also applied to cancer. See W. Symonds, 'What are the Most Probable Causes of Scirrous Cancer and How Can it Best be Treated?', *Diss. RMS,* Vol. 19 (1785–6), 104–13.
104. See a paper by a student listed as Jackson, 'How are we to Explain the Greater Violence of Symptoms Attended on the Variolation Matter Accidently Received Into the System than that of the Same Matter Received by Inoculation?', *Diss. RMS,* vol 11 (1778), 47–58.

105. J. Hill, 'What is to be Understood by the Vis Medicatrix Naturae? What are its Operations?. How are they Performed?', *Diss. RMS,* Vol. 12 (1781–1), 470–82; and W. Robertson, 'Is There a Presiding Power in the Living Human System?: What are the Proofs of its Existence?', ibid, Vol. 19 (1785–6), 16–32.
106. R. C. Mitchell, 'How Far May We Trust to the Operations of Nature in the Cure of Diseases?', *Diss. RMS,* Vol. 17 (1783–5), 378–92; J. Jeffray, 'How Successful is the Doctrine of Critical Days in the Cure of Disease?', *Diss. RMS,* Vol. 14 (1782–3), 404–28.
107. T. Bradley, 'What is the Best Practical Division and Arrangement of Materia Medica?', *Diss. RMS,* Vol. 26 (1790–1), 237–68.
108. W. Barton, 'What are the best Expectorants? How is their Operation to be Explained?', *Diss. RMS,* Vol. 17 (1783–5), 395–407.
109. A. Williams, 'What is the Use of Purgatives?', *Diss. RMS,* Vol. 14 (1782–3), 139–45.
110. J.P. Harris, 'What is the Modus Operandi of Opium and in What States of the System May it be Admitted as Useful?', *Diss. RMS,* Vol. 11 (1778), 221–6; J. Carver, 'What are the Effects of Opium in the Human Body?', *Diss. RMS,* Vol. 14 (1782–3), 129–38; A. Kerr, 'What are the Effects of Opium on the Human Body?', *Diss. RMS,* Vol. 23 (1788–9), 459–65.
111. S. Miller, 'Upon What Principles is the Operation of the Gum Resin, Squills, Etc. as Expectorants to be Explained and in What Cases are Such Properly Indicated?', *Diss. RMS,* Vol. 12 (1780–1), 92–104.
112. J. Lawson, 'What are the Effects of Peruvian Bark?', *Diss. RMS,* Vol. 14 (1782–3), 368–83; J. Craven, 'What is the Action of the Bark on the Human Body, and In What Diseases is it Given with the Greatest Advantage, and Does it Act Specifically in the Cure of Intermittents?', *Diss. RMS,* Vol. 21 (1786–8), 49–58.
113. J. Kutter, 'What are the Best Astringent Remedies that are Employed in Medicine? How Far Can Any Reasonable Explanation be Given of their Modus Operandi on the Living Body?', *Diss. RMS,* Vol. 19 (1785–6), 48–58.
114. W.M. Thackeray, 'What are the Best Diuretics; their Mode of Operation, and in What Disease are they Most Beneficial?', *Diss. RMS,* Vol. 23 (1788–9), 146–57.
115. H.B. Wilson, 'What is the Modus Operandi of Diaphoretics and their Use in Medicine?', *Diss. RMS,* Vol. 14 (1782–3), 145–170.
116. A. MacGilchrist, 'What is the Nature of Antimony? In What Diseases is it Applicable and What is the Modus Operandi in these Diseases?', *Diss. RMS,* Vol. 14 (1782–3), 334–47; W. Jackson, 'What are the Most Useful Preparations of Antimony and in What Diseases are they Most Eligible?',

Diss. RMS, Vol. 17 (1783–5), 178–84.

117. A. MacGilchrist, 'What are the Effects of Bloodletting?', *Diss. RMS,* Vol. 14 (1782–3), 123–8; W. Barton, 'What are the Uses and Advantages Attending the Practice of Bloodletting?', *Diss. RMS,* Vol. 14 (1782–3), 506–16.
118. E. Fairlough, 'What are the Most Effectual Preparations of Mercury as Used in Venereal as Well as Other Diseases?', *Diss. RMS,* Vol. 17 (1783–5), 285–95; E. Bradley, 'On the operations of Mercury', *Diss. RMS,* Vol. 23 (1788–9), 466–81.
119. E. Alexander, 'Can Arsenic be Administered with Advantage in Any Disease?', *Diss. RMS,* Vol. 23 (1788–9), 362–92.
120. E. Goodwyn, 'What are the Effects Arising from Blisters Applied to the Human Body? In What Manner do they Produce these Effects? In What Diseases are they Useful?', *Diss. RMS,* Vol.12 (1780–1), 463–69; W.P. Hayle, 'What is the Nature and Property of Cantharides and in What Disease are Blisters, Principally Required?', *Diss. RMS,* Vol. 17 (1783–5), 91–109.
121. For an overview, S. Shapin, 'The House of Experiment in Seventeenth-Century England', *Isis,* 79 (1988), 373–404; see also M. Nicholson and J. Windram, 'Mathew Baillie Gardiner and the Royal Medical Society and the Problem of the Second Heart Sound', *Proceedings of the Royal College of Physicians of Edinburgh,* 31 (2001), 357–67.
122. G. Blane, 'What is the Nature of Antiseptics and How do they Operate?', reprinted in Royal Medical Society, Edinburgh, *Dissertations by Eminent Members of the Royal Medical Society* (Edinburgh: D. Douglas, 1892), 15–31.
123. J.F. Enders, 'Francis Home and his Experimental Approach to Medicine', *Bulletin of the History of Medicine,* 38 (1964), 101–12.
124. E. Harrison, *op. cit.* (note 41), 188–211.
125. Bard wrote his thesis on this subject. See Samuel Bard, *De Viribus Opii* (Edinburgh: Donaldson & Reid, 1765).
126. T. Skeete, 'What are the Diseases in Which Opium May be Employed With Advantage, and How Far Can its Modus Operandi be Accounted For?', Diss. RMS, Vol. 17 (1783–5), 110–56.
127. S. Fitt, 'Are the Proofs Decisive Which are Brought on by Different Authors to Conclude that the Absorption is Only Determined by the Lymphatic System?', *Diss. RMS,* Vol. 19 (1785–6), 176.
128. See A.H. Maehle, 'The Ethical Discourse on Animal Experimentation, 1650-1900', in A. Wear, J. Geyer–Kordesch and R. French (eds), *Doctors and Ethics: The Earlier Historical Setting of Professional Ethics* (Amsterdam: Rodopi, 1993), 214.
129. *Ibid.*, 222–3. Thomas Percival penned these warnings in his work *A Father's Instructions: Moral and Literary Dissertations* (Warrington: J. Johnson, 1784).

130. P.S., 'On the Necessity of Contracting Cavities and the Ventricles of the Heart', *Diss. RMS,* Vol. 10 (1794), 19–85.
131. Spooner, *op. cit.* (note 84), 234–44.
132. Experimental Committee, 'Experiments with Cold', March 1785, in Diss.RMS., Vol. 8 (1785), 9–25.
133. The possible author of these experiments was S. Thibaud who apparently read a paper titled 'What are the Ties Which Unite the Vegetable to the Animal Kingdom?' during the 1787–8 session.
134. [S. Thibaud?], 'Brief Account of Certain Experiments Made in Consequence of Some Opinions', *Diss. RMS,* Vol. 9 (1777), 22–42.
135. T. White, 'What are the Qualities of Bile and What are the Best Remedies for Checking Morbid Secretions of it?', *Diss. RMS,* Vol. 17 (1783–5), 459–73.
136. 'Experiments to Determine Whether the Fatal Consequences of Respiring Fixed Air are Produced by the Application of that Fluid to the Nose or Fauces or the Internal Surface of the Lungs', *Diss. RMS,* Vol. 8 (1785), 60–84.
137. H. Bowles, J. Jachmann, W. Alexander, 'Experiments on Sugar of Lead to Determine Whether it be a Stimulus', *Diss. RMS,* Vol. 8 (1785), 85–121.
138. E. Goodwyn, *The Connection of Life with Respiration, or An Experimental Inquiry into the Effects of Submersion, Strangulation and Several Kinds of Noxious Airs* (London: J. Johnson, 1788), XI.
139. For an overview of the resuscitation efforts of outwardly drowned persons, see E.M. France, 'Some Eighteenth-Century Authorities on the Resuscitation of the Apparently Drowned', *Anaesthesia,* 30 (1975), 530–8.
140. W. Alexander, 'What are the Effects of Opium Upon the Healthy and Diseased Animal?', *Diss. RMS,* Vol. 19 (1785–6), 204–46.
141. M. Grant, 'What are the Causes, Nature, and Effects of Sleep?', *Diss. RMS,* Vol. 23 (1788–9), 393–413; among other papers J. Allen, 'In What Manner Does the Muscular Fibre Recover its Irritability After Partial Exhaustion?', *Diss. RMS,* Vol. 26 (1790–1), 269–301.
142. See *Medical Commentaries,* 4 (1789), 375–97.
143. J. Clerk, 'Upon What Does the Contractility of the Muscular Fibre Depend, and What are its General Laws?,' *Diss. RMS,* Vol. 26 (1790–1), 192–210.
144. See R. Whytt, *The Works of Robert Whytt, M.D.* (Edinburgh: T. Becket, 1768); Samuel Crumpe, *An Inquiry into the Nature and Properties of Opium* (London: G.G. and J. Robinson, 1793).
145. To further confirm such a hypothesis, Wilson went on to employ tobacco solutions using more frogs with similar results although the tobacco were less effective than the opium. He concluded that opium had two distinct physiological outcomes: an immediate local stimulant or irritating effect

followed by a debilitating or sedative action after reaching the brain through the normal blood supply. See A.P. Wilson, 'Concerning the Action of Opium on the Living Animal Body', *Diss. RMS,* Vol. 9 (1777), 65–98.

146. Rosner believes that students failed to verify experimental findings and therefore made no lasting contributions to medical knowledge. See Rosner, *op. cit.* (note 33), 182–94.

147. The regulations are contained in a letter included among the handwritten documents of this dispute, MSS Collection, RMS, Edinburgh. They were transcribed from the Infirmary Manager's minutes (now missing) of 15 June 1785 and also part of a pamphlet cited by Gray, *op. cit.* (note 18), 78–9.

148. The letter is titled 'The Students of Medicine in the University of Edinburgh Inform the Managers of the Royal Infirmary', in *A Narrative of Some Late Injurious Proceedings of the Managers of the Royal Infirmary Against the Students of Medicine in the University of Edinburgh* (Edinburgh, 1785), 9–21. No copies of this publication have been found. The pamphlet was originally part of the Royal Medical Society' archives, now in the MSS Collection, Edinburgh University Library.

149. 'Robert Boswell for the Infirmary', 4 July 1785, in *ibid.,* 22–7.

150. 'To the Honourable, the Managers of the Royal Infirmary', *ibid.,* 28–38.

151. 'Royal Infirmary', 18 August 1785, *ibid.,* 39–47.

152. 'To the Learned and Respectable Faculty of Medicine of the University of Edinburgh', *ibid.,* 48–54.

153. 'James Gregory, Answer from the Professors to the Address of the Students of Medicine', dated 30 August 1785, *ibid.,* 55–77.

154. 'Thomas Beddoes for the Committee, To the Learned and Respectable Professors of Medicine', *ibid.,* 81–8.

155. See Royal Infirmary Edinburgh, Minutes of Managers, MSS Collection, Edinburgh University Library, Vol. 6, 1 October 1792, 157–58.

156. Wilson, *op. cit.* (note 145), 98; see also his publication *An Experimental Essay on the Manner in Which Opium Acts on the Living Animal Body* (Edinburgh: G. Mudie & Son, 1795).

3

The Royal Medical Society versus Campbell Denovan: Brunonianism, the Press, and the Medical Establishment

During the years 1778–90, the activities of the Royal Medical Society were severely disrupted because of a growing antagonism between supporters of rival medical theories and practices. Bitter confrontations between Cullenians – supporters of William Cullen – and Brunonians – sympathisers of John Brown – shattered the earlier framework of polite disputations. When accounts of the contentious proceedings were published in a local tabloid, the Society, citing issues of professional privacy, filed a lawsuit involving famous local lawyers. The story provides an extraordinary opportunity to assess the contemporary status of Brunonianism, its efforts to demystify medicine, and the growing power of print media to influence broad sectors of the public.

Cullenians and Brunonians: setting the stage for conflict

> It is a misfortune that the students of physic, a science which depends so much upon experiment, should be mislead; first by framing visionary theories in their own brains, and then producing and tenaciously defending them in their public societies; where their object, like their fellow students of the law, is often victory rather than the discovery of truth.
>
> Thomas Newte (1791)[1]

The above comments, written by an English traveller touring Scotland in the 1780s, betray a rather harsh critique of the weekly meetings held by the Royal Medical Society of Edinburgh during a somewhat turbulent period in its history.[2] The Society had traditionally been an important forum for discussions of contemporary medical knowledge and practices. Members were encouraged to summarise and debate views held by their professors and other medical authorities, an early practice endorsed by William Cullen (1710–90), a prominent sponsor (Chapter 2).[3] Cullen had attended Society meetings as a student in 1735–6 and was considered one of its founders. His great popularity with medical students rested on his keen abilities as lecturer and mentor. According to one of his academic colleagues, James Gregory

(1753–1821), Cullen indirectly stoked the fires of debate with his belief that 'ardour' or passion in the pursuit of knowledge was the first and most essential prerequisite for becoming a medical student. In Gregory's opinion, however, 'much labour and ingenuity [was] wasted on frivolous subjects'.[4] Indeed, many of the discussions scheduled by the leadership of the Society generated more passion than reason. 'Let me beg of you, gentlemen, to manage your disputes with candour, discretion and a becoming decency', pleaded George Sutherland, one of the Society's presidents, as early as 1751. 'When you have an opportunity of correcting one another's mistakes, do it in a gentle, friendly manner without the appearance of malice or ridicule which would betray a low, mean spirit', he continued. Sutherland urged students to 'never allow your passions to get the better of your reason.'[5]

By the early 1780s, there were signs that these ritualised debates among 'gentlemen' Society members, including the use of specially appointed 'impugners', were breaking down. Growing partisanship and rancour came to conspire against John Gregory's (1724–73) carefully constructed medical persona – an individual endowed with sensibility, humour, and patience to deal with the ambiguities and paradoxes of the medical profession.[6] A climate of dissension and factionalism came to prevail during meetings. Students became extremely excited, even frenzied: 'their debates on controverted points [were] sometimes conducted with all the violence of party spirit', recalled his son, James Gregory.[7] An unusually bitter and confrontational attitude emerged as the arguments took aim at the established medical theories currently taught at the University of Edinburgh.[8] According to one student, James Mackintosh (1765–1832), 'every mind was in a state of fermentation'. Meetings tended to drift toward 'metaphysical inquiries'. Unfortunately, 'accurate and applicable knowledge was deserted for speculations'; 'speculators could not remain submissive learners' because they wanted to think for themselves and believed themselves to be much more clever than their professors.[9]

'Disputing societies have been established and the members of these societies are no more wise, more learned or better than other people', observed another anonymous critic in 1781. This writer described the evils of allowing such disputes, which appealed mostly to passion and attracted young people with strong opinions. Unfortunately, 'until mankind could divest itself of pride and self-love, it would be vain to think that the situation would change'.[10] The Society's first historian explained that 'the lyceum of social investigation was converted into a turbulent arena where rival factions struggled for superiority and the dispensers of health to others engaged in a sanguinary warfare among themselves.'[11] Even James Gregory came to the conclusion that theoretical speculations and debating skills were not as important in the pursuit of scientific medicine although they had done more good than harm.[12]

At stake in Edinburgh at the time was the growing antagonism between students partial to the ideas of Cullen[13] and those who believed in the newly minted doctrines of his former student, John Brown (1735–88), a long-standing member of the Society since 2 May 1761. The rift between the two men, initiated by Brown's vehement and outspoken public rejection of Cullen's medical system, had the effect of polarising the membership. Henceforth, the Society's traditional framework of polite discourse was periodically disrupted. Some sessions became convenient opportunities for ideological battles between the so-called 'Cullenians' and 'Brunonians' – characterised by Mackintosh as a struggle of the 'Catholic Church' versus the 'Heretics'.[14] Nicknamed 'Old Spasm', Cullen was closely identified with Edinburgh medicine, his reputation widely recognised throughout Britain and Europe, especially after the publication of his *Nosology* (1769) and *First Lines of the Practice of Physic* (1776–9).[15] Cullen had officially retired in 1779 although he still retained an active private practice. The Royal Medical Society together with the Town Council and Lord Provost took up a subscription for the installation of his marble bust at the University. For decades a popular teacher and mentor, Cullen's visibility and popularity among newly arrived students was now ebbing. In an era of significant epistemological shifts, his penchant for systematic arrangements of medical knowledge were increasingly subjected to critical reviews and unfavourable commentaries.[16] As James Gregory put it, Cullen's 'tub' or medical system was being 'knocked to pieces', prompting medicine – 'the whale' – to search for another aquatic habitat to play in: Brown's medical system.[17]

Brown, better known by his Latinised name 'Bruno', openly assailed his former teacher's medical theories and practices after 1778.[18] He exploited Cullen's notions of nervous sensibility and power, seeking to reduce them to a supreme vital quality he called 'excitability' subject to quantification and mathematical formulas. In doing so, Brown aimed at greater certainty in medicine through the employment of a Newtonian-like principle capable of explaining the behaviour of all living organisms. Lacking much clinical experience, his personal sufferings from a gouty illness became an empirical confirmation for his simplified ideas on disease and therapeutics. Brunonianism came to raise a number of important theoretical and practical issues that were intensely debated within the confines of the Royal Medical Society.[19] From a methodological point of view, adherents stressed the inductive nature of their beliefs, which were acquired through bedside experiences. This created a rather simple division among diseases according to the amount of nervous excitability currently present in the body. This distinction rendered complex disease classification systems based on hypothetical causalities or similar symptomatology obsolete.[20]

Brown's attacks on conventional medical therapeutics focused particularly on the so-called 'antiphlogistic' medical approach based on humoralism, the traditional effort to deplete the body of its presumed harmful fluids. He believed that physicians were basically wrong in assuming that all inflammatory diseases resulted from vascular plethora. Instead, Brown argued, sickness usually reflected systemic bodily weakness, not strength. Therefore, the ancient practices of attempting to expel dangerous fluids from the body by means of bloodletting, purges, and emetics was not only ineffective but outright harmful, because they prolonged and exacerbated a patient's disease.[21] Brunonians also discredited the idea of a natural healing power residing in the body, which could ultimately be trusted to assist recovery.[22] Finally, they rejected drugs considered 'specific' to particular diseases and deemed other compounds still listed in official pharmacopoeias totally ineffective.

Brunonianism represented a direct assault on British professional identity and power by challenging both contemporary medical theories and therapies. Conscious of their elite status and energised by the allure of a new and simplified medical system, some of Brown's adherents viewed the Cullenians as members of a conservative and corrupt corporation solely preoccupied with retaining patronage and profits derived from their teaching.[23] By the same token, opponents of Brunonianism judged Brown's medical ideas theoretically incomprehensible and practices clinically reckless. In pursuing his revolutionary quest, Brown tried to include the public in this debate, encouraging unorthodox domestic healing efforts. He stressed the importance for laypersons to use intuition and exercise their freedom of learning with regard to health-related matters.[24] Brown's own preference for large doses of stimulants in the form of opium and alcohol definitely struck a popular cord. He also ranted against the veil of mystery which medical jargon and schools of medicine had placed over the healing art. The inherent simplicity of the Brunonian scheme was 'intended not for the exclusive use of medical readers but also for the public at large' in an expanded medical marketplace.[25] At a time when Britons were becoming virtually obsessed with their own physical wellbeing, Brunonian populism came to be seen as a dangerous encouragement for quackery and do-it-yourself physic.[26]

Barred from graduating at Edinburgh University because of his heretical views, Brown had been forced to take his medical degree in 1780 at nearby St Andrews University, a notorious Scottish diploma mill. Back in Edinburgh, he began offering an extramural private course of lectures based on his new medical ideas, summarised in the *Elementa Medicinae* (1780).[27]

Coincidentally in the same year, Brown, surrounded by a train of pupils and admirers, was elected senior president of the Royal Medical Society.[28] Although such a leadership position provided him with an official forum from which to launch attacks on his former mentor, Brown apparently left such matters in the hands of his students. Two of them, Edward Stevens and John Ford, were junior presidents during Brown's tenure, with Ford assisting in the successful negotiations to obtain a Royal Charter. Relinquishing most of the routine business to other officers, Brown actually chaired only one meeting in 1780. Perhaps he was too preoccupied trying to earn a living as a physician and remain solvent, since he was beginning to be widely ostracised by the Edinburgh medical establishment. Indeed, at a meeting in January 1781, Society leaders had to appoint a special committee to force Brown into surrendering the student dues he had collected during his presidency.[29]

In spite of Brown's lack of personal involvement in the Society's debates that pitted his 'new' medical doctrine against Cullen's 'old' one, the stage was nevertheless set for a series of intense confrontations between the most outspoken Cullenian and Brunonian adherents. Students supporting Cullen's ideas were defined by their opponents as timid and prudent; Brunonians characterised themselves as 'more active and enterprising' than their opponents. Sceptics caught in the middle of the confrontations 'thought it better to practice a lukewarm conformity to the established system than to embrace doctrines somewhat more specious indeed but perhaps equally false.'[30] Looking at the situation decades later, the Society's historian explained that, among medical students, the Brunonian theory was garnering 'a degree of popularity and admiration frequently bordering on fanaticism'. He based this phenomenon on 'the easy perspicuity of [Brown's] doctrine, its mathematical and scientific aspects, the respectable truth which it contained and even the confidence with which it was enforced'.[31] A recurrent subject for discussion at the Society's sessions was the action of opium. Indeed, both Cullen and Brown differed sharply on the perceived pharmacological qualities of this popular drug. Cullenians stressed its sedative actions, while Brunonians perceived its superior stimulating powers. Student presentations on opium thus became a litmus test for defining adherents from both rival camps. Each side tried to employ a similar rhetoric, portraying and justifying their conclusions as being more 'scientific', an argument that necessarily led to extensive epistemological discussions.[32]

In fact, during the 43rd session, a paper read in March 1780 by another of Brown's principal disciples, John W. Howell, laid out some of the basic Brunonian tenets. Howell spoke on rescuing – or at least relieving – the art of medicine from its present state of uncertainty and hypothetical reasoning. Howell admitted that medicine would never provide total certainty or be entirely free of errors. In a thinly disguised reference to Cullen, he blamed 'a bigoted veneration of great names' for much mischief in medicine 'by making men trust more to the hypotheses of others than to their own observation'.[33] During the same session, another favourite student of Brown, James Campbell, explained that reasoning based on hypothetical and erroneous theories was prejudicial to the medical art. 'Presumption may swagger, bustle and quibble and prejudice obstinately will hold its assent', he remarked, but sound reasoning and accurate observation were the preferred paths.[34] Campbell strongly condemned one of the central tenets of medicine, the doctrine of 'morbific' matter. This notion, traditionally linked to classic humoralism, predicated that most diseases were caused by the accumulation of noxious humours within the body, and that natural healing powers should be trusted to expel such substances. The practitioner's role was merely to assist nature by engaging in depleting treatments such as bleeding, purging, vomiting, and perspiration. However, Campbell urged his colleagues to reject this approach, arguing that disease primarily affected the solid parts of the body in the form of imbalances of neuromuscular excitement. With respect to bloodletting practices, Campbell remarked that 'neither Apollo nor any of the other prophetic Gods of Greece ever uttered a more mysterious and incomprehensible response. Loss of blood in a considerable degree weakens the body'.

A year later, the Society witnessed a disagreeable episode involving John R. Martyn, a newly admitted student who, carried away by the intensity of a debate, allegedly threatened 'to settle the differences by appeals to the sword'.[35] After the duelling offer became public, the leadership under the presidency of Thomas Kerr called an extraordinary session for 12 February 1781. At the meeting, the Society decided to expel Martyn. The militant student was accused of endeavouring 'to take away the freedom of debate essential to the wellbeing of the Society'. Moreover, Martyn was denounced for introducing 'anarchy and confusion' into the sessions. His threats were deemed to have exposed the organisation 'to the ridicule of strangers'.[36] Gregory had no doubt after Martyn's challenge 'that some [students] would gladly have died martyrs to their medical faith'.[37] For a society of young gentlemen learning to become reputable practitioners, fears that their status and that of the professors would suffer irreparable harm were well-founded, especially if the behaviour was negatively portrayed to the public. Surrounded by surgeons, apothecaries, herbalists and miscellaneous peddlers of nostrums, elite physicians were still in the minority.[38] Duelling was now widely condemned because it seemed to disregard both divine and human law. It was definitely inappropriate for physicians. Writing in his *Medical Ethics*, even Thomas Percival (1740–1804) found the previously genteel practice repugnant.[39]

Following his ousting, Martyn blamed his expulsion on 'some despotic teachers whose prejudice and self-interest [were] a sufficient reason to do everything in their power for their own ends to keep students in the dark'. In his opinion, these unnamed professors stifled 'liberal inquiry' as well as expressions from the 'honest dictates of the heart'. In Martyn's view, Edinburgh's conservative academics resisted the 'evident superiority of a doctrine founded on the simple laws of the animal economy and the dictates of common sense', an allusion to Brown's controversial new ideas. He expressed contempt 'for the behaviour of a party in the Society who have no spirit to think for themselves' – a parting shot at the Cullenians then firmly in control of the Society. Martyn predicted that his unprecedented dismissal would 'bring disgrace on a Medical School once the most famed in Europe'.

Martyn's threats and subsequent expulsion from the Royal Medical Society caused one Edinburgh publication to recommend that henceforth all debates of the Society be cancelled and the various papers simply circulated among the student members. 'Surely nobody will say that the cause of truth can be promoted by such violent proceedings or that the Medical Society in such condition is calculated for making men wiser or better', concluded the anonymous critic.[40] Unfortunately, the Martyn affair turned out to be only the first skirmish. A series of rhetorical battles ensued in an atmosphere of intolerance.[41] The heated exchanges would soon come to the attention of the reading public in Edinburgh. In the meantime, Brown was being marginalised and snubbed by Edinburgh's medical establishment. The medical faculty banned the official exposition of Brunonian ideas in inaugural dissertations. Although Brown vehemently protested this discriminatory measure, he was forced to take thirteen of his students to the University of Aberdeen in order to have them awarded their medical degrees. As a private tutor, Brown faced a dwindling number of customers since he taught concepts and practices now deemed unacceptable to university officials.

Early hostilities: a chronicle

Under the heading 'Pantheon Intelligence', the *Edinburgh Evening Post*, a local tabloid, carried a short story on 11 January 1783. The publisher of the anonymous article was none other than Campbell Denovan – a sympathiser and friend of John Brown, who would later publish a revised edition of Brown's *Elementa Medicinae*. The newspaper article described in vague detail a debate that had taken place earlier in an unnamed local medical society concerning whether an increase in medical knowledge had decreased the bills of mortality'.[42] Quoting presumed witnesses of the debate, the essay reported that the first discussant at the meeting strongly assailed the traditional depleting therapies still in vogue, recommending instead life-saving, stimulating medicines. The unidentified speaker was quoted as claiming that 'as soon as the Brunonian system and practice should come to be generally known and adopted, the bills of mortality would then decrease in an astonishing degree'.[43] Such opinions, expressed by an obvious adherent of Brown, were, according to the newspaper story, answered 'with an uncommon degree of pleasantry, wit, and good humour' by another unnamed member of Edinburgh's medical establishment. Drawing on his experiences as a naval surgeon, this individual was quoted as saying he considered the use of Brunonian spirits of wine in fevers 'as ridiculous as to make use of oil to quench a fire if one's house were in flames'. Then, a third discussant countered, railing against the 'absurdity of the ordinary practice of medicine' and reading a letter from another 'conscientious' student of physic who had decided to quit medicine altogether 'on account of the thousands annually murdered by the prescriptions of Dr. Bolus, Dr. Clysterpipe, and Professor Arsenick'.[44] Eventually, the article reported, the presiding clerk, who also expressed his disapproval of Edinburgh's 'general mode' of medical practice, terminated the Society's increasingly animated debate. While cloaked in humour, the story's underlying sarcasm expressed strong doubts about the efficacy of contemporary medicine.

One week later, on 18 January 1783, the *Edinburgh Evening Post* once again disclosed that the same medical society had endured another debate about therapeutics. A fierce discussion ensued following the reading of a letter from a naval surgeon currently stationed in Rio de Janeiro and apparently addressed to John Brown. Military personnel and former students often attended sessions as guests and the author may well have been among the latter. This communication, quoted verbatim in the paper, described in highly complimentary terms the superiority of Brown's therapeutic approach in the treatment of 'Bengal fever' through the use of opium and camphor. 'Rest assured that in whatever quarter of the globe, I shall always think on [sic] Johannes Bruno M.D. with veneration', the letter ended. According to the newspaper, the assembled students then called for a vote to endorse the Brunonian approach to medical treatment 'and the question [was] decided in the affirmative by a great majority'.[45] Both newspaper columns prompted a letter to the editor – real or fictitious – under the pseudonym '*Medicinae Studiosus*' – a student of medicine. The note appeared in a subsequent issue of the *Edinburgh Evening Post* expressing approval for the newspaper's accounts praising their 'theatrical strictures'. The author also acknowledged that the publications had attracted considerable attention among medical students hitherto unfamiliar with Brunonian ideas. In fact, at a subsequent meeting of the Society, a group of members unanimously approved a resolution to send weekly accounts of meetings for publication in the newspaper. 'Tho it may not afford so much entertainment as your theatrical intelligence, it would in all probability prove highly useful to the public at large', the students were quoted.[46]

Denovan, publisher of the *Evening Post* promptly responded, characterising the request so reasonable that 'we could not help [but] comply with it'.[47]

Together with the reader's letter, the newspaper printed the first instalment in a separate section entitled *Medical Intelligence*. The article contained a summary of the discussions conducted at the Society a week earlier on 'some of the leading points of the new and old systems'. The initial presenter was George Maxwell, an adherent of Cullen, who spoke on the uses of cold water in haemorrhages. Maxwell categorised such treatments as stimulants, while in his opinion opium and wine were sedatives.[48] According to the newspaper story, Maxwell's ideas were 'vigorously opposed by a number of young gentlemen' who followed Brunonian principles. In fact, one of them was quoted as saying that Cullen 'had not only advanced doctrines contrary to facts but had expressly contradicted himself'. Indeed, the paper claimed that this gentleman, 'expatriated with so much eloquence and strength of reasoning that the majority of the Society were fully convinced of the justice of his remarks and of every fact of the new doctrine that had been delivered that night.'[49]

In the next 'Medical Intelligence' column appearing in the *Edinburgh Evening Post*, the anonymous correspondent admitted that the latest meeting of the Society had witnessed a comeback of the Cullenians. In his view, they had come 'fully determined to overpower their opponents if not by strength of reasoning at least by a multitude of words.' Apparently one by one the student partisans of Cullen rose, delivering 'long studied harangues' and preventing a single Brunonian from taking the floor. This time around, it seemed, Bruno's party had been seemingly 'overpowered by numbers' and the presiding officer would only promise further discussions for the following session.[50] Two weeks later, the newspaper carried another instalment of its medical news. This time, the account recited a fierce debate generated by a presentation on the nature and effects of sleep. The presenter, Robert Cleghorn, was characterised as a former adherent of Cullen's medical system who now voiced his opposition to 'hypothetical explanations', complaining that 'he had been misled by former doctrines'. Cleghorn's empirical leanings were clearly expressed at the beginning of his presentation when he informed his student audience that 'nothing has retarded our progress in science [more] than the vanity of explaining the cause of everything'. To collect and arrange phenomena was a 'dull and inglorious task', abandoned for a much more attractive effort to construct theories.[51] Cleghorn's presentation also lambasted the 'vanity of explaining the cause of everything instead of looking at nature' – a frequent criticism of eighteenth-century medical systems. This student also took Cullen to task for deficiencies in his classification of diseases, especially the lumping together of sleep, syncope, and death as manifestations of a state of nervous 'collapse'.[52] Cleghorn found this notion 'deficient and unsatisfying' although at the same time he had to admit that theory still remained 'the best manner of speaking' because 'it shortens language and connects a great variety of phenomena by one general principle'. In this vein, the discussion after Cleghorn's presentation on sleep considered as another state of indirect or direct debility, became another celebration of Brunonian ideas.[53]

Freedom of the press

Reaction from the leadership of the Royal Medical Society – composed mostly of Cullenians – was quick. As the *Edinburgh Evening Post* reported in its next issue, 'everything we had narrated relative to the business was read and commented upon, paragraph by paragraph' at the last meeting of the Society. 'The opprobrious epithets of scoundrel and villain' were given to the anonymous student who had leaked the information to the press, and, although his identity was not revealed, he was officially expelled from the Society.[54] A statement signed by the Society's paid secretary, John Miller, sought to categorise the newspaper accounts as 'erroneous, illiberal and false', and designed 'to serve the sinister purpose of some interested individuals'.[55] Not only would any future published reports lack authorisation from the Society's leaders, but also the public was urged to treat them 'with that silent contempt which it merits'. Pressured by officers such as John H. Engelhart,[56] one of the contemporary presidents, the entire Society membership focused their discussions on the issue of professional privacy rather than rivalry. After much deliberation, a new rule was approved on 22 February: henceforth any student caught providing information about the Society's proceedings to members of the press would be 'ipso facto expelled'. The membership approved another proposal that no visitors be admitted until the publications of Society debates ceased. Moreover, a small committee was appointed to draft a statement for publication in the *Edinburgh Evening Post* refuting all previously printed accounts. This group was composed of Samuel Ferris, Stephen Dickson, together with John Stark, another president. In addition to changes in their rules, the officers of the Society also began exploring the possibility of prosecuting Denovan, the publisher of the newspaper.

Denovan responded rather defiantly to this legal threat. In an appendix to the same issue of his newspaper, he questioned the authority of the student leaders to sue him. He asked: 'how do they imagine that they have a power in Edinburgh superior to [that] which the constitution allows to the three highest orders of the state, viz, to put a negative on the freedom of the press?' For Denovan, such liberty was readily accepted in England, but in Scotland 'a few great names' exerted their powerful censorship on all printed matter. He also questioned why a society, 'instituted for the purpose of watching over the health of his Majesty's subjects', had the right to conceal from the public 'a business' in which the public was most interested.[57] In addition to general issues of free speech and public disclosure of medical matters, Denovan also focused on the specific controversy between Cullenians and Brunonians. He questioned whether medicine, as taught by the Edinburgh medical professors, had indeed achieved a degree of perfection that allowed no further improvements. Should not the discovery of truth in every department of knowledge actually require 'mutual discussion?', he asked. In Denovan's view, the 'extraordinary tumult' during Society meetings occurred because 'a doctrine which was meant to be suppressed and the followers of it excluded [from] the Society has met with respectable converts to it'.[58] At the end of his editorial, he returned to the question of freedom of the press: 'The medical department in the *Edinburgh Evening Post* shall be carried on', he promised, 'with the same attention to truth and freedom of sentiment as ever'. At the same time, however, Denovan expressed willingness to compromise. He offered to meet with officials of the Society to avoid further misunderstandings while reminding his foes to respect 'the perfect liberty of the press'.

Perhaps to avoid further strife, Denovan desisted from publishing another 'letter to the public' prepared by a contingent of medical students in the 25 February 1783 issue of his newspaper. In their announcement, the Brunonians wanted to reiterate the fact that the previous disclosures to the press were legal and made by respectable members of the Society 'whose only aim is the establishment of truth'. Unmoved by the gesture, the Royal Medical Society approved a motion of Stephen Dickson on 1 March appointing a committee. The group was charged to investigate 'whether any and what legal means may or ought to be pursued for preventing such publications in the future and for bringing to justice the author or abettors of them'. Informed of these developments, Denovan subsequently retaliated by including the Brunonian 'Letter to the Public' in the next issue of his newspaper.[59]

Between 1 March and 12 April 1783, the *Edinburgh Evening Post* printed seven additional articles dealing with the activities of the Royal Medical Society. Some of them focused on a paper already delivered a month earlier by a new student member, Robert D. Willis. Willis strongly railed against 'reasoning beyond the reach of observation', a familiar argument employed by the Brunonians. Instead, physicians needed to be guided by experience in practice.[60] Willis condemned the 'genius of teachers who have generally rejected the evidence of sense and bewildered themselves in explaining the mode by which nature conducts her operations... [who have] attached [themselves] to theory and hypothesis, and have laboured to accommodate every new discovery to the principles of their own imagination.'[61] Another instalment of Willis' presentation came on 19 March, when the newspaper mentioned the student's sharp personal attack on Cullen. Referring to the professor, Willis was quoted saying 'it astonishes me to hear a man daily labouring to instil into the minds of his pupils a theory, which he himself confesses is useless at the bedside.' Cullen's nosology was another frequent target of Brunonians since 'all arrangements of diseases founded on appearances only must be rejected'. Indeed, Willis concluded his polemical presentation with the observation that 'if we attempt to explain all wonders of our system with no better furniture than an imaginary spasm, we shall create innumerable difficulties.'[62]

The newspaper reports were unabashedly partisan. Using humour and satire and describing events through the eyes of an enthusiastic follower of John Brown's system of medicine, Cullen's theories were routinely disparaged.[63] Openly favouring the Brunonian party, the *Edinburgh Evening Post* once more tried to ridicule its opponents under the rubric of 'Medical Intelligence Extraordinary'. The column deliciously revealed that three students, characterised as 'enemies of the New System' and charged with composing the Society's official 'manifesto', had met to discuss the matter in a certain coffeehouse. Called 'to testify their utter *abhorrence* of the *erroneous system'* they promptly 'destroyed six bottles of Dr Brown's *quickly diffusible stimuli!'*[64] Brandy consumption, it seemed, was the great equaliser across Edinburgh's ideological medical trenches. Scattered between lengthy descriptions of the students' sectarian arguments, however, were fears that all the Brunonians were going to be expelled from the Society and indeed the University. On 1 March, the 'Medical Intelligence' column of the newspaper took up this issue. 'If the terror of losing a degree is held up to them, in order to seduce them from the proper method of prosecuting their studies, there is no degree upon earth so respectable as to be put in the balance'. The article ended with the statement that 'we hope the time is not far distant when the Medical Society in particular, and the students of this University in general will esteem themselves obliged to the *Edinburgh Evening Post* for the instruction it has afforded them.'[65]

Unfortunately for Denovan, the leadership of the Royal Medical Society thought otherwise. At their 8 March meeting, a committee composed of four students, Stephen Dickson, Robert Cleghorn, Henry Ainslie, and Robert Willis – the last two identified as Brunonians – was selected to draft a summary of the previous events for possible legal action. While the Society's leadership pondered its next move, a defiant Denovan continued to publish his 'Medical Intelligence' section. In its 15 March issue, the *Edinburgh Evening Post* printed another extensive summary of Willis' paper, applauding especially his critique of medical systems and the backwardness of contemporary medicine.[66] The matter of a possible lawsuit was taken up again on 22 March and a legal opinion sought from two of the most famous legal authorities in Edinburgh: Henry Erskine and Robert Cullen.[67] The queries posed by the Society for their legal opinion revolved around the newspaper's 'Medical Intelligence' articles: could they be considered a libel upon the Society? If so, what proper steps should be taken to punish the author or 'abettors'? If not, how could such publications be prevented in the future? Finally, could the publisher be forced to reveal the identity of the student who had provided the information or was considered the author of the column? [68]

The lawsuit

By the end of March 1783, the confrontation between the Royal Medical Society and the *Edinburgh Evening Post* intensified and took on an increasingly legalistic tone. On 29 March, the newspaper printed a 'Medical Entertainment' section signed by 'Cacodaemon' – an evil spirit – who identified himself as an old member and former president of the Society. Laced with Latin phrases, this diatribe, full of sarcasm, may have been authored by none other than John Brown himself, hiding in the shadows. 'Me, ye cannot injure, for I fill your Hall and ye observe me not. I ride in a misty veil and ye discover not the moving of my chariot', the note stated. 'Facts are my horses, and they are driven by spasm, my invisible charioteer. I sometimes perch upon the cornish of your door and laugh at your folly'.[69] The anonymous writer also strongly criticised two unnamed Society presidents, probably John H. Engelhart and Andrew Fyfe, claiming serious irregularities linked to their election. The author also bitterly complained that the Brunonian minority members selected to consider the need for legal action against the newspaper were totally excluded from a number of secret deliberations sponsored by the Society's leadership.[70]

On that same day, Robert Cullen and Henry Erskine provided their detailed answers to the Society's queries. They determined that 'publishing any account of the transactions of the Society without its consent is an injurious encroachment upon what is undoubtedly their exclusion right'. Moreover, the lawyers agreed that 'the publication is no doubt the more injurious in that it does not convey a fair and true representation of the Society's proceedings'.[71] Indeed, Cullen and Erskine even claimed to detect a 'malicious intention', a 'tendency to expose to ridicule and contempt', that would 'lessen the estimation' of the medical organisation. Therefore, they strongly advised the Royal Medical Society 'to bring action before the Court of Session, not only against the publisher of the newspaper, but also the actual author of the articles'. In closing, they expressed the hope that 'after executing a summons...the publisher of the newspaper will think it prudent to desist from continuing the publication of such articles'. However, to ensure such a course of action, the Society was told 'to apply to the Court immediately by Bills of Suspension... and praying for an interdict to prohibit and discharge the publishing of such articles till the action was brought.'[72] Cullen and Erskine's legal opinion was presented to the full membership of the Society during the 5 April 1783 session. After further discussions just before the summer recess a week later, a resolution to initiate the legal proceedings against Campbell Denovan was passed by a fourteen-vote majority. Quite predictably, a number of Brunonian students, including Ainslie, Willis, Lubbock, together with lesser-known disciples John Lawson, William Thornton, Thomas Pretyman, Robert Batty, and Thomas Hobbes objected to the proposal. A week later, the Society's leadership went on to appoint a special committee to manage the legal process. The group included four presidents from the 1782–3 session, Stark, Evory, Fyfe, and Engelhart, together with Dickson, Wallis, Pringle, and Wilkinson. Denovan immediately took issue with the Society's decision to prosecute him. On 26 April, another editorial appeared in the current issue of the *Edinburgh Evening Post* denouncing the increasingly politicised atmosphere in the Royal Medical Society and its bitter debates as well as despicable backdoor manoeuvring. 'Would there be anything reprehensible or dangerous in point of law in receiving and publishing the favours of correspondents?' asked Denovan. In his view, occasional reports of important medical works in the newspaper could be seen as 'useful information' designed to 'prepare the public for a favourable reception' of new medical knowledge. Any judgement against him, Denovan warned, 'will give a wound to the freedom of the press in this country for which neither the new nor the old system of medicine would ever afford a remedy.'[73] This last statement reflected the publisher's attempt to dampen some of the strident Brunonian partisanship displayed in the newspaper accounts. In fact, Denovan now feared that his journalistic contributions to promote the 'new' theory of John Brown could indeed backfire, accentuating the already deep divisions within the membership of the Royal Medical Society. Some of these 'first aggressors', Denovan observed, 'are now complaining of the effects of their conduct since the exposure of it in our paper, laying the blame obliquely upon their opponents'. In fairness, he conceded, the defendants of the 'old' theory have 'ever been modest, genteel, and honourable'. Printing their responses in the newspaper, Denovan pretended, allowed 'us an opportunity of evidencing our impartiality in exhibiting both sides of the question to the public'.[74] On 2 June 1783, a so-called 'notorial requisition' was made on Campbell Denovan in which the editor of the *Edinburgh Evening Post* was requested to reveal the name of the author of his 'Medical Intelligence' reports. The publisher, however, refused to disclose his sources to the court, prompting a 'summons of declarator and damages' to be filed on behalf of the Royal Medical Society against him. The Society additionally sought five hundred pounds sterling in damages for these newspaper publications which were 'calculated to vilify and injure the Society, to expose it to ridicule and contempt'.[75] On 8 July, the case was first heard before Lord Hailes and the action dismissed. However, the Court allowed the pursuers of the lawsuit to amend their libel.

In the meantime, at the onset of a new academic year, Edward Harrison, senior president of the Society and a student with Brunonian leanings, opened the 47th session on 1 November 1783 with a paper on the effects of opium and alcohol on the human body. For him both remedies constituted the 'basis of modern medicine'. Harrison began his remarks by stating he would only present new information on what was widely perceived to be a controversial topic. Like other members, he emphatically denied engaging in hypotheses. 'My business [is] to collect facts', he explained, 'let others reason on them'. Harrison condemned experimental animal trials with opium and alcohol, especially the pulse measurements, because he thought that they were inherently flawed since these creatures were already compromised (Chapter 2). To remedy this situation, he had personally engaged in a bit of auto-experimentation, swallowing a grain of solid opium and thereafter checking the frequency of his own pulse for several hours at fifteen-minute intervals. Similar testing of the effects of opium on respiration and body heat followed and all were duplicated by one of Harrison's student friends. The results showed no noticeable acceleration (stimulation) or slowdown (sedation) of vital signs in presumably healthy humans – as respectively claimed by Brunonians and Cullenians. In Harrison's view, the findings challenged Cullen's assertions that opium was contraindicated in inflammatory conditions. With respect to alcoholic beverages such as brandy and wine, the student insisted that their stimulating action had to be equivalent to that of opium but he could not offer experimental proof.[76] No matter, his audience undoubtedly was already quite familiar with their effects.

Two weeks later, Lord Hailes ruled on the appeal prepared by the Royal Medical Society against the *Edinburgh Evening Post* and its publisher. To the surprise of student officers, the judge declared that the publication of debates held by the Society, established for the purposes of free scientific inquiries, were lawful. Moreover, Denovan's 'Medical Intelligence' reports were held not actionable since they only contained vague and sometimes unintelligible references to the actual events.[77] As the leadership conferred about another appeal, the meeting of 22 November featured another paper by a Brunonian student, Richard Lubbock. Lubbock offered another rebuttal of older humoral views by discussing human growth in terms of vascular expansion stimulated by excitability instead of blood.[78] On 6 December, Henry Ainslie, read an essay on the best means of preserving health and curing disease. Following Brown, Ainslie postulated that all diseases arose from an excessive or deficient action of the powers creating life.[79] Another speaker, Samuel Hinds, called Cullen's theory 'evidently false', accusing theorists of simply 'juggling words' to generate fame and disciples. 'The idea of a system indeed necessarily excludes all future improvement in as much as it supposes a perfection of our knowledge, and therefore prevents our attention to facts', he observed.[80]

While Brunonians sought to dominate the Society's proceedings, the Cullenian leaders refused to give up on their lawsuit. The court again denied two additional petitions on 29 November and 20 December 1783, even though the student organisation decided to drop its earlier demands for monetary damages. During the legal proceedings, Denovan succeeded in portraying himself a 'poor printer of an Edinburgh newspaper', only trying to obey the law. He assured the court that he had no intention 'of throwing away his time and money upon nice metaphysical disquisitions'. Moreover, Denovan refused to pay for court expenses, categorising them as 'legal punishment'.[81] Further representations by the Royal Medical Society before the Lord Ordinary on 28 January and again 13 February 1784 were equally unsuccessful.[82] Meanwhile, encouraged by the judicial rulings, Brunonian students John Lawson, Thomas Pretyman and James Jeffray presented their provocative and lengthy papers on medical practice, thus re-igniting the controversy. On 24 January 1784, Lawson attacked the credibility of contemporary therapeutics, characterising the current articles of materia medica as 'relics of the doctrine of Asclepiades and Themison'.[83] In reviewing the effects of Peruvian bark, he questioned the notion that this popular drug was specifically indicated for the treatment of particular diseases, especially the ague or intermittent fever (Chapter 5). In the Brunonian world of therapeutics, all stimulants were believed to exert the same action: increase bodily excitability. After a brief paper by Pretyman on haemorrhages,[84] Jeffray spoke on 14 February 1784 on the classical doctrine of 'critical days'. A valuable prognostic tool for ancient physicians was the notion that the evolution of most febrile diseases was punctuated by some crucial clinical turns, occurring at particular and predictable times during the process. Traditionally, these critical days were attributed to the actions of an unknown but widely accepted natural healing power in the body – the '*vis medicatrix naturae*'. However, following the Brunonian system, Jeffray strongly rejected its existence; instead, he characterised the concept as a chimera, 'pardonable in the dark ages of ignorance but at present in this enlightened era of true philosophy, altogether without excuse'. Jeffray believed that expectant therapy, based on trust in such an 'evil genius', could be deceiving, even dangerous, and lead to fatal results. He explained that the human body was always in a state of flux, depending on applied stimuli. The degree and duration of stimuli, in turn, relied on 'a thousand contingent circumstances'. Practitioners needed to be aware of this complex dynamic by making an inventory of stimuli instead of trusting in a mystical power. Such insights transformed Brunonian therapeutics into an activist, even aggressive form of treatment.[85]

After such presentations and in the ongoing backlash against public discourse over such matters, members of the Society were invited to discuss the plan to approve a non-disclosure rule concerning the content of the Society's sessions. A motion prepared by Thomas A. Emmet suggested that every gentleman in this Society 'pledge his word of honour – as part of his obligation when signing the laws – that he will not anytime communicate to any printer or publisher'. The motion was extensively debated and eventually approved at a special meeting scheduled for 1 March 1784.[86] In the meantime, the Society, with the aid of Robert O. Cullen, had presented another petition to the court for a review of the case. Again, the main argument in the document was that 'no person against their will and without their consent has a right to print and publish to the world even a fair and just account of their [the Society's] transactions and proceedings'.[87] Based on a number of specific legal cases, Cullen asserted that even students, allowed to take notes on the lectures of their professors, could not legally publish them. Newspaper accounts would rob the Society or the individual authors of the benefits and advantages they could derive from the publication of their papers and transactions;[88] nobody wanted unauthorised leaks of their ideas and arguments before they could be systematically presented in books and monographs. Moreover, the petition stressed that public disclosure of papers and discussions would subvert the very nature of the Society, which traditionally was a forum for 'hasty' student presentations and 'youthful' debate, all arranged for 'their mutual improvement'. With the Society's functions impaired, the lawyer argued, reputation of the Edinburgh Medical School would be at stake. In his final summation, Robert O. Cullen relied on a recent case of the Society of Solicitors of Edinburgh, which had successfully prosecuted a printer for a single publication in a newspaper. 'The publications in the present case were not only much more injurious, but also continued and repeated', Cullen concluded, 'calculated to expose the Society to ridicule'.[89]

But on 15 July 1784, the Court of Session rejected the Society's final petition to reconsider the matter and no further representations were attempted.[90] Denovan, on the other hand, had won a Pyrrhic victory. The expenses incurred in the legal battle had brought him to the brink of bankruptcy and hastened the demise of the *Edinburgh Evening Post.* Ostensibly designed to promote Brown's medical ideas, its 'Medical Intelligence' reports had been more fluff than substance, full of innuendo and sarcasm, keen on rumour and cryptic on information. In their indignation about repeated leaks to the press, concerned members of the Royal Medical Society had rallied against students identified as Brunonians because they were suspected of violating the confidentiality of the Saturday evening meetings. Presumed to have provided leaks to the press, the students were cast in the role of villains trying to discredit the Royal Medical Society, injure its elite student body, and by implication, challenge the authority of the Edinburgh Medical School.

Conclusion

In subsequent years, Brunonian students continued to make presentations to the Society. During the 1784–5 session under the leadership of senior president Jeffrays, Charles Throckmorton (a founding member of Brown's Masonic lodge),[91] William Spooner[92] and George Bachmetieve, relied on predictable Brunonian arguments in their papers. Bachmetieve repeated his teacher's metaphor meant to describe human physiology: 'at the close of the day, the living frame, like the lamp, which has long been burning, approaches towards the state of exhaustion'.[93] But the ultimate goal of the Society was recognised: 'the candid discussion, which every paper has a right to claim in this Society, affords the best opportunity of investigating truth and detecting error'.[94] Yet, even after Brown's departure to London in 1786, the Society, under the senior presidency of another Brunonian, Edmund

Goodwyn, experienced further partisan wrangling.[95] Impressed by the claims of Brown's excitability, Goodwyn himself felt motivated to study the essential qualities of life with the help of animal and human experiments, hoping to discover a general vital principle.[96] Another president during that 1786–7 session, James Mackintosh, used the opportunity of presenting a case of tertian fever to contrast the Cullenian and Brunonian systems. He spoke for many when he hailed the latter because of its simplicity but condemned it for being narrow. Mackintosh admitted that 'the praise of elegance and precision cannot be denied by its enemies', but its application tempted partisans to 'torture facts...difficult to resist'. By contrast, Mackintosh characterised Cullen's doctrine as comprehensive, embracing 'incomparably more facts and principles that prove repugnant to that simplicity in causes and variety in effects which philosophy discovers and advances in the works of God'.[97]

During the 1789–90 session, one of the presidents, Robert Gray, discussed the causes of hysteria in terms compatible with Brown's ideas, followed a year later by William Belcher who used his own clinical exposition on the same disease to summarise Brown's fundamental ideas.[98] Another talk by William Alexander on the effects of opium was based on a series of animal experiments demonstrating – not unexpectedly – its stimulating instead of sedative qualities. Addressing his Cullenian opponents, Alexander suggested that 'the partisans for this absurd hypothesis' should finally 'confess that they have sacrificed the dictates of truth in support of absurd theories and vain imaginations'.[99] In the 1790s, as the original partisans on either side graduated or left town, the extreme partisanship gradually subsided in the Society, although a few less strident papers sympathetic to Brown's ideas continued to be delivered. In Gregory's use of metaphors, Brown's 'tub' had 'drifted over to the Continent' where it 'afforded infinite amusement and full employment' especially among German physicians.[100] After the death of Cullen and Brown, the new crop of students joining the Society seemed untouched by the bitter battles. Yet, a guide for medical studies at the University of Edinburgh, published in 1790, still cautioned that 'young men, unacquainted with the extent of knowledge necessary for medical practitioners' could 'often be led astray into intriguing fields of fancy and speculation'.[101] In a reference to Brown, this manual warned newcomers that 'in a political view, no private teacher ought to be preferred to the professor' since 'the gentleman who had attended *eminent teachers* will always be preferred by the judicious part of mankind'.[102]

William Stroude, the Society's historian, characterised this period of time as one of 'mutual bigotry and intolerance between detached parts of a common system'.[103] Gregory was more outspoken, branding the entire episode as 'the most complete and ludicrous specimen of the importance of debates'.[104] The Society's traditional approach to truth had been based on unfettered collective argumentation in an atmosphere of collegiality, reason and moderation. 'These debates might, no doubt, be laughed at by a spectator', recalled the former Brunonian, James Mackintosh, 'but if he could look through the ridiculous exterior, he might see that they led to serious and excellent consequences'. In fact, Mackintosh went so far as to admit that 'such debates were the only public examination in which favour could have no place and which never could degenerate into mere formality; they must always be severe and always just.'[105] When some of the contents of these internal debates were leaked to the Edinburgh press, Society members and their university mentors realised that exposing the public to their theoretical and therapeutic disagreements could be potentially quite harmful to their professional image and the cultural authority. In bringing legal action, the students anticipated Percival's ethical injunctions of professional *esprit du corps* and the argument that disputes should not be communicated to the public at large. Indeed, such disclosures could be personally injurious to individual physicians and could 'hardly fail to hurt the general credit of the faculty'. For Percival, there existed a 'tacit compact not only to submit to the laws but promote the honour and interest of the association so far as they [were] consistent with morality and the general good of mankind'.[106] The Society's proceedings were not to be compared with frequent parliamentary debates reproduced in newspaper accounts, which served to inform the public about Britain's political business. The Edinburgh disclosures appeared to question the very foundation of contemporary medical knowledge – espoused by the local medical school – thus threatening its reputation and by extension, potentially harming student enrolments. Stressing the issue of professional privacy, the student organisation attempted to muzzle the local press and forbade the publication of reports about its proceedings in the *Edinburgh Evening Post.*

In dealing with this crisis, the Society's Cullenian-leaning leadership passed new stringent rules, forbidding its members, under threat of expulsion, from divulging any details of their weekly deliberations. The newspaper's publisher argued vehemently that, in addition to the need for free speech and open disclosure of medical matters, the public was entitled to learn about any and all new medical information that promised to benefit the sick. After protracted negotiations and an accusation that the newspaper reports were libellous, a legal battle ensued, involving the most famous lawyers in Edinburgh working *pro bono* for the Royal Medical Society. Although the case was eventually dismissed, and a number of appeals were rejected, the episode brought into sharp relief the eighteenth-century tensions between professional secrecy and the public's desire to share the theoretical and practical ambiguities of medical knowledge. The events also disclosed the contemporary power of print media to potentially reach broad sectors of the public and influence local culture.[107] Above all, the RMS versus Campbell Denovan case exposed the fragile nature of eighteenth-century medicine's professional authority.

Notes

1. T. Newte, *Prospects and Observations on a Tour in England and Scotland: Natural, Oeconomical and Literary* (London, 1791), 365–6.
2. A valuable source is J. Gray, *History of the Royal Medical Society 1737–1937* (Edinburgh: University Press, 1952).
3. Further information can also be obtained from L. Rosner, 'The Royal Medical Society', in *Medical Education in the Age of Improvement* (Edinburgh: Edinburgh University Press, 1991), 119–34; and T.N. Bonner, *Becoming A Physician: Medical Education in Britain, France, Germany, and the United States, 1750–1945* (New York: Oxford University Press, 1995).
4. J. Gregory, *Memorial to the Managers of the Royal Infirmary* (Edinburgh: Murray and Cochrane, 1800), 209–10.
5. See the presidential address dated 9 November 1751: G. Sutherland, 'A Congratulatory Address to the Medical Society', in *Dissertations Read to the Royal Medical Society, Edinburgh* (*Diss. RMS*) 95 vols (Edinburgh: 1751–1833), MSS Collection, Edinburgh University Library, Vol. 1 (1751), 65–9.
6. L. Haakonssen, *Medicine and Morals in the Enlightenment: John Gregory, Thomas Percival and Benjamin Rush* (Amsterdam: Rodopi, 1997), 46–93.
7. Gregory, *op. cit.* (note 4), 210.
8. J. Christie, 'Edinburgh Medicine in the Eighteenth Century: The View From the Students', *Social Society of the History of Medicine Bulletin,* 19 (1976), 13–15.
9. R.J. Mackintosh (ed.), *Memoirs of the Life of Sir James Mackintosh,* 2nd edn, 2 vols (Boston: Little Brown & Co, 1853), Vol. I, 29–30.
10. 'On Disputing Societies in General, the Pantheon and Medical Society of Edinburgh', *The Weekly Mirror,* No. 22, 16 February 1781, 393–5.
11. [W. Stroude], 'History of the Medical Society of Edinburgh', in *List of Members, Laws, and Library Catalogue of the Medical Society of Edinburgh* (Edinburgh: W. Aitken, 1820), LXXXI.
12. Gregory, *op. cit.* (note 4), 11.
13. For Cullen's system of medicine, see L.S. King, *The Medical World of the Eighteenth Century* (Chicago: University of Chicago Press, 1958), 139–43 and 214–19; Brown's ideas are summarised in G.B. Risse, 'The Brownian

System of Medicine: Its Theoretical and Practical Implications', *Clio Medica,* 5 (1970), 45–51; and an extensive presentation of eighteenth-century medical systems is G.B. Risse, 'Eighteenth-Century Medical Systems', in *The History of John Browns's Medical System in Germany During the Years 1790-1806*, Ph.D. thesis, University of Chicago, 1971, 3–67.

14. Mackintosh, *Memoirs, op. cit.* (note 9), Vol. 1, 25. See also Gray, *History, op. cit.* (note 2), 50–61.
15. Consult the essays in A. Doig *et al.* (eds), *William Cullen and the Eighteenth-Century Medical World* (Edinburgh: Edinburgh University Press, 1993).
16. Gray, *op. cit.* (note 2), 64. See also King, *op. cit.* (note 13), 193–226.
17. Gregory, *op. cit.* (note 4), 21.
18. One of the reasons for this rift was Brown's personal experience with gout after 1771. He followed Cullen's medical advice and started a standard vegetarian diet and 'antiphlogistic' or depleting regimen. However, instead of being rewarded for his efforts, Brown suffered several more incapacitating gouty attacks. Perhaps Cullen's 'cure' had made matters worse. Depressed and frustrated, Brown went on to test this hypothesis and resumed his hearty meals and alcohol drinking. Contrary to prevailing clinical experience, the gout apparently subsided for the next six years.
19. [Stroude], *op. cit.* (note 11), XXX. See also M. Barfoot, 'Brunonians Under the Bed: An Alternative to University Medicine in Edinburgh During the 1800s', in W.F. Bynum and R. Porter (eds), *Brunonianism in Britain and Europe* (London: Wellcome Institute for the History of Medicine, 1988), 22–45.
20. Risse, 'Brownian System', *op. cit.* (note 13), 45–51.
21. See [J. Brown], *The Elements of Medicine of John Brown,* trans. from Latin by the author, 2 vols (London: J. Johnson, 1795).
22. A contemporary judgement by James McKintosh, a prominent Brunonian disciple, summarises the contemporary dilemma: 'In science as in human life, it is impossible to separate excellencies from a tendency to their neighbouring faults. Of a doctrine which derives diseases from increase or diminution of action, the excellence is simplicity and the defect narrowness', *Diss. RMS*, Vol. 20 (1786–7), 214.
23. For background, R.L. Emerson, 'Scottish Universities in the Eighteenth Century, 1690–1800', *Studies on Voltaire and the Eighteenth Century,* 114 (1977), 453–74.
24. R. Porter, 'Spreading Enlightenment: The Popularisation of Medicine in Georgian England and its Paradoxes', in R. Porter (ed.), *The Popularisation of Medicine, 1650–1850* (London: Routledge, 1992), 215–31.
25. W. Cullen Brown, *The Works of Dr John Brown*, III vols (London: J. Johnson, 1804), Vol. II, 129.

26. A. Digby, *Making a Medical Living: Doctors and Patients in the English Market for Medicine, 1720–1911* (Cambridge: Cambridge University Press, 1994).
27. J. Brown, *Elementa Medicinae*, 2 vols (Edinburgh: Denovan, 1780); see G.B. Risse, 'John Brown', in D. von Engelhardt and F. Hartmann (eds), *Klassiker der Medizin*, 2 vols (Munich: C. H. Beck, 1991), Vol. 1, 24–36.
28. [Stroude], *op. cit.* (note 11), LXXXII.
29. Royal Medical Society, Minutes of Meetings, sessions 31 January/10 February 1781, MSS Collection, Royal Medical Society, Edinburgh. Brown apparently returned the money at the 17 February session.
30. Mackintosh, *op. cit.* (note 9), Vol. I, 25.
31. [Stroude], *op. cit.* (note 11), LXXX.
32. See, for example, J.P. Harris, 'What is the Modus Operandi of Opium and in What State of the System May it be Admitted as Useful?', *Diss. RMS,* Vol. 11 (1778), 221–6. Harris presented his essay on 12 December 1778 stressing the sedative and narcotic effects of the drug.
33. J.W. Howell, 'What are the Likeliest Means of Rescuing or at Least Relieving the Art of Medicine from its Present State of Uncertainty and Error?'. *Diss. RMS,* Vol. 12 (1780–1), 59–64. Howell was another important disciple of Brown. He was admitted to the RMS on 19 December 1778.
34. J. Campbell, 'What Objections May be Made to the Doctrine of Morbific Matter?', *Diss. RMS,* Vol. 11 (1778), 37–87. Campbell may have been related to the Campbells of Inverrary. Matriculated at the University since 1775, he became one of Brown's students and a faithful friend forced to seek his medical degree at St Andrew's University where he received his diploma on 17 October 1781. A year later, Brown named his last child in Campbell's honour, but the boy died apparently of whooping cough in 1786.
35. Martyn had been admitted to the Society on 9 December 1780. He apparently never had the opportunity of presenting a paper so that his opinions on the contending medical systems is unknown although there are suggestions that he was a Brunonian sympathiser.
36. The story is told in Gray, *op. cit.* (note 2), 57–8.
37. Gregory, *op. cit.* (note 4), 210.
38. For details consult R.A. Houston, *Social Change in the Age of Enlightenment, Edinburgh 1660–1760* (Oxford: Clarendon Press, 1984).
39. C.D. Leake (ed.), *Percival's Medical Ethics* (Baltimore: Williams & Wilkins, 1927), 142–6.
40. *Weekly Mirror, op. cit.* (note 10), 394, also quoted in D.D. McElroy, *Scotland's Age of Improvement* (Pullman, WA: Washington State University Press, 1969), 134.
41. [Stroude], *op. cit.* (note 11), LXXXI.

42. The session described in the newspaper seems to have taken place on Wednesday, 8 January 1783. Whether this discussion was based on a particular paper remains unclear. The published dissertations for the 1782–3 session do not mention an essay on this topic.
43. 'Pantheon Intelligence', in the *Edinburgh Evening Post*, No. 279, from Saturday, 11 January to Wednesday, 15 January 1783. MSS Collection, Scottish Record Office, Edinburgh. This newspaper had begun publication in May 1780, sponsored by a 'society of independent gentlemen'. Denovan's 1783 Edinburgh address was listed as Turks Close, Lawnmarket. More information can be found in W.J. Couper, *Edinburgh Periodical Press*, 2 vols (Sterling: E. Mackay, 1908), Vol. 2, 159–60. Except for the issues specifically involved in the 1784 lawsuit, no issues of this newspaper could be found in Edinburgh archives and libraries.
44. *Ibid.*
45. Attached to the newspapers is a separate hand-written and undated account of the controversy with the Royal Medical Society (possibly composed by Denovan himself), MSS Collection, Scottish Record Office, Edinburgh, 11–14.
46. *Ibid.*, 15. See also a letter to the editors, published in *Edinburgh Evening Post*, No. 282, 22–5 January 1783.
47. [Denovan], *op. cit.* (note 45), 17–18.
48. G. Maxwell, 'What is the Use of Cold Water in External and Internal Hemorrhages?', *Diss. RMS*, Vol.14 (1782–3), 78–83.
49. [Denovan], *op. cit.* (note 45), 16–17; and *Edinburgh Evening Post*, No. 282, 22–5 January 1783.
50. *Ibid.*, 19–20; and 'Medical Intelligence', in the *Edinburgh Evening Post*, No. 283, 25–9 January 1783,
51. R. Cleghorn, 'What is the Nature and What are the Effects of Sleep?', *Diss. RMS*, Vol. 14 (1782–3), 36–49. The paper was delivered on 11 January 1783. Robert Cleghorn (1755–1821) had been admitted to the RMS on 8 December 1781, and he became a president during the 1783–4 session. A year later, Cleghorn set up practice in Glasgow. For details, see F.A. Macdonald, 'Reading Cleghorn the Clinician: The Clinical Case Records of Dr. Robert Cleghorn, 1785–1818', in C.W.J. Withers and P. Wood (eds), *Science and Medicine in the Scottish Enlightenment* (East Linton, Scotland: Tuckwell Press, 2002), 255–79.
52. Cleghorn, *ibid.*, 48.
53. [Denovan], *op. cit.* (note 45), 21–5; see also 'Medical Intelligence', in *Edinburgh Evening Post*, No. 288, 12–15 February 1783.
54. *Ibid.*, 25–6.
55. *Edinburgh Evening Post*, No. 290, 19–22 February 1783.

56. Engelhart had been admitted to the Society on 1 December 1781. His essays suggest that he was a supporter of Cullen's ideas.
57. Denovan contended that 'we mean to give our countenance to the liberty of our fellow citizens, whether civil, ecclesiastical, or moral, and to encourage every improvement and discovery which to us shall appear beneficial to the country.' See *Edinburgh Evening Post*, No. 290, 19–22 February 1783.
58. *Ibid.*
59. [Denovan], *op. cit.* (note 45), 27–8.
60. R.D. Willis, 'Do the Inquiries After the Modus Operandi of Causes Improve the Practice of Physic?', *Diss. RMS,* Vol. 14 (1782–3), 70–7. Willis had been admitted to the RMS on 15 December 1781.
61. *Ibid.,* 70.
62. *Ibid.*, 77.
63. [Denovan], *op. cit.* (note 45), 29–32.
64. 'Medical Intelligence Extraordinary', in the *Edinburgh Evening Post*, No. 292, 26 February–1 March 1783.
65. *Ibid.*
66. 'Medical Intelligence', *Edinburgh Evening Post*, No 296, 12–15 March 1783.
67. Erskine, the third son of the Earl of Buchan, was a prominent Whigg known for his pro bono work and advocacy of the poor. Robert O. Cullen was a son of William Cullen. He had practised law from 1764 and was appointed Lord of Sessions in 1799.
68. Memorial of Queries for the Royal Medical Society, MSS Scottish Record Office, Edinburgh.
69. *Edinburgh Evening Post*, No. 300, 26–29 March 1783.
70. *Ibid.*
71. Answers to the Memorial of Queries for the Royal Medical Society of Edinburgh, MSS Scottish Record Office, Edinburgh. See also [Denovan], *op. cit.* (note 45), 33–6.
72. *Ibid.*
73. *Edinburgh Evening Post*, No. 308, 23–26 April 1783.
74. *Ibid.*
75. Summons of Declarator and Damages. The Royal Medical Society vs. Campbell Denovan. Against Nos 288, 290, 294, 296, 297, 300, 303, 304, 308 and other numbers of the *Edinburgh Evening Post* under the title 'Medical Intelligence', 7 June 1783. MSS Scottish Record Office, Edinburgh.
76. E. Harrison, 'What are the Agreements and Differences in the Effects of Opium and Alcohol on the Human Body in Health and Disease?', *Diss. RMS,* Vol. 14 (1782–3), 188–211.

77. 'It is lawful for every one to publish an account of the inquiries and debates of a society instituted for the purpose of free inquiry and debate concerning matters of science unless such account be of a libelous nature', and the offending articles 'consist of unmeaning declamation of things altogether unintelligible, and therefore not actionable'. Interlocutor of 15 November 1783, in *The Petition of the Presidents and Other Members of the Medical Society of Edinburgh*, 27 February 1784 (Edinburgh: RMS, 1784), MSS Scottish Record Office, Edinburgh, 5.
78. R. Lubbock, 'How is the Increment of the Human Body Effected?', *Diss. RMS,* Vol. 14 (1782–3), 229–55. Lubbock had been admitted to the RMS on 15 December 1781.
79. H. Ainslie, 'How Shall We Best Preserve Health and Cure Disease?', *Diss. RMS,* Vol. 14 (1782–3), 274–94. Ainslie's admission to the RMS had occurred on 1 December 1781.
80. S. Hinds, 'Has the Investigation of Proximate Causes Benefited the Practice of Medicine?', *Diss. RMS,* Vol. 19 (1785–6), 93–103.
81. Representation of Campbell Denovan about the Interlocutor of 15 November 1783. The Court refused to waive fees on 2 December 1783. MSS Scottish Record Office, Edinburgh.
82. See the 13 February 1784 note: 'Judge Lord Ordinary Hailes will receive no more representations in this cause', MSS Collection, Scottish Record Office, Edinburgh. On 12 February, Denovan had made some representations regarding expenses to alter the interlocutor of 28 January.
83. J. Lawson, 'What are the Effects of the Peruvian Bark', *Diss. RMS,* Vol. 14 (1782–3), 368–83. Both Lawson and Jeffray had been admitted to the RMS on 30 November 1782.
84. Pretyman had been admitted to the RMS on 30 November 1782. His essay was titled 'What is the Indication of Cure in Idiopathic Hemorrhagy?', *Diss. RMS,* Vol. 14 (1782–3), 397–403.
85. J. Jeffray, 'How Far Useful is the Doctrine of Critical Days in the Cure of Diseases?', *Diss. RMS,* Vol. 14 (1782–3), 404–28.
86. Thomas Emmet had been admitted to the RMS on 7 December 1782.
87. *The Petition of the Presidents and Other Members of the Medical Society of Edinburgh*, 27 February 1784, 13. This pamphlet is also in the possession of the Scottish Record Office, Edinburgh.
88. *Ibid.*, 7. The document argued that 'the apprehension that their productions may, without their leave, be instantly conveyed to the public in a newspaper necessarily destroys that freedom and ease so essential to the encouraging of their literary efforts.'
89. *Ibid.*, 13.

90. See 'Answers for Campbell Denovan, printer in Edinburgh, defendant, to the Petition of the Presidents and Other Members of the Medical Society of Edinburgh', 18 June 1784. Scottish Record Office, Edinburgh.
91. Throckmorton was a member of the RMS from 21 December 1782. His paper was titled 'What are the Changes the Blood Undergoes in Diseases?', *Diss. RMS,* Vol. 17 (1783–5), 31–40.
92. W. Spooner, 'What are the Effects of Cold Upon the Human Body?', *Diss. RMS,* Vol. 17 (1783–5), 234–44. He had been elected to the Society on 6 December 1782.
93. G. Bachmetieve, 'What is the Cause of Ordinary Sleep and What is its Use?', *Diss. RMS,* Vol. 17 (1783–5), 306–12. He had been admitted to the RMS on 20 December 1783.
94. W. Alexander, 'To What Cause Can the Production of Hectic Fever be Most Probably Attributed?', *Diss. RMS,* Vol. 17 (1783–5), 261–84. Alexander was a member of the RMS from 13 December 1783 and became a junior president for the 1786–87 session.
95. Goodwyn was elected to the RMS on 16 December 1780. He gave a paper critical of traditional humoralism in 1782 titled 'What are the Effects Arising from Blisters Applied to the Human Body?', *Diss. RMS,* Vol. 12 (1780–1), 463–9.
96. E. Goodwyn, *The Connection of Life with Respiration, or An Experimental Inquiry into the Effects of Submersion, Strangulation and Several Kinds of Noxious Airs* (London: J. Johnson, 1788).
97. J. Mackintosh, 'Case of Tertian Fever', *Diss. RMS,* Vol. 20 (1786–7), 214–5.
98. R. Gray, 'Hysteria', *Diss. RMS,* Vol. 24 (1789–90), 1–22; and W. Belcher, 'Hysteria', *Diss. RMS,* Vol. 25 (1790–1), 229–45.
99. W. Alexander, 'What are the Effects of Opium Upon the Healthy and Diseased Animal', *Diss. RMS,* Vol. 19 (1785–6), 204–46.
100. Gregory, *op. cit.* (note 4), 211; see also G.B. Risse, 'Scottish Medicine on the Continent: John Brown's Medical System in Germany, 1796–1806', in *Proceedings of the XXIII International Congress of the History of Medicine,* 2 vols. (London: Wellcome Institute for the History of Medicine, 1974), Vol. 1, 682–7; N. Tsouyopoulos, 'The Influence of John Brown's Ideas in Germany', in Bynum and Porter, *op. cit.* (note 19), 63–74.
101. [J. Johnson], *A Guide for Gentlemen Studying Medicine at the University of Edinburgh* (London: Robinson, 1790), 2.
102. *Ibid.*, 42.
103. Stroude concluded that 'the ill effects of the Brunonian controversy were transient, while the advantages resulting from its leading principles for nearly a quarter of a century could not fail to be considerable.' [Stroude], *op. cit.* (note 11), LXXXI-II. Among well-known students with Brunonian leanings

were William H. Yates, member of the RMS from 19 December 1789, who went to practice in India and wrote *A View of the Science of Life* in 1797, and Alexander P. Wilson, an experimentalist and president of the 1792–3 session. An informal count reveals at least twenty-five prominent Brunonian disciples elected members of the RMS between 1778 and 1792, with fourteen of them (56%) obtaining MD degrees from Scottish universities. This statistic dispels notions that their studies were seriously jeopardised because they adopted John Brown's ideas.

104. Gregory, *op. cit.* (note 4), 211.
105. Mackintosh, *op. cit.* (note 9), Vol. 1, 26.
106. Leake, *op. cit.* (note 39), 104–5.
107. See H.M. Dingwall, 'To be Insert in the *Mercury*: Medical Practitioners and the Press in Eighteenth-Century Edinburgh', *Social History of Medicine,* 13 (2000), 23–44. For more on this topic, J. Barry, 'The Press and the Politics of Culture in Bristol, 1660–1775', in J. Black and J. Gregory (eds), *Culture, Politics and Society in Britain, 1660–1800* (Manchester: Manchester University Press, 1991), 49–81.

PART II:
HEALTH AND DISEASE

4

In the Name of Hygieia and Hippocrates: A Quest for the Preservation of Health and Virtue

Besides random self-help, medicine considered health preservation among its loftiest goals since Antiquity. Body, mind and environment appeared inextricably linked. Lifestyle advice, formulated within the Galenic framework of the 'six non-natural things', included air, food and drink, sleep and wakefulness, exercise, bodily evacuations, and emotions. Such pursuits were ideally suited to the social realities of the Enlightenment. This inquiry reveals the recommendations made by a prominent Scottish physician, William Cullen, to improve the health of his patients. The information is based on unpublished essays and consultation letters, focusing on his clients' constitution and temperament, climate and seasons, lodgings, diet and bodily functions, as well as emotional states.

Introduction

> The care of health, of the fortune, of the rank and reputation of the individual, the objects which his comfort and happiness in this life are supposed principally to depend, is considered as the proper business of that virtue which is commonly called Prudence.
>
> Adam Smith (1790)[1]

In a letter dated 10 February 1777, the prominent Scottish physician William Cullen (1710–90) sought to address the concerns of Robert Ligerwood, Esq., who was seeking his advice by post for 'debility'. Nothing is known about the patient's original consultation, but Cullen's frank response concentrated on a series of lifestyle issues designed to restore strength and preserve health. After telling his correspondent that he had got 'into a very relaxed state of nerves', the doctor chided him for eating a rich diet and drinking an entire bottle of claret every day after dinner. 'I readily believe that chocolate may be too heavy a breakfast', Cullen continued, suggesting that he take up cold bathing and 'going on horseback as often as weather allows'. 'You have been much hurt, I am persuaded, by venery', he concluded, 'but you do not say how you are going to guard against it now.'[2] The exchange exemplified Cullen's role as 'hygienist', a label applied to most contemporary physicians who, in addition of prescribing remedies, also counselled their patients about living healthier lives.

For Cullen and other Enlightenment physicians, health was not just the achievement of a particular bodily state, but a quest for a new philosophy of life. 'The art of health like the art of moral prudence should be known to all mankind who have a daily and hourly occasion for the use of it,' Cullen wrote, insisting that such knowledge resulted from 'the general experience of mankind'. Cullen's basic views on a natural, healthy life were described in an unpublished text 'An Essay on the Preservation of Health'. The manuscript can be dated to the early 1780s[3] and was cited by his disciple, the famous American physician Benjamin Rush (1745–1813) in a letter to Cullen dated 22 December 1784.[4] Another unpublished tract on the subject of health preservation and its linkage to a condition called 'hypochondriasis' (Chapter 9) contains further detailed suggestions.[5] Both original documents and excerpts from Cullen's voluminous medical correspondence conducted as part of a private consultation practice while living in Edinburgh between 1755 and 1790 constitute the basis for this study.[6]

Managing the 'non-naturals: a perspective

In human experience, body, mind, and environment are inextricably linked. Medicine has long included within its boundaries habitat and life-style factors considered influential in maintaining individual health or personal 'hygiene'. Many of the Hippocratic treatises, notably *Airs, Waters, and Places,* provided prescriptions for healthy living. Even the ancient cult of Asclepius, the god of healing, increasingly developed the divine role of his daughter Hygieia – protector of health and prosperity – in an attempt to expand the worship and make it more approachable to women and healthy supplicants.[7] Against the backdrop of a speculative humoralism that defined health as an ideal harmony of bodily fluids influenced by environmental factors, Galen's lifestyle medicine identified six 'non-natural things' capable of affecting the regular balance.[8] These included air, linked to concerns about environmental purity or pollution, sleep and wakefulness, and exercise or bodily movements, including bathing and massage. In addition, there was the issue of bodily intake and output centred on diet and proper discharge of wastes, and finally control of the mind and its passions.[9] Since Antiquity, physicians relied on these 'non-naturals' to inform their recommendations on health maintenance. The information was directed to their primary clients, elite patients from the upper ranks of society who had the literacy, leisure and fortune to follow this advice.[10]

During the Renaissance, life-style became linked with Christianity. In a popular treatise written by the octogenarian physician Luigi Cornaro (*ca.* 1467–1566) of Venice, moral virtue, and longevity were exalted against the horrors of intemperance and premature death. Entitled *A Treatise About a Sober Life* (1558), this work was translated into many languages and reprinted even up to the twentieth century.[11] Like today, preoccupation with one's own physical wellbeing provided an inner-directed outlook in a period of rapid political and social change. For Cornaro and his followers, the best medicine was a temperate and orderly life, to be achieved by simple living in accordance with nature. In fact, Cornaro insisted that man could 'have no better doctor than himself and no better medicine than the temperate life.'[12] Like many physicians in previous eras, Cornaro promoted living in ventilated places, eating and drinking in moderation and getting enough sleep. He also warned against excessive exposure to wind and sun. Cornaro recommended that urban dwellers travel to the countryside during spring and autumn, where they were told to walk or ride horses and contemplate the beauty of nature. For wealthy individuals who had the means to shape their own quality of life, old age was purportedly a coveted time of life without sickness, ultimately ending with a peaceful and natural death. Essentially, Cornaro promoted an idyllic life, orderly and virtuous, which contributed not only to a better understanding and enjoyment of God's wisdom and divine goodness but would ensure eternal life.[13]

Based on its classical roots, the doctrine of the six non-naturals was ideally suited to the intellectual climate as well as the social realities of eighteenth-century Enlightenment, including the growing commercialisation of health.[14] During this time, health and physical wellbeing became framed as civic duty and key instrument of political power (Chapter 1).[15] Discipline and control of the human body became antidotes against the temptations of sloth and luxury. The rewards of personal responsibility were extolled. Buffeted by the effects of a demographic explosion, and living in a climate of profound social and political changes, individuals strived towards retaining a measure of power and control over their own bodies and personal lives. This mood was fuelled by increased anxiety about the prospects of ageing and dying. A decline in religious comforts made self-improvement the primary coping mechanism. For this reason, all literate sectors of society sought to acquire an elementary body of knowledge about what constituted a healthy environment and proper nourishment.[16]

Thanks to the Cartesian conception of the body as machine, physicians came to be viewed as mechanics capable of keeping all parts of the human apparatus in working order. Health maintenance was viewed as an eminently achievable strategy; indeed, it was often represented as a moral duty. The task was made more urgent, as prominent physicians such as Britain's George

Cheyne (1671–1743) painted a vivid picture of a population in declining health: 'with the world's decay, vicious souls and putrefied bodies have in this age arrived to their highest and most exalted degrees.'[17] Mankind had originally been healthy and sound, he opined, but personal high living and environment now seemed to be corrupting the bodily solids and juices, burdening the present and subsequent generations with higher incidences of disease. Under such circumstances, Cheyne preached, 'he who wantonly transgresseth the self-evident rules of health is guilty of a degree of selfmurder.'[18]

Cheyne further discussed what Continental Europeans pejoratively identified as the 'English Malady,' a protean 'nervous' disorder enfeebling civilised Britons of the 'better sort'. While engaged in sedentary occupations, affluent people lived in ever-growing large, polluted, and unhealthy cities such as London and Edinburgh known for their moist air and variable weather.[19] The 'wasting' condition reflected excessive use of food, drink, and sexual intercourse. In an ironic twist of fate, prosperous consumers were being devoured by a condition broadly categorised as 'consumption' (Chapter 7).[20] Based on his own recurring obesity and health problems – caused by gluttony, alcohol and inactivity – Cheyne set out to convince readers of the importance of sobriety and physical exertion: 'It will be eternally true… that only Temperance and Abstinence, Air, Exercise, Diet, and proper Evacuations can preserve Life, Health and Gayety.'[21]

Cheyne's dietary and lifestyle recommendations were based on current iatromechanical notions of bodily functioning. Faced with the temptations of opulence, his contemporaries had failed in the quest to follow the traditional 'Rule of Celsus' which suggested moderation and individual responsibility. Instead, in an increasingly more complex and civilised world, Cheyne wished to seize the initiative and come to their assistance, particularly since as a past victim of similar excesses, he now considered himself an authority. Expertise was asserted by combining scientific medical knowledge with his credentials as a wounded healer; his counsel was based on rhetoric of common sense and personal virtue.[22] Thus, the new medical strategies of health preservation became private 'hygiene'; an individualised approach based on personal initiative, knowledge, determination, and experience. The term hygiene, literally 'health' in Greek, echoed Galen's classical division of medicine into hygiene and therapeutics. For example, writing for the influential *Encyclopédie*, one author suggested the term hygiene 'serves to designate the first of the two parts of medical methods concerning the conduct necessary to follow for the conservation of health'.[23]

Indeed, it seemed easier to sustain health than to recover it, a concept already forcefully expressed by Cheyne and others. The greatest danger was, of course, apathy. Those who felt fine 'at the peak of their powers' seldom sought advice about how to stay fit until it was too late to do something about it, usually in old age. The familiar calculus of living shorter but 'voluptuous' and 'unthinking' lives, rather than longer and more boring existences, made sense to many. Those interested in adjusting their lifestyles, however, needed to be properly indoctrinated in the rules of healthy living. For this purpose, a comprehensive system of hygiene had to be constructed and shared with the public at large. A number of publications ranging from advertisements and pamphlets to manuals and books gradually disseminated basic health-related information.[24] Cheyne's goal expressed in his 1725 work *An Essay on Health and Long Life*, was to instruct the reader 'in the best manner... to preserve his health and lengthen out his life'.[25] The Scottish physician and poet John Armstrong (1709–79) expressed similar sentiments in a popular poem entitled *The Art of Preserving Health* originally published in 1744.[26] How far life could be extended was another matter. 'Let us by a virtuous course of life and the practice of such rules as the experience of the ages has established, endeavour to preserve health of the body and soundness of mind', wrote James Mackenzie (1680–1761), 'until we arrive at the boundaries which Providence seems to have nearly marked out for our respective constitutions.'[27]

The commodification of health within the framework of Britain's eighteenth-century consumer society took place foremost among the upper and 'middling' layers of society.[28] 'Health is so important a blessing that people are entitled to the best information they can get concerning it,' wrote the English physician John Leake (1729–92).[29] Amidst new forms of advertising and marketing, medicine rediscovered an ancient niche: a role for the physician as consultant and educator, ready to teach rules for keeping healthy as well as point out the dangers of certain detrimental living habits. This medical hygiene was part of a traditional professional and social identity that ranged from friend and advisor to therapist.[30] Thus the physician's role as hygienist came to buttress his growing professional power.[31] But this function also had its detractors. Discussing personal hygiene, the German physician, Friedrich Hoffmann (1660–1742) proclaimed that 'to live in a medical fashion, that is according to the strict and academic rules of the physicians, is to live miserably and uncomfortably'.[32] In his view, commitment to 'an overtly precise mode of living' under rigid rules would become oppressive.

Paradoxically, the opulent sector of society was portrayed as being in great need of sound medical advice, not because its members were able to pay for the information but because of their notoriously erratic and injurious lifestyles. Echoing Cheyne, later authors such as Thomas Beddoes

(1760–1808) – an Edinburgh graduate – asserted that 'the unhealthiness of families' was 'in inverse proportion to their wealth'.[33] Blaming luxurious living for ailments such as pulmonary consumption, hysteria and hypochondriasis, gout, as well as female troubles became a favourite strategy for eighteenth-century practitioners (Chapters 7, 8 and 9). Beddoes went so far as to declare that he had specifically written his book *Hygeia* for the 'middling and affluent' classes. In his view this sector of the population had the 'leisure for study, necessary degree of intelligence and the means of carrying good counsel fully into effect'.[34]

Given the uncertainties of contemporary professional knowledge and competence, eighteenth-century physicians operated in an ever-expanding medical marketplace in which eclectic consumers usually played the dominant role.[35] Health-related advice was eagerly sought from a broad array of sources that included family and friends, popular books, magazines and pamphlets, folk and religious healers, irregulars, apothecaries, surgeons and physicians.[36] In the matter of wellness, distrust and suspicion prevailed over the intentions of medical professionals. Patients who summoned healers to their homes or sought written advice usually obtained more than one opinion. In the *Encyclopédie,* its medical author had already complained that 'with regard to rules of health, they appear to have been totally neglected by the masters who have developed medicine'. He admitted that,

> 'the majority of physicians today do not commit themselves to the service of medicine but use medicine to their own ends, since they apply themselves little to the study and prescription of those rules which are necessary to observe for the conservation of health.[37]

Were physicians simply neglecting to provide or deliberately withholding health-related information?

Specificity was one of the hallmarks of professional identity. Indeed, who was more suited than a medical person to know and explain the dynamics between the environment and the forces operating within the human body and mind? Moreover, who could provide specific advice carefully tailored to a particular person by taking into consideration constitutional factors, gender, family background, occupation, climate and lifestyle? 'Seasonable care, urged Beddoes, 'should be taken to provide each individual with a set of ideas, exhibiting the precise relation in which his system and the several organs of which it is compounded stand with external agents, particularly to those with which he is likely to come most in contact.'[38] Mastery over this knowledge provided physicians with additional moral legitimacy as well as economic advantage and social status – all-important goals for British practitioners who were dependent on the patronage of the wealthy.[39] Wrote Leake:

> Valetudinarians would therefore act a friendly part to themselves in supporting a physician as much entitled to reasonable gain for laying down rules towards the preservation of health as he who should prescribe medicines with a view to restore it.[40]

The 'common sense of mankind': William Cullen, 'hygienist'

Within this milieu of the Enlightenment views on health, the prominent Scottish physician William Cullen (1710–90) emerged as a mentor for his aristocratic and middling patients. Cullen was famous as an academic physician, medical systematist, and superb clinician. His role as 'hygienist', intimately linked to his efforts to battle disease, has never received much attention from historians.[41] Yet in offering advice to the healthy and the sick, Cullen and other eighteenth-century physicians always focused on their clients' bodily constitution and temperament within the context of social and environmental conditions. These included lodging, diet, and changes in bodily functions at different ages, seasons and climates.[42] Cullen's health views and management of the 'non naturals' were expressed in an important work, his 'Essay on the Preservation of Health' that can be dated to the early 1780s. This manuscript consists of an introduction and two separate sections. The first presents an overview of the 'animal economy' based on Cullen's physiological ideas; while the second on health preservation examines the several powers acting on the body. Unfortunately, Cullen apparently never developed this second part beyond one chapter concerned with the qualities and effects of air but worked on an alphabetical index for the planned work that stretched from ale and billiards to winter and youth. Cullen's views on health were also reflected in another tract, composed in the form of a letter to a private client.[43] Although both, the 'Essay' and the letter were never published, many of their detailed suggestions appeared in the voluminous medical correspondence Cullen conducted as part of a private consultation practice while he lived in Edinburgh between 1755 and 1790.[44] His numerous opinions emerged from his extensive clinical experience as well as his personal philosophy and lifestyle.[45]

Cullen belonged to a generation of Edinburgh literati that included David Hume (1711–76), Adam Smith (1723–90), Thomas Reid (1710–96), and his colleague John Gregory (1725–73).[46] Within a climate of moderate Presbyterianism, these individuals confronted the perils of an increasingly commercialised world that threatened to destroy traditional values. As a result, they sought to establish the foundations for a new moral society. The aims of this ideology of 'improvement' were political, intellectual, economic, and social. At its core was the ideal of a rational, sensitive and virtuous man operating within a cohesive community. A widely accepted ethic of virtuous personal conduct, promoted by contemporary Scottish philosophers, stressed self-control and physical as well as mental balance, a pursuit by which human moral development was to be supplemented.[47] In his *Theory of Moral Sentiments*, Cullen's old friend Adam Smith declared that 'the preservation and healthful state of the body seem to be the objects, which Nature first recommends to the care of every individual.'[48] Anxious not to squander his endowed advantages, Smith's 'prudent man' was told not to expose his health to known hazards and to be guided in his lifestyle choices by following the trustworthy 'voice of nature'. Smith depicted health preservation as a critical component of private virtue based on the tenets of Christianised Stoicism. Such conduct was considered a personal quest and moral responsibility. Wrote Smith: 'every man, as the Stoics used to say, is first and principally recommended to his own care, and every man is certainly, in every respect, fitter and abler to take care of himself than any other person.'[49]

Cullen was ideally positioned to play an influential health advisory role. Given his broad clinical experiences and medical reputation in Europe and America, 'I have fancied that there was room for my labour upon it', he admitted in his 'Essay'.[50] Cullen's experiences as a widely travelled ship surgeon, apothecary's apprentice, town magistrate, general practitioner and hospital attendant had provided a wealth of opportunities to deal with individuals from all walks of life. He shared his patients' ethics, language and culture. Eighteenth-century practitioners relied more on their social rather than medical skills to prosper. They embedded themselves into networks of influence and patronage to build their lucrative private practices.[51] In Cullen's case, honours such as Physician to His Majesty in Scotland, President of the Royal College of Physicians of Edinburgh, and Fellow of the Royal Medical Society of London provided sufficient professional *gravitas* and authority. Already a much sought-after medical consultant, Cullen led by example. His friendly and discreet manner impressed even the most fickle and demanding clients, many of them living in Edinburgh, a centre of affluence, culture and conspicuous consumption. He insisted that health information 'should be readily acquired by every person of observation and reflection'.[52] Cullen was aware that an ideal lifestyle based on Enlightenment values appealed primarily to members of the polite and affluent classes who possessed sufficient education, resources, and leisure to learn and follow the principles of personal hygiene.[53] Among his patrons were military officers, merchants, housewives – as well as 'gentlemen' and local aristocrats 'relieved from servile labour or very assiduous employment'.[54]

By contrast, Cullen conceded that 'the greater part of mankind' was 'doomed to constant labour'. By their own circumstances, workers were less capable of that study and reflection necessary to learn the principles of healthy living. But labour and the simple life were considered healthy: 'Happily their manner of life and even their very hardships are the best means for preserving their health', Cullen asserted (Chapters 7 and 8).[55] Much as been written recently about the professional medical ethos of Cullen's time. His academic colleague, John Gregory (1724–73), portrayed the ideal Enlightenment physician as being well-born and 'genteelly' educated, a person of 'liberal and ingenuous manners' as well as humanity.[56] Gregory's practitioner was conceived as possessing sensibility and sympathy to engage with his patients and build trusting relationships. 'Sympathy produces an anxious attention to a thousand little circumstances that may tend to relieve a patient,' he wrote, adding that it 'naturally engages the affection and confidence of a patient, which, in many cases is of the utmost consequence to his recovery.'[57]

Cullen attempted to tutor his clients regarding the rules for keeping healthy within a similar ethical and sympathetic framework. This regimen included climate changes, dietary recommendations for food and drink, sexual moderation, exercise, and mental stimulation. There were always 'inequalities of constitution' and 'manners of life' that could not be placed into a single and uniform straightjacket of health rules. Responding to Hoffman's critique of strict medical guidelines, Cullen admitted that 'a study of the due measure may be useful' because 'there may be a variety in the situations of persons which the duties of life may require, but which may be rashly pushed further than necessary.'[58] For Cullen, therefore, medicine's contribution to the search for good health was clear. Preserving it was an important part of the healing art because it would lead to the prevention of disease.[59] Thus, cast in a decidedly medical fashion as opposites, health and disease needed to be understood as dynamic bodily and mental states, their boundaries subject to shifts that demanded constant vigilance.

All health preservation efforts were based on basic medical knowledge regarding the essential dynamics of bodily functioning. While prudence suggested that all persons should avail themselves of this vital information, it was clear that only a few individuals possessed the necessary knowledge, skill, and discernment to practice the art of health on their own.[60] For Cullen, the laws of the animal economy together with knowledge of bodily structures and functions were 'part of the system of physic and therefore only known to persons who have studied it'.[61] In 1780, Cullen admitted to one of his private patients 'as I cannot teach you physic it is not very easy for me to obviate all your doubts.'[62] However, Cullen promised assistance to those persons who were genuinely interested in health-related matters even when they feared that understanding such basic medical knowledge was beyond their capacities for 'laborious research.' 'We cannot possibly render the knowledge of our subject satisfying or useful', he wrote, 'without giving the reason of the several opinions or advice we are to deliver.' In fact, Cullen urged his patients to examine the rationality of his general principles and judge for themselves the propriety of his doctrines.[63]

But there was a downside to the acquisition of rudimentary health-related knowledge. Referring to previous concerns, Cullen warned about obsessive pursuits of health that could transform his clients into 'frivolous, unsociable, contemptible and selfish' persons. Studying physic was instructive for understanding the underpinnings of a healthy life but also 'apt to fill the mind with many learned but often groundless fears and apprehensions'.[64] 'In the present age where writing is so easy and so much encouraged, there is a great ground for suspecting facts which the vanity of making a book or the interest of vending one give occasion to,' Cullen cautioned.[65] Armed with a smattering of information, some individuals already endowed with a 'melancholic' temperament were believed to be in danger of 'sinking' into what was then categorised as 'hypochondriasis' – a morbid condition of perennial anxiety and fear of illness and death.[66] Women, for their part, were susceptible to symptoms of 'hysteria' (Chapter 9).

Like others before him, Cullen was aware that many practitioners expressed little interest in the art of health, since their 'profits arise chiefly from curing diseases'.[67] While some physicians appeared reluctant to enter the business of lifestyle management, health advice became an opportunity for many to claim professional control over domestic practices and self-help attempts, thus contributing to the Enlightenment's medicalisation process.[68] Cullen tried to position himself within the tradition of eminent past physicians who had taken time to teach the art of preserving health and preventing diseases. At the same time, he was aware of the danger of sharing too much medical knowledge with laypersons, a double-edged sword that could either enhance but also discourage the business of doctors. Cullen admitted that 'it is possible that the gentlemen of my profession may allege that I am endeavouring to give a great part of the system of physic to all men promiscuously.' This would produce 'a set of smatterers in physic who may presume upon their imperfect and incomplete knowledge to prescribe for themselves and others.'[69] Moreover, Cullen understood the power and control exercised by his private patients whose prejudices, circumstances, and behaviour could clash with even the best-intentioned medical advice.[70] He complained about persons' 'utmost impertinence to dispute with physicians and turn aside their best advice'. To avoid such an outcome, Cullen planned to provide only 'general views as necessary for the conduct of health' without going into greater detail. He tried to stress the need for practitioners to tailor the rules of healthy behaviour, adjusting them to fit a client's basic endowments or 'peculiarities' of constitution and temperament.[71]

While much of Cullen's health information was based on traditional, common sense conduct transmitted orally for centuries – if not millennia – he nevertheless carefully framed and dispensed the advice according to rationales derived from his own medical theories. Another source was his personal health regimen. Like Cheyne before him, Cullen occasionally reminded readers of his status – he apparently suffered from chronic gout and turned vegetarian. Both the traditional and personal aspects were essential for legitimising his expertise, thus persuading clients through the employment of a rhetoric that combined scientific and polite language.[72] To explain the workings of the body, Cullen presented a vitalistic physiology that tried to re-interpret bodily events as mechanical and chemical actions performed under the direction of the nervous system. The fundamental premise was that thanks to nerves, the human body was capable of interacting with the physical and social environment. The body's basic solids, the fibres, were elastic and flexible, endowed with sensibility and motion. Brain, soul and the body were interconnected.[73] Oddly, Cullen insisted that the ancient doctrines grounded in classical humoralism 'should be entirely deserted' in favour of a new scheme focused on the state of the 'moving powers'. Yet, most of Cullen's culturally constructed human body remained centred on the fluid balances of a 'porous' organism, perhaps in deference to traditional notions still guiding the health practices of his potential eighteenth-century clientele.

In Cullen's time, sensibility had become a key physiological concept. Defined as an essential property of the nervous system, it was described as the ability of perceiving and responding to sensory impressions. Since nerve transmissions were considered to occur through vibrations of an ethereal fluid, the quality of such perceptions was in part dependent upon the state of the nervous fibres. In Cullen's system, there was a nerve-mediated 'sympathy', or dynamic between the various organ systems that insured the integrity of the human body. Concepts such as sensibility and sympathy, moreover, played important roles in the establishment of Scotland's 'common-sense' philosophy and social intercourse. Natural sensibility was considered a mark of civilised social life, capable of enhancement and refinement that allowed individuals to sharpen their perceptions and feelings.[74]

As the body gradually matured, its solid parts became increasingly denser but decreased in mobility. The peak of life and greatest strength and sensibility occurred around the age of thirty-five, gradually declining toward the fifties and further until the solids became too rigid for sustaining vital functions due to vascular obstructions and impaired blood circulation.[75] Thus, age and sex were key factors to consider when providing advice. Many of Cullen's clients were affluent and ageing individuals who were told they faced a natural and inexorable process of deterioration of their bodily frames that could only be slowed down and made more comfortable through significant changes in lifestyle. 'If the body begins to decline or is already affected with any clinical disease, I think it is then advisable and even necessary to fall into a regimen and a strict manner of life and to be very obstinate in keeping it', counselled Cullen.[76]

While Cullen's health advice seemed to be primarily directed at males, he nevertheless also dealt briefly with gender differences. Like many other contemporary medical authors, Cullen suggested that the majority of women were endowed with softer, lax bodily solids, delicate and elastic nerves, as well as a fuller arterial system and a nervous power endowed with greater sensibility expressed by a 'changeable temper'. In his view, the exquisite female temperament 'suits them to the haemorrhages to which nature has intended'; these menses properly occurred because of arterial plethora. The result was a more delicate yet equally feeble female constitution in even greater need of health advice and maintenance (Chapters 8 and 9).[77] Reflecting widespread contemporary views about female vulnerability, John Leake confirmed Cullen's concerns. 'Were women as attentive to the inestimable blessings of health as the capricious extremes of novelty and fashion, it would be fortunate for themselves and their offspring', he wrote.[78] Leake tried to enlist female vanity to achieve compliance with his hygienic rhetoric. 'The great secret of improving beauty consists in the art of preserving health', he declared, because it 'animates and lights up the countenance with expressive smiles, which touches the lip with vermilion and diffuses over the cheeks a freshness and vivid glow surpassing Circassian bloom.'[79]

Airs, waters, and places

Cullen offered unique health advice. Like other contemporary physicians, he preferred to conceive Galen's 'non-natural things' as powers acting on the human body and thus potential causes for disease.[80] For example, Cullen suggested to his patients that they become more aware of the linkages between climate and health. Within traditional humoralism, air was not only essential for life but it affected human bodies by its changing qualities of heat, cold, dryness, and moistness. In the new mechanical physiology, air gravity and elasticity played additional important roles, helping to compress the human body by keeping the fibres tight and fit. To Cullen, this action preserved the balance between the solids and fluids and assisted in respiratory mechanics. In his new bodily paradigm, solid fibres were governed by the central nervous system, with heat contributing to the relaxation of the solids by increasing their elasticity.[81] Daytime air was warm and dry, which weakened and relaxed bodily fibres and promoted perspiration; at nightime, however, cold and moist air made the body sluggish and heavy. Direct exposure to the sun was to be avoided when temperatures in the shade were above sixty-four degrees Fahrenheit. Too much heat was problematic. People were believed to be healthier and more active in colder climates.

Air movement in the form of winds was particularly important for shaping the weather, depending on the time of day, season, and geographical location. Cullen discussed the seasonal variations experienced in Scotland and the rest of Western Europe and the vicissitudes of heat and cold on the human constitution, humoral mix and nervous energy.[82] Country air was deemed quite healthy, especially during summers and thus therapeutic for incipient cases of phthisis (Chapter 7). The exception were localised sea marshes where putrefying vegetable or animal matter could produce vapours or 'miasma' responsible for 'ague', a crippling periodic fever (Chapter 5).[83]

For Cullen, pure mountain air possessed a beneficial cleansing action. Sea breezes were equally desirable, often leading to recommendations for sailing.[84] In a letter to a colleague dated 13 April 1779, Cullen observed that,

> the air on the coast of Fife is as pure as can be but when the wind sets in from the Northeast as it does in April and May, the air is very bleak. I advise [her] to go to some distance from the seacoast. She will probably be better off passing June in the Highlands.[85]

On other occasions, Scotland's dampness and moisture triggered this injunction: 'set off for some of the southern parts of Europe to pass the winter there.'[86] Because of its western exposure to the Atlantic Ocean and cooler summers, Cullen considered France the most healthy country in Europe.[87] This was particularly true for individuals with propensities for gout.[88] While country air was beneficial, the air in towns was dangerous, filled with smoke billowing from hundreds of chimneys – Edinburgh was later known as 'Auld Reekie' – and with stench emanating from countless latrines, dunghills, stables, slaughterhouses, cemeteries, and other receptacles of putrefaction. In Cullen's view, paved streets prevented the health-bringing perspiration from the earth.

Indoor air, preferred by people of fashion, was also hazardous, polluted by the constant smoke from fireplaces, burning candles, and cigars.[89] Smoking tobacco was to be avoided; excessive heat was similarly undesirable in the home environment. Cullen recommended that bedchambers be kept at forty-five to fifty degrees, never over sixty-four degrees fahrenheit. 'Persons living very constantly in heated chambers will even be relaxed and weakened more than persons exposed frequently to cooler air', he declared.[90] Thus, it was important to get out of bed every morning and expose oneself naked to a source of cold air, a ritual that would provide all the benefits of cold bathing and increase the tone of the entire bodily system.[91] Always attentive to climatic conditions in Scotland, Cullen emphasised the importance of wearing woollen clothing to dispel dampness and moisture. He was also partial to flannel nightshirts because they could absorb sweat. Legs and feet had to be kept warm and dry by wearing worsted understockings and thick shoes.[92]

Standards of health: sleep and exercise

Sleep and wakefulness suggested to Cullen that the animal spirits were 'alternatively exhausted and recruited' during the diurnal cycle.[93] He seemed to possess a clear understanding of our biological clock when making suggestions about the amount of sleep needed, proposing an average of six to eight hours for keeping the body strong and healthy.[94] When bodily perspiration decreased in the evening, it was time to sleep. Retiring to spacious and well-ventilated bedrooms, individuals were told to lay on their sides with limbs slightly bent, the body well covered but not oppressed by heavy bed clothing, their minds at ease. Elderly persons of dry constitutions benefited from a good deal of sleep, allowing their spirits to hopefully reconstitute and readily flow on first awakening. Sleeplessness dried and wasted the body, while excessive rest relaxed the fibres and dulled the mind. To keep this nervous energy in motion, Cullen suggested that his patients should immediately get up upon awakening, and move about. 'Late hours and lying in bed in the morning are very hurtful to weak nerves', wrote Cullen to a Mrs Wallis in April 1782, adding that 'she must do more for herself by proper regimen than can be done by medicine'.[95]

Exercise was judged absolutely necessary and deemed the best health prevention. In fact, for Cullen, both the human frame and mind were made for action. Here again, he skilfully combined views concerning bodily humoral balances with nervous harmony. Exercise provided agility and vigour to the body's solids, promoted blood circulation, digestion, and secretions, especially perspiration, while stimulating the spirits and rendering the mind cheerful. For its part, indolence rendered the mind 'peevish, splenetic and unhappy'.[96] For physical success, Cullen insisted exercise be moderate, continued until a glowing warmth came over the whole body and the person broke out in a sweat, but avoiding overheating and fatigue. Regular exercise could be achieved by walking 'briskly' or dancing, even playing golf. While strengthening the limbs, arms and chest, the latter also had the advantage of being played in open fields. Cullen similarly found swimming in cold water a healthy summer endeavour, coupled with ice skating during winters. In a letter to the Earl of Mornay, Cullen used the patient's presumed 'relaxed' state of nerves to observe that 'my Lord is so very unable and little disposed to exert himself – our machine must go far wrong if it is allowed to stand still. I wish my Lord would stir a little more than he does.'[97]

Tennis and fencing were considered delightful but too strenuous for older folks.[98] Cullen's favourite exercise for elderly persons who could afford it was horseback riding, ideally on days without rain and wind and during mornings and forenoon or about four to five hours following dinner during afternoons. The indoor alternative was swinging on a rope, or using a 'chamber horse' or exercise machine.[99] Riding opened the chest and strengthened respiration; it sharpened appetite, assisted the digestion, and promoted perspiration without totally exhausting the body. Cullen observed that 'riding straight out for some miles is much better than a circuit in the same air as the change of scene and air will recreate the spirits.'[100] The proper riding season in Scotland was between 1 April and 1 November. The next best thing was sailing or riding in an open carriage. To compensate for the diminished physical involvement, Cullen insisted that, in proper weather, his clients travel virtually all day, alternating horseback with carriage – riding in successive stages and finishing their excursions before dinner.[101] In fact, on 15 July 1760 a seemingly exhausted Adam Smith wrote to Lord Shelburne following a partial recovery from a three-week long and recurrent cold. According to Smith, Cullen, his physician, 'thought it his duty to inform me plainly that if I had any hope of surviving next winter I must ride at least five hundred miles before the beginning of September.'[102]

As a supplement to exercise, cold bathing and massage were considered powerful stimulants of nerves and muscles that invigorated the bodily system by conveying physical strength and stamina. 'For strengthening, there is nothing more effectual than cold bathing with a handful or two of salt into the water before using it', wrote Cullen to Lord Gardenstone in 1777.[103] Routine bathing was advised to begin with two-month old infants, employing a washtub in the bedchamber.[104] As evidenced in one of his consultations, his bathing instructions could be quite detailed.[105] Nearby spa towns like Scarborough and Moffat could be visited with benefit. They were traditionally considered watering-holes for affluent invalids and hypochondriacs.[106] Writing to another female patient whose nervous system and soft muscular fibres were said to be extremely delicate from an early period of life, Cullen suggested she try the curative effects of the baths at Harrogate in Yorkshire and those of Buxton in Derbyshire.[107] Bath was another popular destination for Cullen's patients.[108] Responding to inquiries from France and the West Indies, Cullen even recommended swimming in the sea. For those interested in travelling to various contemporary European spas, he wrote a twelve-page letter in September 1784 discussing their water temperatures and chemical compositions.[109] In addition, massage was to be performed with a flannel cloth or 'flesh brush', gently rubbing the body each morning but especially after evening baths for about fifteen minutes.[110]

Diet and bodily discharges

The body's incorporation of food and drink and its natural evacuations represented another key interaction with the environment. Diet – from the Greek *diaita* – originally represented a person's manner of living, including food and drink, dress, maintenance, board and lodging. Cullen was aware that prevailing British culture believed that consumption of hearty and abundant food and drink conveyed the needed energy and stimulus to all bodily systems. However, as the extremely obese Cheyne had previously pointed out, this invigorating 'cult' of roast beef and alcoholic beverages was proving to be a growing liability. Stomach, liver and bowel disorders were ubiquitous. Food and drink in moderation and variety became part of the new chant for staying healthy. Physicians insisted that foodstuffs needed to be considered within the total physical and social environment of an individual. For Cullen, therefore, dietary management became a cardinal aspect of health preservation, adjusted to ease digestion and promote perspiration.[111] In a 1787 letter to James Ogilvy, the Earl of Findlater, Cullen recommended a moderate regimen to alleviate this patient's chronic indigestion, blaming 'a certain delicacy and weak nerves' for the problem.[112] Cullen sensibly distributed food intake into three separate meals beginning with a moderate breakfast of tea with bread and butter, followed by a heartier dinner at noon, and ending with a very light supper to be taken several hours before bedtime. For breakfast, grains were desirable, including rye, barley, oats, and medium wheat. Soft eggs were easily digestible – poaching the best way of preparing them.[113] Light and tender animal food – including chicken and veal were preferred over wildfowl, venison, beef and pork that were more difficult to digest. Cullen recommended boiled or moderately roasted meat, rather than backed or fried, heavily salted, smoked and dried meats. Fish could be easily digested but failed to enhance perspiration. On one occasion, however, he observed that 'the chicken and fish dishes in Italy are too rich'.[114] Rice, barley, and potatoes were desirable; fruits such as apples and pears could be baked or boiled. Shallots and onions were ideal in promoting perspiration and urine while vinegar, pepper, pickles and spices were to be avoided.

Perhaps because of his gout, Cullen sanctioned a popularly promoted asceticism and partial vegetarianism.[115] Meat, the scourge of refined life, was considered an unnecessary stimulant. If they could afford it, only labourers working hard in the outdoors under cold conditions benefited from eating it. Designed primarily for wealthy, indolent males, Cullen's regimen was meant to be a remedy as well as a preventative for contemporary maladies of civilisation.[116] Most people in other parts of the world lived happily on an essentially vegetarian diet that purified the blood. In a 1784 letter to William Bayliss, physician to the King of Prussia, Cullen recommended that Mr Heynitz, Director of Mines, should avoid strong tea and coffee, consume breakfast cereals, occasionally a soft-boiled egg, some butter and dry toast. For dinner, the diet called for light white fish or meat in great moderation, boiled or roasted together with rice, barley, or potatoes. However, fat, fried or baked meat – pork, bacon – with heavy, greasy sauces or herring and salmon together with flatulent vegetables, such as cabbage and lettuce were to be avoided.[117]

Cullen recommended drinking common or bottled mineral water from Brixton, Bristol, or Scarborough with meals. Wells near Edinburgh at Leith also furnished a pure product. Cow or goat's milk for potential consumptives should be taken warm, but Cullen was concerned about adulterated products.[118] Chocolate loaded the stomach and was not easily digested or perspired. Strong tea and coffee relaxed and weakened the stomach and, by consent, the entire nervous system causing tremors and fainting spells. For their part, ales and beers could be constipating, but they helped the digestion of meats and additionally promoted urinary discharge. In his frequent comments about wine, Cullen acted like a true connoisseur: he preferred wines with little acidity. He rejected Rhenish and other weak-bodied German labels, while approving of fuller Spanish and Portuguese red wines including Lisbon and Madeira sherries which he considered stronger and better than the French and Hungarian products. In Cullen's opinion, small quantities of wine – two or three glasses per meal – were adequate because they temporarily stimulated the spirits. Excessive wine drinking was pernicious, eventually wearing out the nervous system. This was especially the case with all heavy and strong-bodied red wines routinely adulterated with lead acetate to give them strength and sweetness.

Overindulgence caused gastrointestinal symptoms – constipation and cramps – suggestive of lead poisoning as well as what was then known as 'irregular gout' (Chapter 6).[119] To persons who consulted him, Cullen steadfastly maintained that the consumption of all malt liquors as well as rum and brandy was 'improper'. In his opinion, these products possessed a certain viscidity that made them difficult to digest. To be sure, all alcoholic beverages were powerful stimulants generously imbibed during Scotland's winter season, but Cullen warned that when their invigorating action dissipated, the bodily system would become more feeble and susceptible to cold and disease. If indulged in, 'spirits' should be mixed with water to preserve sobriety. When prepared with frequently adulterated rum, punch could be further weakened with lemon syrup rather than fresh fruits, thus promoting both perspiration and urine.[120]

Cullen preached the need for a proper internal fluid balance. He insisted that the health of the body depended on regular sensible perspiration, especially because of its links with digestion.[121] As in earlier times, eighteenth-century physiology continued to uphold humoral views, claiming that any obstruction to the flow of perspiration would have nefarious consequences, leading to the putrefaction of bodily fluids and appearance of a number of illnesses. Following particular diurnal and seasonal patterns, perspiration – mostly the insensible kind – represented about half of the volume in discharges. After seven to eight hours of sound sleep, such bodily exhalations were more profuse in the morning, diminishing towards mid-day and early afternoon, only to rebound and flow freely towards evening before diminishing once more around bedtime. Sweat could be promoted through thicker clothing as well as the intake of light, nourishing food – neither fat nor viscid – and warm, stimulating drinks.

Men were believed to have a more efficient insensible perspiration than women do although not enough to prevent traditional fluid imbalances characterised as 'plethora'. Since they did not have a periodic menstrual evacuation to rid themselves of excess bodily fluid, males experienced similar monthly crises of urinary secretion to compensate for the female menses. Alternatively, both sexes could shed blood in the form of nosebleeds and haemorrhoidal discharges to rid themselves of excessive fluid.[122] Sweating was also more profuse in young rather than older people, more abundant in sanguine and choleric temperaments than in phlegmatic and melancholic ones. Summertime allowed for the highest perspiration output, wintertime the lowest. Moreover, perspiration increased during moments of joy, cheerfulness, and during all physical activities and pleasant sensations. For Cullen, cold air was the most common culprit in arresting perspiration and creating a fluid imbalance by causing a spasm that diffused to the whole surface of the body. The result of such a blockage was bodily sluggishness, lack of appetite, and higher excretion of urine. Some people complained of swelling or hoarseness in the throat, a plugged nose, cough, and even difficulty breathing, while others fretted about gripes and purging in the lower belly or rheumatic pains among muscles and joints. Perspiration could be restored in phlegmatic and melancholic persons through exercise and stimulating drinks, while those of robust, sanguine, or consumptive constitutions had to be placed on a cooling regimen and subjected to bloodletting.

Ideally, urinary discharges were nearly equal in quantity to perspiration. However, the seasonal patterns were almost inverted, with urine exceeding sweat during the winters. Again, there was less voiding or urine during mornings than afternoons, although variations were closely linked to the volume of fluid intake. Heat diminished urinary excretion while its colour and acrimony increased because of greater concentration. Large quantities of limpid urine could be suddenly voided in connection with emotional turmoil such as hysteric fits (Chapter 9). All warm liquors promoted perspiration while all fermented liquors promoted urine. On average, older people seemed to void more urine and less sweat. In the end, Cullen admitted that 'urine indeed does not fall much under our observation and the management of it is little in our power.'[123] For Cullen, the regularity of stool excretion was a function and consequence of perspiration and urinary discharges. In his letters of advice he recommended that his patients go to stool at least once a day. However, given the widespread gluttony and lack of exercise among his affluent clientele, constipation was perceived as a common and chronic condition. Cullen blamed it on the ingestion of smoked, dried or baked meats, cheese and milk, unripe fruits, as well as spirituous liquors and rough wines. Cold and grief could also be implicated. Without recourse to purgatives, stool was promoted by the ingestion of animal broth, ripe fruits or sweets such as honey, figs, sugar, and warm drawn whey. Salt, malt liquors, and gentle bodily exercise – especially walking – could also be helpful. In this regard, Cullen also expressed concern about another bodily fluid – saliva – 'a liquor very necessary to our digestion'. In fact, Edinburgh physicians played an important role in the physiology of digestion when Benjamin Rush and Edward Steven performed experiments on animals and humans concerning the roles of saliva and gastric juices (Chapter 2). According to Cullen, 'some persons make a very great waste of saliva' through their use of tobacco.[124]

Finally, Cullen dealt with the emission of genital fluids, primarily the ejaculation of semen. Such 'solicitations of natural vigour' were deemed healthy since the climax also promoted much needed perspiration and stimulated the spirits. Cullen was no prude. His treatment of Samuel Johnson's and his 'female friend's' venereal complaints was quite explicit and devoid of moral undertones.[125] However, frequent emissions could easily squander a man's strength and health. Like his contemporaries, Cullen believed in the vitality of sperm and expressed concern about 'excesses of venery' by urging moderation in sexual relations. 'Pleasure of all kinds wastes the spirits, relaxes and weakens the body and as this is the highest pleasure of sense, so it must weaken the body more than anything else,' he preached.[126] Cullen even indicated that abstinence would not hurt his elderly but still lustful male clients.[127] He explained that when sex 'is indulged without any cravings of the body and to gratify a lecherous fancy rather than a natural appetite, when it is done in drink after fatigue or a full meal in an unease posture, in all these cases it does great mischief.'[128] To another patient, Cullen explained that 'you have been much hurt, I am persuaded, by venery', adding that 'I cannot give you any positive rule but you should abstain as much as you can.'[129] Even a melancholic minister was urged to curb his conjugal rights: 'avoid frequent communication with your wife', Cullen wrote, 'as I suspect that too [much] venery has been the chief cause for your complaint.'[130] Following the sexual act, indigestion and heartburn could ensue, eventually affecting the nervous system, and even promoting the dreaded 'hypochondriasis' (Chapter 9).

Balancing the mind

The last Galenic 'non-natural' was the most difficult to manage. According to Cullen, the mind played a key role in human physical and mental health, and physicians, as moral philosophers, were entrusted with the management of the passions. He was keenly aware that 'soul and body mutually affect one another'.[131] In fact, every bodily temperament was accompanied by a certain set of passions, virtues and vices. Cullen wrote that 'such is the connection between virtue, the health of the soul and the health of the body that all the virtuous and moderate passions contribute to the health of the body and all the vicious and excessive [ones] are very hurtful to it.'[132] The passions could 'sensibly affect indeed every fibre and function of the body', with love, joy, anger and chagrin capable of invigorating all systems. Anxiety and fear stopped circulation, weakened the body and produced trembling and coldness.[133] Cullen believed that courage was a 'natural consequence of a state of vigour in the body' while physical debility caused timidity.[134]

The environment was responsible for a certain 'tone of mind' – meaning a balanced stimulation – necessary for proper somatic sensibility and mental functioning. 'There is hardly any state of mind more uneasy than that of vacancy of thought,' asserted Cullen, adding that 'no mortal can bear it and the whole business of a great part of mankind is to avoid it'.[135] Fear and dread were common among civilised people who lived within protected environments. Isolation stifled their sense of cheerful conversation, the most lasting and safest of all amusements. To keep their heads occupied, the poor were believed to cheerfully embrace toil and labour while the rich were constantly prodding their exhausted minds to find something to fill up their idle time and prevent boredom. Most people, however, including weary and idle persons of means, failed to have a natural disposition to entertain themselves and thus were forced to seek enjoyment from a great variety of shows and diversions. Playing fashionable indoor games such as billiards and bowling was salutary but could be dangerous if engaged in too passionately. Cullen asserted that 'variety must be necessary in amusements, study, and indeed, in the whole of life.'[136]

For Cullen, storytelling excited the motions of the spirits without exhausting them. So did the process of learning the arts and sciences unless one obsessively 'pushed' such healthy inquiries. During youth, this motion of the spirits was considered to be brisk and unfettered the mind therefore kind, humane, generous, and bold. Because of progressively sluggish circulation, the mind in old age became sullen, peevish, full of fears and doubts, even despondent.[137] In dealing with mental stimulation and the passions, Cullen stressed the importance of self-confidence and hope for peace of mind and bodily health: 'no man can be easy if he is ashamed of himself or if he cannot flatter himself on some piece of worth or excellence'.[138] When the mind became completely engaged in 'one particular subject' for prolonged periods of time, the nervous system weakened and the body could be rendered 'languid and unfit for action'.[139] Responding to a request, Cullen advised a client that 'long application to business will do harm', suggesting instead that he 'intermix business, relaxation and exercise'.[140] 'A very solitary life is certainly bad…and a little society would certainly be of good service', Cullen asserted in another letter, adding that 'when the season will allow it, a journey with a change of scene and air may be highly useful'.[141] In 1778, he followed his own advice by purchasing the Ormiston Hill estate in Kirknewton just outside Edinburgh, a refuge and 'hobby, a scheme of pleasure' away from his main residence in the crowded Old Town.[142]

Replying in the same year to a minister who had tired of his burdensome pastoral duties, Cullen recommended that he 'seek company and amusement, take a few glasses of wine but never approach to the least intoxication'. In fact, the entire nervous system often needed to be rebalanced through stimulation to shake it out of its languor. Exercise, change of place and climate, could lead to the 'possible interruption of thought or train of thinking' that had caused those sullen feelings.[143] Besides a vigorous program of exercise and diet to prevent languor, Cullen suggested avoidance of sudden and strong emotions. He was especially emphatic in calling for the 'management of the mind' of patrons who were believed to be susceptible to fits. The passions could be responsible for triggering a common female disease: 'hysteria', especially in 'women of refinement' who were believed to have very delicate feelings (Chapter 8). Management of these fits required much discretion from family members. To one patient Cullen advised: 'I would avoid everything that can disturb her and if she likes it give her some amusement'.[144]

In one episode toward the end of his own life, Cullen received a letter from a brother of Lord Torphicken, hastily dispatched from Newcastle in 1789. The man, after leaving Edinburgh, had become increasingly restless and despondent, spending his nights sitting in a chair and 'indulging certain extravagant but very harassing thoughts', possibly suicide. A prompt answer from the doctor was demanded, mailed to a house in Stamford, Lincolnshire. Cullen's immediate response sought to reassure his client that 'this love of solitude' was distressing but not especially dangerous, although if such a state of depression continued, it would indeed negatively affect his general health. Since it arose from a 'general languor' of the nervous system, Cullen recommended vigorous exercise and felt that companionship was essential.[145] The very next day, Cullen answered another cry for help from a minister. Fearful of being attacked by strangers, the clergyman admitted feeling melancholic. Cullen promptly diagnosed the condition as 'hypochondriasis' and suggested multiple outings on horseback as the most effective cure, excusing his brief answer because of a 'very infirm state of health which my time of life necessarily brings on' (Chapter 9).[146]

Indeed, in a commentary on ageing and health preservation, Cullen had previously confided in a colleague from Newcastle-upon-Tyne. Writing in October 1789, he admitted that 'the infirmities of age have been gradually coming on for years past and I don't find that they advance faster than in proportion to my years'. However, Cullen conceded that 'they diminish the action of my body and mind, but as I judge, more in the former than in the latter'. In accordance with his own efforts to follow a balanced lifestyle, Cullen disclosed that 'for many years past I have taken very little strong drink and always found myself hurt by the smallest excess in it'. His intake of wine for the year 1789, he insisted, was identical to that in previous years and only occurred at dinner, never exceeding two or three glasses when eating in company.[147] Cullen died several months later, on 5 February 1790, at the age of seventy-nine.

Conclusion

History does not specifically record the level of compliance with Cullen's multifaceted health advice. There was a contemporary toast making the rounds in London establishments: 'may no English nobleman venture out of the world without a Scottish physician' – possibly a tribute to the ubiquity of Edinburgh medical graduates.[148] Perhaps it was fashionable for Cullen's patrons to seek counsel when they believed themselves to be in trouble but equally appealing to flaunt it when their condition improved. In presenting such a comprehensive program of health preservation, Cullen clearly anticipated that some of his clients would 'conclude that our accounts are fanciful and that all caution and reserve in these reports are unnecessary'.[149] Although he was forced to admit that individual health 'abuses' might not have immediate and readily discernible consequences, Cullen predicted that their deleterious and cumulative effects would eventually 'sap and undermine the constitution' of his clients, triggering numerous diseases at a more advanced age. He also conceded that a minority of 'remarkably robust and strong' persons would get away with their patently unhealthy habits for extended periods of time. However, he urged that such constitutional exceptions should not be used as excuses to reject all health advice. This tendency, he warned, 'has killed more young people than half the apothecaries of England'.[150]

The opposite stance was equally dangerous. Plagued by morbid fear of becoming ill, people 'acquainted with the powers of the non-naturals' became, according to Cullen, 'extremely scrupulous in their manner of life', dreading the emergence of diseases 'in every cloud'. Some individuals 'even sometimes imagined themselves affected with many [diseases] that they never dreamed of or felt before they unluckily engaged in this study'. In fact, as historian Roy Porter has pointed out, the new health trade drastically increased the scope of disease and demand for medical attention.[151] Cullen tried to reassure potential hypochondriacs that although 'caution and reserve [could] be very commendable', a very scrupulous and exact manner of living was the most likely thing to affect a person. Perhaps this basic ambiguity about the potentially deleterious consequences of sharing significant medical knowledge with the public was responsible for Cullen's hesitation to complete his text and publish it. On the other hand, there was already a glut of similar publications on the market, notably William Buchan's popular *Domestic Medicine* and numerous anonymous tracts. Moreover, Cullen remained quite busy attending to his consultation practice through the mails. Already in his seventies, the last decade of his life found him still answering nearly two hundred letters per year.[152] Cullen's former student, Benjamin Rush, encouraged him to finish the project. In a letter Rush wrote:

'I shall not cease to pray that you may not only live to finish your work upon the "art of preserving health" but that you may stamp a value upon it that shall ensure, not its sale only but its immortality, by living till you are a hundred years old, and much longer if it shall please God.'[153]

Cullen's detailed health advice, displayed in this essay, signalled a profound lifestyle shift away from stout and sluggish robustness to more trim, leaner and active bodies. His texts reveal an eclectic human physiology still largely based on the tenets of classical humoralism that sought to balance bodily fluids through dietary intakes and natural evacuations. Superimposed on this model were newer notions of nervous excitability demanding adjustments in stimulation for the proper functioning of the various organ systems as well as the mind. In both instances, Cullen skilfully linked the optimum functioning of this composite body and mind to the surrounding physical and cultural environment of Scotland. His views disclose the basic motivations and strategies employed by eighteenth-century physicians to deal with Britain's affluent classes. The contemporary lifestyle of the rich and famous was proclaimed risky to life and limb, in need of discipline and change. Under such circumstances, health preservation became an important medical marketing tool. Physicians proffered their advice to pampered and often sceptical clients by exposing deleterious linkages between environment, human behaviour and physiology. Political arithmetic also suggested that in the aggregate, private health or hygiene became public health, ultimately making the nation stronger and safer (Chapter 1). Cullen characterised this knowledge as 'the common sense of mankind' and he consistently included such advice in dealing with sufferings and ailments of his clients.[154] To Cullen, an educated, virtuous Scot, the art of health was a key component of the practical morality that needed to guide polite contemporary culture in its response to the perceived excesses of luxurious living. Given his status as an ageing and periodic gout sufferer, most recommendations also mirrored his own fashionable Stoicism and spartan lifestyle. Ultimately, Cullen's general rule aimed 'to keep a due medium between an absolutely irregular life and one too scrupulously exact'.[155] Decades later, medicine's gradual concentration on the effects of disease – Galen had called them 'preternatural things' – came to eclipse the physician's traditional role as 'hygienist'. As a result, the importance of health preservation as a prominent aspect of medical intervention would become overshadowed by a narrower focus on bodily pathology and the gradual expansion of effective therapies.

Notes

1. K. Haakonssen (ed.), A. Smith, *The Theory of Moral Sentiments*, 6th edn (Cambridge: Cambridge University Press, 2002), 249. For details about Smith's ideas, see N. Phillipson, 'Adam Smith as Civic Moralist', in I. Hont and M. Ignatieff (eds.), *Wealth and Virtue: The Shaping of Political Economy in the Scottish Enlightenment* (Cambridge: Cambridge University Press, 1983), 179–202.
2. Letter to Robert Ligerwood, in Cullen's consultation letters. They will be quoted as Cullen's Correspondence, XXI vols (Edinburgh, 1755–90), MSS Collection, Royal College of Physicians, Edinburgh. The letter to Ligerwood can be found in Vol. VIII.
3. W. Cullen, 'An Essay on the Preservation of Health', parts I-II (Edinburgh, undated), Thomson/Cullen Papers, MSS Collection, Glasgow University Library.
4. L. H. Butterfield (ed.), *The Letters of Benjamin Rush*, 2 vols (Princeton: Princeton University Press, 1951), Vol. I, 346.
5. W. Cullen, 'An Essay on the Hypochondriac Disease (in a letter),' Thomson/Cullen Papers, MSS Collection, Glasgow University Library.
6. For more details, G.B. Risse, '"Doctor William Cullen, Physician, Edinburgh": A Consultation Practice in the Eighteenth Century,' *Bulletin of the History of Medicine,* 48 (1974), 338–51.
7. M.T. Compton, 'The Association of Hygieia with Asclepios in Graeco-Roman Asklepieion Medicine', *Journal of the History of Medicine,* 57 (2002), 312–29.
8. S. Jarcho, 'Galen's Six Things Non Natural: A Bibliographic Note and Translation', *Bulletin of the History of Medicine,* 44 (1970), 372–7. Owsei Temkin considered the concept 'one of the most enduring contributions of Galenism to medical thought'; see his *Galenism: Rise and Decline of a Medical Philosophy* (Ithaca, NY: Cornell University Press, 1973), 180.
9. See L.J. Rather, 'The "Six Things Non-Natural": A Note on the Origins and Fate of the Doctrine and a Phrase', *Clio Medica,* 3 (1968), 337–47, and P.H. Niebyl, 'The Non-Naturals,' *Bulletin of the History of Medicine,* 45 (1971), 486–92. The most recent discussion can be found in L. Garcia Ballester, 'On the Origin of the "Six Non–Natural Things" in Galen', *Sudhoffs Archiv,* 32 (1993), 105–15.
10. An early medieval work stressing health preservation and longevity was written by Roger Bacon and published in 1243. An English translation from the Latin version is *The Cure of Old Age and Preservation of Youth* (London: Flesher and Evets, 1683). For an overview, see A. Wear. 'The History of Personal Hygiene', in W.F. Bynum and R. Porter (eds), *Companion Encyclopedia of the History of Medicine,* 2 vols (London: Routledge, 1993),

Vol. 2, 1283–1308.

11. L. Cornaro, *The Art of Living Long*, trans. from Italian (Milwaukee, W. F. Butler, 1903). Also available is a eighteenth-century edition, *Discourses on a Sober and Temperate Life*, trans. from Italian (Philadelphia: T. Dobson, 1791).
12. *Ibid.*, 58.
13. R. Palmer, 'Health, Hygiene and Longevity in Medieval and Renaissance Europe', in I. Kawakita, S. Sakai, and I. Otsuka (eds), *History of Hygiene* (Tokyo: Ishiyaku EuroAmerica, 1991), 75-98. Further details are in H. Mikkeli, *Hygiene in the Early Modern Medical Tradition* (Helsinki: Finnish Academy of Sciences and Letters, 1999).
14. W. Coleman, 'Health and Hygiene in the Encyclopédie: A Medical Doctrine for the Bourgeoisie', *Journal of the History of Medicine,* 29 (1974), 399–421.
15. See M. Foucault, 'The Politics of Health in the Eighteenth Century', in C. Gordon (ed.), *Power/Knowledge, Selected Interviews and Other Writings 1972–1977* (New York: Pantheon, 1980), 166–82.
16. For modern England, A. Wear, 'Making Sense of Health and the Environment in Early Modern England', in A. Wear (ed.), *Medicine in Society: Historical Essays* (Cambridge: Cambridge University Press, 1992), 119-47.
17. G. Cheyne, *An Essay on Health and Long Life*, 2nd edn (London: Strahan, 1725), 231. For details, R. Porter, 'Civilization and Disease: Medical Ideology in the Enlightenment', in J. Black and J. Gregory (eds), *Culture, Politics and Society in Britain 1660–1800* (Manchester: Manchester University Press, 1991), 154–83.
18. *Ibid.*, 5. For a recent biographical account, see A. Guerrini, *Obesity and Depression in the Enlightenment: The Life and Times of George Cheyne* (Norman, OK: University of Oklahoma Press, 2000).
19. G. Cheyne, *The English Malady: Or a Treatise of Nervous Diseases of All Kinds* (London: S. Powell, 1733).
20. R. Porter, 'Consumption: Disease of the Consumer Society?', in J. Brewer and R. Porter (eds), *Consumption and the World of Goods* (London: Routledge, 1993), 66.
21. Cheyne, *English Malady, op. cit.* (note 19), 254; see also G.S, Rousseau, 'Medicine and Millenarianism', in his *Enlightenment Borders: Pre-and Post-Modern Discourses, Medical, Scientific* (Manchester: Manchester University. Press, 1991), 78–117.
22. S. Shapin, 'Trusting George Cheyne: Scientific Expertise, Common Sense, and Moral Authority in Early Eighteenth-Century Dietetic Medicine', *Bulletin of the History of Medicine,* 77 (2003), 263–97.

23. Hygiene was more important than therapeutics because it contributed to the wellbeing of humanity, thereby 'achieving the strongest state of health that the nature of human life will allow, and to preserve this state' See A. d'Aumont, 'Hygiene,' in D. Diderot and D'Alembert (eds), *Encyclopédie ou Dictionnaire Risonné des Sciences, des Arts et des Méteiers*, new ed., XXXVI vols (Geneva: 1777–9), Vol. XVII, 919.
24. W. Buchan, 'Introduction', in *Domestic Medicine*, 9th edn (London: T. Cadell, 1786), XV-XXVIII; see C. Lawrence, 'William Buchan: Medicine Laid Open', *Medical History*, 57, 1 (1983), 22–42; and R. Porter, 'Lay Medical Knowledge in the Eighteenth Century: The Evidence of the Gentlemen's Magazine', *Medical History*, 29, 2 (1985), 138–68.
25. Cheyne, *op. cit.* (note 17), XVIII.
26. J. Armstrong, *The Art of Preserving Health: A Poem* (London: Millar, 1757).
27. J. Mackenzie, *The History of Health and the Art of Preserving It* (Edinburgh: W. Gordon, 1759), 436; see also H. Mikkeli, 'Legitimizing a Discipline: James Mackenzie's History of Health (1758)', in D.R. Kelley (ed.), *History and the Disciplines: The Reclassification of Knowledge in Early Modern Europe* (Rochester: University of Rochester Press, 1997), 277–95.
28. For more details, see N. McKendrick, J. Brewer, and J.H. Plumb, *The Birth of a Consumer Society: The Commercialization of Eighteenth-Century England* (Bloomington: Indiana University Press, 1982).
29. J. Leake, *Practical Observations Towards the Prevention and Cure of Chronic Diseases Peculiar to Women*, 7th edn (London: Evans, Murray and Egerton, 1792), 36.
30. See H.J. Cook, 'Good Advice and Little Medicine: The Professional Authority of Early Modern English Physicians', *Journal of British Studies*, 33 (1994), 1–31; and T. Broman, 'Rethinking Professionalization: Theory, Practice, and Professional Ideology in Eighteenth-Century German Medicine', *Journal of Modern History*, 67 (1995), 835–72.
31. Foucault, *op. cit.* (note 15), 177.
32. F. Hoffmann, *Fundamenta Medicinae*, trans. L.S. King (New York: American Elsevier, 1971), 103–4.
33. T. Beddoes, *Hygeia or Essays Moral and Medical on the Causes Affecting the Personal State of our Middling and Affluent Classes*, III vols (Bristol: J. Mills, 1802), Vol. I, 72.
34. *Ibid.*, Vol. I, 8-9.
35. For an analysis, N.D. Jewson, 'Medical Knowledge and the Patronage System in Eighteenth-Century England', *Sociology*, 8 (1974), 369-85.
36. For detailed analysis of the medical marketplace, see D. Porter and R. Porter, *Patient's Progress, Doctors and Doctoring in Eighteenth-Century England* (Stanford, Calif.: Stanford University Press, 1989), especially 33–69. For

further detail concerning patients' experiences with illness based on their own narratives, R. Porter and D. Porter, *In Sickness and Health: The British Experience 1650–1850* (London: Fourth Estate, 1988.)

37. Aumont, *op. cit.* (note 23), 919; consult also A. Emch–Dériaz, 'The Non-Naturals Made Easy', in R. Porter (ed.), *The Popularization of Medicine, 1650–1850* (London: Routledge, 1992), 134–59. This essay deals with the work of S. Tissot, especially his *Advice to the People in General with Regard to their Health*, trans. from French (Edinburgh: A. Donaldson, 1768).
38. T. Beddoes, *op. cit.* (note 33), Vol. I, 26–7.
39. R. Porter, '"A Little Learning": Knowledge and Health in the Eighteenth Century,' *Gut*, (1989), 75–80; and A. Digby, *Making a Medical Living: Doctors and Patients in the English Market for Medicine, 1720–1911* (Cambridge: Cambridge University Press, 1994).
40. Leake, *op. cit.* (note 29), 42.
41. A brief biographical sketch is R.W. Johnstone, 'William Cullen', *Medical History* 3, 1 (1959), 33–46. More recently, refer to the contributions in A. Doig *et al.* (eds), *William Cullen and the Eighteenth-Century Medical World* (Edinburgh: Edinburgh University Press, 1992). An article devoted to Cullen's clinical skills in that publication is G.B. Risse, 'Cullen as Clinician: Organization and Strategies of an Eighteenth-Century Medical Practice', 133–51.
42. B. Parr, 'Hygienistes,' in *The London Medical Dictionary*, 3 vols (Philadelphia: Mitchell, Ames & White, 1819), Vol. I, 778.
43. Cullen, *op. cit.* (note 5).
44. Cullen's consultation letters were written to patients and their physicians in Scotland and other parts of the world. See details in Risse, *op. cit.* (note 6).
45. R.M. Stott, 'Health and Virtue: Or, How to Keep Out of Harm's Way – Lectures on Pathology and Therapeutics by William Cullen *c.*1770', *Medical History*, 31, 2 (1987), 123–42.
46. Details in A. Broadie, *The Tradition of Scottish Philosophy: A New Perspective on the Enlightenment* (Edinburgh: Polygon, 1990).
47. See J. Dwyer, *Virtuous Discourse: Sensibility and Community in Late Eighteenth-Century Scotland* (Edinburgh: J. Donald Publ. 1987), 95–116; and M.B. Becker, *The Emergence of Civil Society in the Eighteenth Century: A Privileged Moment in the History of England, Scotland and France* (Bloomington: Indiana University Press, 1994).
48. Smith, *Theory of Moral Sentiments, op. cit.* (note 1) 248. More details in T. L. Beauchamp, 'Common Sense and Virtue in the Scottish Moralists', in R. Baker, D. Porter and R. Porter (eds), *The Codification of Medical Morality* (Dordrecht: Kluwer, 1993), 99–121.

49. Smith, *op. cit.* (note 1), 256; see also K. Tribe, 'Adam Smith: Cultural Crtitic?', *Journal of Economic Literature,* 37 (1999), 609–32.
50. Cullen, *op. cit.* (note 3), I, 2.
51. In this regard, Cullen had a long experience since his early days with the Duke of Hamilton and later Lord Kames. Porter and Porter, *op. cit.* (note 36), 117–44. A recent biographical sketch of Cullen was written by E.M. McGirr, *Cullen in Context,* Stevenson Lectures in Citizenship 1990 Series (Glasgow: University of Glasgow, 1990).
52. Cullen, *op. cit.* (note 3), I, 15.
53. *Ibid.,* I, 22.
54. In a letter to Lady Roxberry dated 26 December 1786, Cullen provides the following advice for a debilitated constitution: 'A very solitary life is certainly bad for such a constitution and a little society... would certainly be of great service, and when the season will allow of it, more or less a journey with a change of scene and air may be highly useful.' Cullen, *op. cit.* (note 2), Vol. XIX.
55. Cullen, *op. cit.* (note 3), I, 21.
56. J. Gregory, *Lectures on the Duties and Qualifications of a Physician* (London: W. Strahan, 1772), 11–2.
57. *Ibid.*, 19–20. For details, Lisbeth Haakonssen, *Medicine and Morals in the Enlightenment: John Gregory, Thomas Percival and Benjamin Rush* (Amsterdam: Rodopi, 1997), 46–93; see also C.J. Berry, 'Sociality and Socialisation', in A. Brodie (ed.), *The Cambridge Companion to the Scottish Enlightenment* (Cambridge: Cambridge University Press, 2003), 243–57.
58. Cullen, *op. cit.* (note 3), I, 8.
59. 'When there is some defect in the constitution – some bias and tendency towards disease, and it is only by preventing this tendency, by correcting these defects that is by preventing disease that we preserve health', Cullen explained to his students around 1770; see W. Cullen, 'Lectures on Physiology', 5 vols., Edinburgh, *c.*1770, MSS Collection, Royal College of Physicians, Edinburgh, as quoted in Stott, *op. cit.* (note 45), 128.
60. V. Smith, 'Prescribing the Rules of Health: Self-help and Advice in the Late Eighteenth Century', in R. Porter (ed.), *Patients and Practitioners: Lay Perceptions of Medicine in Pre-Industrial Society* (Cambridge: Cambridge University Press, 1985), 249–82; and L.R. Murphy, *Enter the Physician: The Transformation of Domestic Medicine, 1760–1860* (Tuscaloosa: University of Alabama Press, 1991).
61. Cullen, *op. cit.* (note 3), I, 19.
62. The letter was dated 16 October 1780. See Cullen, *op. cit.* (note 2), Vol. XIII.
63. Cullen, *op. cit.* (note 3), I, 23.

64. Cullen, *op. cit.* (note 5), 1.
65. Student transcription of a series of Cullen's 1772 clinical lectures were collected in two notebooks entitled 'Medical Tracts I and II' (attributed to John Unthank) and in my personal possession.
66. The literature on the history of hypochondriasis is extensive. A broad introduction is S. Baur, *Hypochondria: Woeful Imaginations* (Berkeley: University of California Press, 1988).
67. Cullen, *op. cit.* (note 5), 1.
68. G.B. Risse, 'Medicine in the Age of Enlightenment', in Wear (ed.), *Medicine and Society, op. cit.* (note 16), 149–95; R. Porter, 'Spreading Medical Enlightenment: The Popularization of Medicine in Georgian England and its Paradoxes', in R. Porter (ed.), *The Popularization of Medicine, 1650–1850* (London: Routledge, 1992), 215–31.
69. Cullen, *op. cit.* (note 3), I, 25.
70 . 'In private practice it is often difficult to act agreeably to one's judgment, as it is often necessary to pay attention to the prejudices of the people who are unacquainted with the nature of the attending circumstances,' J. Sherwyn, *Medical and Philosophical Commentaries,* II (1793), 396
71. Cullen, *op. cit.* (note 3), I, 27–8. See also S. Pilloud and M. Louis–Courvoisier, 'The Intimate Experience of the Body in Eighteenth Century: Between Interiority and Exteriority', *Medical History,* 47, 4 (2003), 473–92.
72. On the rhetoric of illness, see W. Wald, 'Medicine by Post in Eighteenth-Century Britain: The Changing Rhetoric of Illness in Doctor–Patient Correspondence and Literature', PhD dissertation, Brandeis University, 2001 and his article 'Doctor-Patient Correspondence in Eighteenth-Century Britain: A Change in Rhetoric and Relationship', *Studies in Eighteenth-Century Culture,* 29 (2000), 47–64. For a discussion of the historiographic issues, D. Harley, 'Rhetoric and the Social Construction of Sickness and Healing', *Social History of Medicine,* 12 (1999), 407–35.
73. For an overview, W.F. Bynum, 'Cullen and the Nervous System', in Doig, *op. cit.* (note 41), 152–62; see also R, Rey, 'Vitalism, Disease and Society', in R. Porter (ed.), *Medicine in the Enlightenment* (Amsterdam, Rodopi, 1995), 274–88
74. 'The nerves and nervous fibers of the body have all a sympathy and consent with one another', Cullen, *op. cit.* (note 5), 20. For details, C. Lawrence, 'The Nervous System and Society in the Scottish Enlightenment', in B. Barnes and S. Shapin (eds), *Natural Order: Historical Studies of Scientific Culture* (Beverly Hills: Sage Publications, 1979), 19–40; J. Mullan, *Sentiment and Sociability: The Language of Feeling in the Eighteenth Century* (Oxford: Clarendon Press, 1988), 18–56. For France, A.C. Vila, *Enlightenment and*

Pathology: Sensibility in the Literature and medicine of Eighteenth-Century France (Baltimore: Johns Hopkins University Press, 1998). For notions regarding ether see J.R.R. Christie, 'Ether and the Science of Chemistry, 1740–1790', in G.N. Cantor and M.J. Hodge (eds), *Conceptions of Ether: Studies in the History of Ether Theories, 1740–1900* (Cambridge: Cambridge University Press, 1981), 85–110.

75. Cullen, *op. cit.* (note 5), 102.
76. *Ibid.*, 43.
77. Cullen, *op. cit.* (note 3), I, 120.
78. Leake, *op. cit.* (note 29), 17.
79. *Ibid.*, 18.
80. Cullen, *op. cit.* (note 5), 42–3.
81. 'The air affects human bodies by its changeable and sensible qualities of heat, cold, dryness and moisture, by its properties of gravity, elasticity and by the steams with which at different times and in different places it may be impregnated,' *ibid.*, 43. For details, J. Arbuthnot, *An Essay Concerning the Effects of Air on Human Bodies* (London: Tonson & Draper, 1733)
82. Cullen explained that the West Coast of Europe remained much warmer in winter than places on the same latitude on the East Coast of America. In the British Isles, south and west winds brought warmth and moisture, while north and east ones were cold and moist, thus potentially harmful. See *ibid.*, 47.
83. Cullen, *op. cit.* (note 5), 43.
84. See E. Gilchrist, *The Use of Sea Voyages in Medicine*, 2nd. edn (London: Millar, 1757).
85. Letter dated 13 April 1779, Cullen, *op. cit.* (note 2), Vol. XI.
86. *Ibid.*, Vol. XVIII. The letter was dated October 1785.
87. 'The gay, cheerful lively temperament of the people which has been the same in all ages, shews that the climate is fitted to give a greater flow of spirits,' *ibid.*, 48–9. Spain's Mediterranean coast was also a popular destination to escape from the rigours of Scottish winters, but their summers could be excessively hot and a return to Britain desirable as acknowledged by one of Cullen's patients: 'By your directions, my dear Sir, I have taken a berth in a London tracker that will sail before the first of May for London. Had you not advised this, I assure you Sir, nothing would have tempted me to leave this mild and agreeable atmosphere so soon.' Letter from Cadiz, Spain, dated 27 April 1784, in Cullen, *op. cit.* (note 2), Vol. XVII.
88. See Cullen's 1786 letter to George Ramsey, the Earl of Dalhousie, in *ibid.*, Vol. XIX.
89. Cullen, *op. cit.* (note 3), II, 52. 'People of fashion pass much of their time in crowded rooms full of people and candles; renders them liable to diseases'.

90. *Ibid.*, 33.
91. *Ibid.*, 104.
92. Letter to George Burnett, dated 16 October 1780, Cullen, *op. cit.* (note 2), Vol. XIII.
93. Cullen, *op. cit.* (note 5), 15.
94. 'There is a tendency in the economy to regular and periodical movements with regard to most of the phenomena of the system', and 'we are exposed to certain causes that produce a regular diurnal revolution in our system.' W. Cullen, Clinical Lectures (Edinburgh, 1773), MSS Collection, Royal College of Physicians, Edinburgh, 199–200.
95. Cullen, *op. cit.* (note 2), Vol. IX.
96. Cullen, *op. cit.* (note 5), 52–3.
97. In consultation with Drs Monro and Stedman. Cullen, *op. cit.* (note 2), Vol. I.
98. Cullen, *op. cit.* (note 3), II, 98. In a letter dated 2 April 1789, Cullen also prescribed exercise to an obese lady, a Mrs Ludford, for gradual weight loss; she was first to walk across her room twice a day, gradually lengthening the distance by a few yards. See Cullen, *op. cit.* (note 2), Vol. XXI.
99. Cullen, Hypochondriac Disease, *op. cit.* (note 5), 68. For details, F. Fuller, *Medicina Gymnastica or Treatise Concerning the Powers of Exercise*, 3rd edn (London: R. Knaplock, 1707).
100. *Ibid.*, 69.
101. Letter of Cullen, dated 24 August 1779, Cullen, *op. cit.* (note 2), Vol. XII.
102. See M. Barfoot, 'Dr William Cullen and Mr Adam Smith: A Case of Hypochondriasis,' *Proceeding of the Royal College of Physicians, Edinburgh,* 21 (1991), 204–14.
103. Letter dated 30 August 1777, in Cullen, *op. cit.* (note 2), vol IX.
104. G.B. Risse, 'William Cullen and Child Care: A 1788 Letter,' *Clio Medica,* 8 (1973), 65–7.
105. 'I begin with a tempered water by putting to four parts of spring water of about 50 F one part of boiling water, and with this giving hardly a feeling of cold, I wash the whole body over. This I repeat every second day, by I keep back one eighth part of the boiling water until I bring it to the temperature to that of the spring water needed for sponging head and shoulders.' Letter dated July 1788, Cullen, *op. cit.* (note 2), Vol. XX. See also W.N.B. Watson, 'Early Baths and Bagnios in Edinburgh', *Book of the Old Edinburgh Club,* 34 (1974), 57–67.
106. For details, R. and F. Morris, *Scottish Healing Wells* (Sandy: Alethea Press, 1982).
107. Letter dated 19 February 1781, Cullen, *op. cit.* (note 2), Vol. XIII; also check C.F. Mullett, *Public Baths and Health in England, 16th–18th Century*

(Baltimore: Johns Hopkins Press, 1946).
108. See R. Porter (ed.), *The Medical History of Waters and Spas* (London: Wellcome Institute for the History of Medicine, 1990).
109. N.G. Cooley, 'Physicians and the Chemical Analysis of Mineral Waters in Eighteenth-Century England', *Medical History*, 26, 2 (1983), 123–44.
110. Cullen, *op. cit.* (note 5), 71.
111. As Cullen explained, digestion of our aliments occurred because 'for the performance of this, stomach and intestines are endowed with a constant, gentle motion whereby they agitate and push forward their contents. On this account, they are furnished with a great number of nerves and probably require a great quantity of animal spirits.' Cullen, *op. cit.* (note 5), 21; see also J.W. Estes, 'The Medical Properties of Food in the Eighteenth Century', *Journal of the History of Medicine*, 51 (1996), 127–54.
112. Cullen, *op. cit.* (note 2), Vol. XX.
113. Cullen, *op. cit.* (note 5), 53–4. For details, R. Passmore, 'William Cullen and Dietetics', in Doig, *op. cit.* (note 41), 167–85.
114. Letter to William Batt, dated 19 July 1788, in Cullen, *op. cit.* (note 2), Vol. XX.
115. See A. Guerrini, 'A Diet for a Sensitive Soul: Vegetarianism in Eighteenth-Century Britain', *Eighteenth-Century Life*, 23 (1999), 34–42.
116. R. Porter, 'Gout: Framing and Fantasizing Disease', *Bulletin of the History of Medicine*, 68 (1994), 1–28, and more recently R. Porter and G.S. Rousseau, *Gout: The Patrician Malady* (New Haven: Yale University Press, 1998).
117. This consultation was carried out between September and November 1784 with a British physician, William Baylies, living in Berlin. Cullen, *op. cit.* (note 2), Vol. XVII.
118. In a letter dated 9 July 1779, Cullen recommended a half English pint of goat's milk for breakfast, remarking however that 'milk is always hurt by being carried from any distance'. Therefore, Cullen suggested patients lodge near a goat's pasture and 'let the goats be brought as near as possible to the door' for milking, *ibid.*, Vol. XII.
119. R.P. Wedeen, 'Irregular Gout: Humoral Fantasy or Saturnine Malady', *Bulletin of the New York Academy of Medicine*, 60 (1984), 969–79.
120. In a letter written to Lord Gray and dated 26 June 1779, Cullen provided very precise indications for the consumption of drinks to assure proper digestion and avoid washing down the food: one quarter English pint increasing to a full one in divided draughts half hour intervals before breakfast, followed with half a pint in the afternoon and evening. See Cullen, *op. cit.* (note 2), Vol. XII.
121. Cullen, *op. cit.* (note 5), 23.

122. G. Pomata, 'Menstruating Men: Similarity and Difference of the Sexes in Early Modern Medicine', in V. Finucci and K. Brownlee (eds), *Generation and Degeneration: Tropes of Reproduction in Literature and History from Antiquity to Early Modern Europe* (Durham: Duke University Press, 2001),109–52.
123. *Ibid.*, 97.
124. Cullen, *op. cit.* (note 5), 102.
125. See a series of letters between January and March 1785 in Cullen*, op. cit.* (note 2), Vol. XVII.
126. *Ibid.,* 103.
127. 'In young people the want of this excretion may be hurtful but this is seldom the case of persons more advanced and I believe that elderly persons can seldom be hurt by abstinence in this matter.' Cullen, *op. cit.* (note 5), 103.
128. *Ibid.*, 104.
129. See letter to R.L., Esquire, dated 10 February 1777, Cullen, *op. cit.* (note 2), Vol. VIII.
130. Letter to Reverend K.G. dated 7 December 1778, *ibid.*, Vol. XI.
131. Cullen, *op. cit.* (note 5), 72. For a recent analysis of Cullen's ideas concerning the nature of the mind see J.P. Wright, 'Materialism and the Life Soul in Eighteenth-Century Scottish Physiology', in P. Wood (ed.), *The Scottish Enlightenment: Essays in Reinterpretation* (Rochester, NY: Rochester University Press, 2000), 177–97.
132. *Ibid.,* 74.
133. *Ibid.,* 14.
134. Cullen, Lectures on Physiology, in Stott, *op. cit.* (note 45), 138.
135. Cullen, *op. cit.* (note 5), 79–82.
136. *Ibid.*, 83.
137. *Ibid.*, 15.
138. *Ibid.,* 77.
139. *Ibid.*, 15.
140. Letter to Mr. Bailey dated 10 Sep 1777, Cullen, *op. cit.* (note 2), Vol. IX.
141. Letter to Lady Roseberry dated 26 Dec 1786, *ibid.,* Vol. XIX.
142. J.Thomson, *An Account of the Life, Lectures and Writings of William Cullen MD*, 2 vols (Edinburgh: Blackwood, 1832), Vol. I, 564.
143. Letter dated 23 November 1789, Cullen, *op. cit.* (note 2), Vol. XXI.
144. Letter dated 5 May 1779, *ibid.*, Vol. XI.
145. Letter to Alexander Sandilands, dated 10 November 1789, *ibid.*, Vol. XXI.
146. Letter dated 11 November 1789, *ibid.*, Vol. XXI.
147. *Ibid.*, Vol. XXI.
148. Extracted from A. Carlyle's autobiography, in J.G. Fife (ed.), *Scottish Diaries and Memoirs, 1746–1863* (Stirling: Mackay, 1942), 152.

149. Cullen, *op. cit.* (note 5), 108.
150. *Ibid.*, 110.
151. Porter, *op. cit.* (note 17), 179.
152. Risse, *op. cit.* (note 6) 345.
153. Rush, *op. cit.* (note 4) 346.
154. Cullen, Lectures on Physiology, in Stott, *op. cit.* (note 45), 129.
155. Porter, *op. cit.* (note 17), 111–2. See also R. Porter, 'Flesh and Form', in *Flesh in the Age of Reason* (New York: W.W. Norton, 2003), 227–43. He characterised the new cult of bodily slimness and sensibility as a 'new puritanism'.

5

Ague in Eighteenth-Century Scotland?: The Shifting Ecology of a Disease

Each age and society reveals a unique set of biological and cultural circumstances responsible for the appearance of particular diseases. The study of ague in eighteenth-century Britain, including Scotland, suggests that this condition can generally be included under the current concept of malaria. The analysis is based on a variety of sources, including parish reports, institutional records, and the writings of prominent physicians. A careful review of the evidence concludes that ague in Scotland was mostly an import and its eventual disappearance linked to the country's geography and climate, as well as the agricultural and industrial revolutions that took place on its soil.

Introduction

> Agues are occasioned by effluvia from putrid stagnating water. This is evident from their abounding in rainy seasons and being most frequent in countries where the soil is marshy, as in Holland, the fens of Cambridgeshire, the Hundreds of Essex, etc.
>
> William Buchan (1786)[1]

The awareness of the waxing and waning of disease in historical times prompts questions such as why did a number of conditions erupt in certain localities and at particular periods; and, what and who were to blame? Long an interest of historians of medicine, disease now has become the target of multidisciplinary inquiries. These studies have a venerable tradition stretching back to Antiquity, beginning with the Hippocratic treatise *Airs, Waters, and Places.* That text, from around 450BC, conveys a number of ecological notions regarding relationships between humans and their physical and cultural environment that were conducive to the disease.[2] Since classical times, a number of writers – mostly physicians – have continued to furnish us with numerous accounts, from mere chronologies to complex stories that speculate about the causes and dynamics of disease distribution.[3]

Until recently, disease manifestations were considered in isolation from human ecology. The focus was on sick individuals or groups, thus neglecting a wider environmental viewpoint. However, to achieve a better understanding of changing patterns, both past and present, scholars need to employ models that allow the detection and integration of factors currently known to be involved in the emergence of disease. Such a dynamic relationship between the biological, social, and cultural environments can help explain the appearance, spread, and waning of specific health problems. The challenge is clear: can we identify and employ a spatial and temporary framework that would allow the integration of scientific and cultural information? To be meaningful, a paleoecology of health and disease must be based on current pathological and other scientific criteria. Scientific insights and conclusions are of course subject to future revisions as further information becomes available, but so are all historical interpretations.[4]

Historical ecology provides a distinctive and holistic perspective on human societies because its objective is the study of relationships between humans and other elements of the biosphere, focused within specific temporal, regional, cultural and biological contexts. Multidisciplinary in nature, historical ecology fosters collaboration between social sciences such as anthropology, geography, and history with the physical and biological sciences. Its essential premise posits that humans are both biological and cultural entities; their relationship with the surrounding environment is dialectical. Indeed, all human activity takes place in particular contexts or environments and historical events in turn are responsible for shaping such relationships between societies and their milieu.[5]

To date, historians and scientists have already established a number of intriguing webs of causality, with attention focused on the biological and cultural contexts – how human activities predispose or inhibit such dreadful events. In truth, no one ever lived in purely 'natural' environments. All individuals exist in human-shaped habitats, no matter what level of social organisation.[6] Each society and time period reveal a unique blend of circumstances and social responses to disease that can only be understood within specific geographical, social, political, economic, and cultural contexts.[7] Thus, an in-depth exploration of one particular health problem may reveal the full web in which disease moves. This discussion focuses on 'ague' which afflicted the inhabitants of Scotland's lowlands in the last third of the eighteenth century.[8]

'Ague' was a popular term in the British Isles for centuries. It is a word perhaps derived from the French 'aigu' meaning acute. In Chaucer's time, the name was used to categorise an acute or violent fever. Later, this meaning gradually shifted to a series of symptoms distinguished by fits or paroxysms of fever. In Antiquity high fevers had already drawn attention from physicians who bestowed different names on them such as 'quotidian', 'tertian', or 'quartan' because the attacks would occur with predictable regularity every twenty-four, forty-eight, or seventy-two hours.[9] Moreover, 'ague fevers' were also linked with abdominal swellings representing enlargements of the liver and spleen. Since the sixteenth century, the salty marshlands of Kent and Essex in England, notorious for their lack of salubrity and high levels of mortality, were singled out for the frequency of 'marsh fever' or 'ague' among its inhabitants. Beyond these core areas the disease was also present in the fens of Lincolnshire, Cambridgeshire, and Norfolk which acquired similar deadly reputations.[10]

Ague was an old construction of disease that certainly must have included a number of other acute and chronic conditions. Even before the eighteenth century, however, the contemporary medical literature increasingly restricted the term 'ague' to brand a type of fever that had distinctive intermittent characteristics. Names such as 'tertian-ague', 'quartan-ague', or 'intermittent fever', began to appear in the medical writings of the period.[11] Easily detected by healers and lay persons in Britain, the abdominal tumour was popularly referred to as 'ague-cake'.[12] Historians must usually exert great caution when equating vague and shifting past disease constructions and nomenclatures with modern ones. In this case, however, the rather typical and rhythmic manifestations of the disease and current scientific understanding of environmental factors involved in its spread has encouraged scholars to make an exception. Venturing into the hazardous currents of retrospective diagnosis,[13] 'ague' has indeed been equated in most instances with what now is known as malaria.[14] 'Mal'aria' – the Italian word for 'bad air' – had already been coined in the sixteenth century to designate a similar febrile condition that prevailed in the marshlands surrounding the cities of Rome and Venice. Following the bacteriological revolution, malaria came to be defined as a debilitating disease caused by a microscopic organism called plasmodium that could be transmitted to humans by bites of an anopheline species of mosquitoes.[15] Since then, historians have documented the widespread occurrence of malaria in England and Northern Europe from the seventeenth to the twentieth centuries. Holland, Denmark, and other Baltic States, including Russia, certainly had extensive areas of endemic malaria during the 1700s.[16]

Given its harsher Nordic climate, eighteenth-century observers surprisingly insisted that ague was also 'one of the scourges of Scotland', passing indeed through the country 'like a blight'.[17] Then, around 1800, similar sources suggested the disease had apparently vanished, never to return. Should one therefore consider the possibility that ague and malaria were not synonymous in Scotland? Was the Scottish ague another disease altogether? Or, could malaria possibly have been present in certain regions of Scotland? If malaria was present, how could one explain its rise and apparent retreat?[18] The discussion examines a number of original eighteenth-century sources in an attempt to answer these questions and solve the ague puzzle. Together, the sources support a reconstruction of particular events that evince the presence of malaria in Scotland and reveal the social and economic conditions of eighteenth-century Scotland as well as the biological characteristics of a complex disease.[19] Thus, the sickness which afflicted many Scots during the late-eighteenth century was the expression of a distinctive ecology of disease, a product of the unique geography, microclimates, and the organisation of the Scottish Lowlands.[20]

Ague and the Parishes of Scotland

The first and oft-quoted evidence for ague comes from the *Statistical Account of Scotland* assembled by John Sinclair (1754–1835) and published in 1794. This account was a collection of parish reports composed by their respective ministers who addressed standard questions of agricultural development, trade, population changes, climate, and disease. Although in his analysis Sinclair emphatically asserted that 'there is no country in Europe whose inhabitants are more distinguished by their healthiness',[21] he nevertheless described a number of health problems believed to be connected to geography and climate, diet and lifestyle. Not surprisingly, among the most prominent was ague, a disease Sinclair called 'enfeebling to the constitution', and one which, according to the author, 'formerly prevailed over a large proportion of Scotland'.[22] However, from Sinclair's references to individual reports, it appears that only limited salty marshes in the Northeast, near the Firth of Tay and lower course of the River Tay in Perthshire, were affected, along with similar areas in Berwickshire on the Tweed near the English border. According to these sources, the disease usually appeared in the spring and autumn, affecting local servants and labourers to the extent that 'farmers found it difficult to carry on the various operations of husbandry' without proper help.[23]

Writing in the 1790s, Sinclair emphatically remarked that such unhealthy conditions were now almost history. The ague, he asserted, 'has become less common', indeed 'entirely banished from a number of districts'.[24] In his view, the ostensible causes for this favourable turn of events were improvements in agriculture, including the enclosure and draining of wastelands newly converted to cultivation. With pride, Sinclair contrasted the emaciated and jaundiced-looking Scots of yesteryear, rarely reaching the age of seventy years, with new, robust individuals attaining the advanced age of ninety to one hundred. 'Such are the triumphs of cultivation', he boasted.[25] A study of the individual reports seems to confirm Sinclair's conclusions. A chronicle from the parish of Peterhead, on the coast north of Aberdeen, disclosed: 'no instance of a real intermittent fever or ague being hatched in this parish. Many people have agues but they bring them from Holland, the seaports in the Baltic, the fenny counties in England or the south of Scotland.'[26] Further south, in Angus, however, the reports regarding the frequency of agues had become more common. Parishes such as Kirkden, Tannadice, Careston, and Barrie on or near the Rivers Esk and Tay retell the story of earlier and more frequent encounters with ague, but virtually non-existent in the early 1790s because of 'draining of the grounds' and disappearance of 'stagnated water'.[27] Another area often mentioned as having ague was the Carse of Gowrie in Perthshire, a tract of alluvial meadow that remained an extensive marsh until drained and brought under cultivation before the end of the eighteenth century. Located between Perth and Dundee, the Carse was cited in several parish reports, including the frequently quoted 1793 account from Abernyte. 'Thirty years ago if a farmer in the spring wanted four of his cottagers for any piece of work, he generally ordered six knowing the probability that some of them, before the work could be finished, would be rendered unfit for labour by an attack of ague', read the chronicle.[28]

In the south, a number of parishes along the banks of the Tweed River in Berwickshire and Roxburghshire provided similar descriptions. In Eccles, for example, marsh miasma was blamed for ague. It was said to have been almost epidemic among 'the lower classes of people', but spared the gentry and more opulent farmers.[29] The parish of Roxburgh reported 'troublesome spring agues in two or three places which lie low and damp.'[30] Decades earlier, Kelso, Earlstoun, and Dunse recorded similar visitations of ague. In these accounts all parishes boasted in detail their notable improvements in agriculture since about 1780, especially the draining of marginal, marshy lands, the practice of crop rotation, and the growth of their cattle herds, now often left on the range year round. As Christopher Douglas, Kelso's physician and reporter wrote, 'since the introduction of turnip husbandry, the market is plentifully supplied with the very best-fed cattle during the whole year'.[31] Moreover, significant population gains between 1755 and 1795 in market towns like Berwick and Kelso reflected the new agricultural prosperity at a time when most rural Scottish parishes showed deficits, signalling a steady exodus of unemployed farmhands into manufacturing towns and cities or to permanent emigration across the Atlantic. Such were the paradoxes of efficiency and progress.

A final parish report should be mentioned. Although it was received from Kirkbean in south-east Galloway, and therefore located away from the areas most frequented by ague, it nevertheless confirmed the contemporary perception regarding the imported nature of this disease. The local minister writing his account repeated the assertion that ague was more frequent in earlier times; its decline attributed to agricultural improvements that drained the land and instituted an intensive system of crop rotation. According to the minister, however, knowledgeable individuals in the parish had another explanation: 'formerly many of the inhabitants went into Lincolnshire for employment during the harvest and returned infected with this disease.' Near the end of the century, however, these workers had found employment in their own parishes and therefore ague was no longer imported into the country.[32]

Medical views of ague

Like their colleagues in previous centuries, eighteenth-century practitioners were also fascinated and puzzled by the appearance and manifestations of this disease. The Italian physician Giovanni M. Lancisi (1655–1720) had already studied the marshes around Rome and published an influential treatise on the subject in 1717. Scottish physicians accepted the traditional linkage of ague with 'marsh *miasmata*', 'vapours' or 'effluvia' arising from fenny places where the shallow ground was excessively wet or marshy. The stagnant waters, a mixture of salt and rainwater, contained vegetable and animal matter prone to dissolve and putrefy under the influence of heat and moisture. It triggered a form of fermentation with release of noxious gases and contagious particles at small distances from the source, then rendered inert when carried further over land by winds.[33] Once inhaled, these vapours were believed to act as sedatives within the body. According to William Cullen, the leading medical academic in Edinburgh, the miasma actually caused enough debility in the neuromuscular system to allow the onset of vascular spasms which in turn triggered the initial cold stage of the ague fever, which was characterised by intense and prolonged chills.[34]

All British medical authors apparently were aware of the prevalence of ague fevers in south-eastern England. James Lind (1716–94) blamed this state of affairs on the evaporating qualities of the easterly winds that supposedly created the cold and debilitating foul air. Yet, individual predisposition remained an important factor for the miasma to affect the body. As widespread and serious sickness in the marsh country continuously created opportunities for employment, 'unseasoned' – meaning not acclimatised – newcomers came to the area ready to take the place of ailing natives, especially during harvest time. 'Many people who were formerly in the yearly habit of repairing to the eastern part of this country as reapers, imported this disorder on their return', wrote one practitioner in 1795.[35] However, the fever was far less common than formerly known, a circumstance arising either from earlier harvests or more probably 'the country being more cleared and better drained',[36] a development which Sinclair's nearly contemporary reports from Scottish parishes also stressed.

Its physicians duly noted the presence of ague in Scotland. William Cullen (1710–90) remarked in 1772 that 'very seldom a spring season passes in this part of Scotland [the lowlands] without more or less of the appearance of intermittents, especially among the vulgar'.[37] Even Edinburgh, with its neighbouring lakes and lochs, appeared similarly affected.[38] This vernal ague was described as being a mild disease, easily cured if left to nature while the autumnal fever could be quite severe and frequently fatal. Another Edinburgh professor, James Gregory (1753–1821) blamed the easterly winds blowing from the North Sea for the occurrence of ague and especially for the recurrence of febrile attacks.[39] Most of these fevers remained erratic in their pattern of fits, especially those appearing during the spring which were 'not of the same malignant nature as they are in the more southern parts of Europe'.[40] On occasion, the 'ague' was eventually discovered to be a manifestation of pulmonary consumption (Chapter 7). In 1785, one Edinburgh medical student justified his presentation on ague to members of the Royal Medical Society because of 'the intricate and dangerous nature' of the disease.[41] Scots seemed more prone to catch the ague when they visited Holland than did the Dutch themselves who lived in a moist environment.[42] However, in the Netherlands the sickness was generally autumnal, starting toward the end of August or early September, just like in the fens of southeastern England.[43] Indeed, in the opinion of James Gregory, most ague cases in Scotland were imported from England. Even Cullen in his clinical lectures admitted that before going to Edinburgh he had not seen a single patient suffering from ague in his twenty years of practice near Glasgow.[44]

Based on their clinical course, Cullen divided all fevers into two fundamental types: continuous and intermittent. The former was classified 'according as they show either an inflammatory irritation, synocha or typhus'.[45] Intermittents, for their part, were characterised by intense episodes of fever, each event separated from the next by regular intervals in which the affected individuals returned to normal temperatures and felt better. Following previous authors, Cullen distinguished a 'quotidian fever' in which febrile paroxysms occurred daily. More common, in his view, was the 'tertian intermittent' with intervals of forty-eight hours between fits, thus affecting patients every other day. Another form, the 'quartan intermittent', showed a seventy-two hour intermission between attacks. When these febrile peaks failed to display such a regularity, medical authors proposed the existence of other varieties, including a 'double tertian', with daily fever but serious paroxysms on alternate days. Furthermore, they created a 'quartan duplex' with two-day intermissions and a 'triple quartan' with daily fever but intermittent and irregular paroxysms. A host of other diagnostic categories such as a 'semi-tertian fever', 'sleepy tertian', 'convulsive tertian', 'partial quotidian', 'remitting quartan', tried to account for a host of erratic clinical pictures.[46] Some of Cullen's colleagues and students, however, strongly criticised such definitions, claimed they had the potential of limiting bedside observations. Nosological labels were thought to be no more than 'terms of art invented to reconcile the hypotheses of physicians' based on a perceived regularity that failed to prevail in nature (Chapters 7, 8 and 9).[47]

Such earnest efforts to characterise the varied symptomatology of ague and establish specific types attests to the clinical ambiguity and fluidity of its disease manifestations as witnessed by eighteenth-century practitioners. One contemporary way of explaining the erratic behaviour of the fever was to accept the idea that at the onset of febrile attacks the disease was still 'imperfectly formed'. Thus, it needed days or weeks before 'settling down' and finally 'revealing itself' as a genuine tertian or quartan variety to the attending physicians.[48] In many ways, the intermittent fever or ague was an ideal disease in which to observe and study the mysterious phenomenon of fever. Cullen, in fact, was so intrigued by the apparent patterns that he built his entire physiopathology around the clearly-marked stages of intermittent fever: cold, hot, and sweating phases.[49]

Eighteenth-century medical treatment of ague was cautious and empirical, dictated by practical considerations instead of an application of speculative theoretical principles. 'The only useful remedies with which we are acquainted are the offspring of empiricism', admitted Samuel Hinds, an Edinburgh medical student presenting a paper in 1785.[50] In fact, Cullen insisted the disease was 'most difficult to cure by art but most easily by nature'.[51] Populations affected by the scourge tended to medicate themselves, using strong spirits, pepper, as well as an infinite variety of folk charms and nostrums. Some tried to rid themselves of the scourge through magical rituals designed to transfer the fever to particular objects. Others ingested cobwebs and spiders based on archaic views that they represented useful antidotes capable of neutralising the poisonous nature of the disease. Opium in the form of laudanum was popularly believed to shorten and abate the recurring hot fits and so were drinks containing alcohol.[52]

Others, however, preferred cinchona or Peruvian bark, a bitter-tasting powder that could be mixed in water, juice, or alcoholic beverages. Hinds gave credit to the 'casual experience of an uncivilised people' – the natives of Peru – and 'the influence of a great religious society' – the Jesuits – for this specific febrifuge. Without the latter, Hinds added, 'this valuable medicine though brought to Europe might have remained in obscurity, unknown and useless'.[53] Although somewhat inhibited by Herman Boerhaave's (1668–1738) strong condemnation of stimulants, many medical practitioners also prescribed opiates freely. Physicians, however, were somewhat hesitant to administer the unpalatable Peruvian bark, giving it only in very small dosages to avoid upsetting their patients. Moreover, they feared that the bark infusion, if given too soon after the onset of a fit, would 'degenerate' the ague and transform it into a potentially dangerous and continuous fever.[54] Indeed, given its bitter flavour and indigestibility, most unhappy ague sufferers would only take this medication for three or four days, then discontinue its use and consequently suffer a relapse.

In Edinburgh, there was strong medical consensus that, for agues, the cinchona or Peruvian bark powder was the drug of choice, especially when given in higher dosages; Cullen remained cautious, claiming he lacked enough experience to fully evaluate the remedy. Its therapeutic action was explained as both astringent and tonic, and therefore, capable of overcoming the vascular weakness and spasms believed responsible for cold fits.[55] Not surprisingly, Cullen's employment of two stimulating remedies such as opium and the bark openly contradicted his theoretical notions about the nature of so-called 'phlogistic' diseases, including fevers. These ailments were usually considered effects of a systemic overstimulation rather than weakness of the vascular system, subject to bodily depletion measures such as bloodletting and the use of emetics and purgatives. Such fundamental inconsistencies between Cullen's theory and practice became a favourite target for a drumbeat of criticisms, especially at lively debates held at the Royal Medical Society. Further disputes arose among practitioners centred on the optimal timing of Peruvian bark administration, with Francis Home (1719–1813) carrying out a number of clinical trials between May 1769 and January 1779 at the Edinburgh Infirmary. Home's published conclusions revealed that the bark was more effective in stopping paroxysms when given at the end of a fever fit. Whether this was linked with the patient's ability to retain the bitter infusions of cinchona powder was not mentioned.[56]

Practitioners were cautioned that the recurrence of febrile paroxysms could not solely be stopped by the use of Peruvian bark, a notion similarly widespread among the public. Relapses of the disease were indeed common; especially when the doses prescribed or tolerated by the patients remained low. Another student member of the Royal Medical Society reminded his audience that 'in the fens of Lincolnshire, not withstanding the use of the bark in every form, the endemic often proves fatal'. [57] But the problem was not only dosage but also drug purity. Unfortunately, the eighteenth-century bark came in different colours – pale brown (official), yellow (flatus), and red (rubella), all obtained from different parts of the tree or from other species of cinchona.[58] All types of bark were imported from the New World and therefore quite expensive and limited in supply; the sale of substitutes was rampant. Another problem was to determine at any particular time which type of bark had a greater concentration of the active principle. Late in the century, some physicians selected the red bark as possessing superior, more potent qualities. Moreover, in an attempt to ameliorate the intense shivering of ague sufferers, contemporary physicians frequently prescribed opium before the fits and gave the bark later when the sweating ended and continued it until the start of another paroxysm. Employment of such drug mixtures made it even more difficult to ascertain the therapeutic effects of individual items of the materia medica. Bleeding was always an option for physicians who dealt with a fever, although many did not recommend it with ague. 'Would not the physician be thought insane who should attempt to cure intermittents by venesection?' questioned one Edinburgh student.[59] To cleanse the digestive system, purgatives and emetics were strongly encouraged. Practitioners also advocated the controlled use of wine and liquors, already widely used by the public. Between fits, exercise and a full diet featuring meat was desirable. In the end, most eighteenth-century physicians considered this therapeutic regimen highly successful, since it often lead to a considerable cessation of the fits and apparent recovery. The exceptions were patients already extremely weakened by recurrent bouts of ague, poor diet, and weeks of rough travel over primitive roads.[60] Incompletely cured intermittent fevers often led to other ailments, including the dreaded pulmonary consumption (Chapter 7).

Ague in Kelso

What can be learned about ague in Scotland from institutional records? In this regard a closer look at the frequently quoted statistics from the Kelso Dispensary is quite informative. Located in the Scottish Lowlands, this charitable institution had been established at the town of Kelso in 1777.[61] In addition to the institution's printed annual reports, a register of patients for the years 1777 to 1785 remained intact, providing important information on the incidence of ague in the entire region. From its inception, physicians and surgeons attending the Kelso Dispensary began to see an ever-increasing number of cases labelled as ague. In fact, this disease assumed truly epidemic proportions in 1781, gradually receding during the later 1780s.[62] While the average number of patients seen each year at Kelso was around six hundred men, women and children, individuals suffering from ague in the early 1780s comprised nearly twenty percent of the entire case-load. In 1781, for example, almost a third of all institutional visits were from persons believed to suffer from ague.[63] Patient registers shed further light on consultations related to ague. Nearly forty percent of those suffering from this disease came from the village of Kelso proper. The rest came from the parishes of Roxburgh, Eccles, Ednam, Earlstoren, Smalholm, Nenthorn, Sprouston, and Gordon – in order of decreasing frequency – all located in the adjacent counties of Roxburgh and Berwick. At times, the sick showed up at the Dispensary in families – parents in their early thirties or late twenties, accompanied by their children who were between the ages of four to thirteen. Among the 'recommenders' – those who were subscribers to the Kelso Dispensary and had the right to send patients – the registers listed a number of local landowners, parish ministers, and Kirk session organisers. For Kelso, the attending medical practitioners themselves often recommended individuals to the institution. Not too infrequently, the selected patient was simply a 'stranger' arriving from a number of more distant points in Scotland such as Edinburgh, Carlyle, Aberdeen, Dalkieth, Banff, and Fort George. From the town of Kelso, for example, the document lists, in 1781, 30-year-old George Anderson, his 40-year-old wife Isabel, together with their 5-year-old son Thomas, all seen on 2 March and pronounced cured by 2 April. Then, there were the Harts from Nenthorn, 21-year-old John, 18-year-old Thomas, 15-year-old Alex, and 10-year-old James, who arrived on 13 April of that same year. They were all listed as cured by 13 May and 8 June.[64] According to dates in the registers, most cases labelled as ague were seen during the spring, beginning early in March and extending into late June, with May being the peak month, an optimum time for relapses. Virtually no cases were recorded during the autumn although a few presented themselves in January and February. Those patients who presented with ague in the winter tended to remain under treatment longer. Both the printed annual reports and the surviving patient registers from the Kelso Dispensary document a steep rise in the incidence of ague in and around that town during the early 1780s. From the available evidence, the disease appeared to have been relatively mild, was easily managed, and even yielded 'cures' within two to four weeks.

Ague at the Edinburgh Infirmary

Beginning with the year 1770, another important source of information was the *General Register of Patients* from the Royal Infirmary of Edinburgh. The Register designated a number of individuals as suffering from ague who were sick enough to actually be hospitalised.[65] The Infirmary was quite famous in its time as a training institution for the local medical school, and it attracted patients from all over Scotland. Indeed, the hospital's status and its ability to negotiate contracts with the Royal Army and Navy drew a substantial number of teaching cases, among them servants, soldiers and seamen, as well as farmers who were brought into specially outfitted wards. However, admission of charity patients was restricted to those considered to be 'deserving', or, 'industrious' poor, willing to work and be responsible for their own economic independence and that of their families (Chapter 1). Contagious and terminally ill individuals and children were usually barred from entrance. All those seeking to enter the institution had to secure letters of recommendation from official sponsors. Admission forms were distributed to official hospital patrons who pledged yearly subscriptions or made other donations. Armed with such documentation, the sick presented themselves at the Infirmary's admissions room for screening and possible entry by the attending physicians.[66] Surviving folios of the Infirmary's *General Register of Patients* contain the name, entry date, and in-house destination for each patient. Clerks responsible for keeping these books later filled in the diagnosis, date of release, and discharge status. Between the years 1770 and 1794, a total of 903 cases of ague were recorded. The registers are incomplete from 1794 to 1800.[67] The data reveal that 70% of the patients diagnosed as suffering from ague were males. Regarding the seasonality of these hospital admissions, the highest month accounting for virtually 20% of all entries was May, followed by April (15%), June (13%), and March (11%). Indeed, taken together, these four months of spring were responsible for nearly two-thirds of all hospital admissions classified as ague. Moreover, if one follows the frequency of ague admissions per year, it becomes immediately clear that the Edinburgh Infirmary admitted a substantially greater number of cases between the years 1780 and 1785, thus mirroring the statistics compiled for the Kelso Dispensary in the Lowlands. In Edinburgh, however, the peak year for ague admissions was actually 1784, when a total of 116 patients diagnosed with this condition were allowed to enter the hospital. In spite of these impressive numbers, ague only represented 6.6% of all hospital admissions for that year.

Once admitted, patients suffering from ague were immediately assigned to specific hospital wards, a destination duly noted in the Register. The bulk – 64% – went into the general medical ward, while about 10% were transferred to the teaching unit placed under the direction of university professors. Nearly 14%, mostly soldiers and recruits, went to the soldiers ward. Finally, 11% ended up in a specially outfitted ward for servants. Such recorded patient destinations provide important clues about the types of persons affected with ague.[68] In the peak year 1784, for example, close to 40% of male admissions were members of Britain's armed forces. Moreover, in the early 1780s, a significant number of servants swelled the numbers of those who came to the Infirmary with ague. The median length of stay in the hospital for all patients diagnosed with ague remained relatively brief:

sixteen days. No important variations in hospital stay could be ascertained between male and female patients, except for a small group of men who remained in the establishment for more than eight weeks. When the length of stay was separately plotted for each hospital destination, only the teaching ward showed an important deviation from the average. Indeed, the median stay in that unit for ague-related symptoms was almost three weeks. This suggests that perhaps teaching cases tended to be more physically compromised or hospitalisation was extended for didactic reasons by the professors in charge.[69] A final word about mortality. The Edinburgh Infirmary's *General Register* overwhelmingly listed ague patients as being discharged as 'cured'. In fact, only four deaths were reported among the 903 patients recorded in the folios, all of them occurring in the 1770s. From other sources, however, it appears that a small number of teaching ward cases did actually succumb to the disease, but the information was conveniently omitted from the Register. In spite of occasional documentary tampering for political reasons – low mortality statistics made the hospital look successful and attracted donations (Chapter 1) – it seems fair to conclude that ague or intermittent fever must have been a relatively benign disease, successfully controlled during a two-week average institutional stay.[70]

Ague in Edinburgh casebooks

A final but extremely important piece of information regarding ague also derives from the Edinburgh Infirmary. The information consists of detailed case histories for thirty-one patients admitted to the institution's teaching ward with a diagnosis of ague between the years 1771 and 1799. These individuals were managed between November and April since this ward was only open during the academic year under the direction of a university professor. All the cases were extracted from medical student notebooks. Students visiting the Edinburgh Infirmary were allowed to copy individual clinical cases from the available ward journals. Because the original hospital ledgers are no longer available, these student notebooks furnish some key and unique information about patients' medical progress and management. Each case begins with a brief history of the circumstances regarding the patient's complaints, followed by a description of the most striking symptoms, length of suffering, and prior treatments. Next, the clinical condition and daily management of the patient was recorded along with a list of dietary recommendations, drug prescriptions, and orders for other treatments such as massage, bleedings, and even electrification. In addition to daily progress notes, each case finished with a discharge category that reveals the perceived level of recovery: 'cured', 'relieved', 'improper', or 'incurable' (Chapter 7).

With the exception of two individuals with incomplete histories, most cases of so-called ague or intermittent fever extracted from the notebooks had one thing in common: the patients had fallen ill while temporarily working in the fens of Lincolnshire, Cambridgeshire, Norfolk, or Kent during the previous autumn harvest. Many became so disabled that they had to be conveyed home by carts or wagons. Ten of the eighteen male patients could be identified as labourers. No occupational label was given to the thirteen female patients, but in their clinical histories they also admitted participating in harvest work. Another inmate, a soldier, had returned from the south of France, a region where malaria was also endemic. A middle-aged female, revealed that she had resided in Holland for fourteen years during which she suffered two separate bouts of the disease.[71] The average age of the male patient was thirty-two while the women inmates were somewhat younger, around twenty-seven years of age. Case histories of male patients indicated the average duration of their feverish complaints was about six and a half weeks. Close to half of them had already received some form of treatment. By contrast, female patients had been sick for almost eleven weeks on average, twice as long as the men, with less than a third of them getting any form of relief.

Once admitted to the Infirmary, male and female patients who were suspected of suffering from ague remained about four weeks in the institution and had an eleven to fifteen percent mortality rate. All were subjected to a so-called stimulating regimen of treatment, which involved the administration of tonics, including the popular Peruvian bark. More than half of them also received purgatives, still a staple of traditional humoral medicine. No patient was bled, but a handful was subjected to small electrical sparks between fits in an attempt to generate additional perspiration and thereby possibly pre-empting the next paroxysm. The rationale for electric treatment was equally humoral: the dramatic bouts of ague fever suggested a state of internal poisoning with the body's natural healing forces attempting to eliminate the venom via the skin through profuse sweating. If physicians could imitate and actually anticipate these natural discharges, further fits would no longer be necessary and the patient could be cured. Practitioners also recommended generous diets, supplemented with meat, wine, and even gin punch to further support the ailing bodies. From the clinical histories it seems clear that the final outcome of hospitalisation was very much influenced by the general condition of the patients before admission. For example, Kenneth Stewart, a 20-year-old labourer, had contracted the ague in England six weeks before returning to Scotland. After becoming very sick, both he and his brother, who also suffered from the disease, attempted to return home in an open wagon. The brother, unfortunately, died on the way. The sick young man, upon admission to the Edinburgh Infirmary on 6 October 1781, was described as quite pale, with abdominal pain and swelling over the region of the spleen. Diagnosed with a fully developed tertian type of fever, he died a month later in spite of all medical efforts to save him.[72]

In early February 1795, Leslie Campbell, a 22-year-old married woman and her 3-year-old child, Margaret, were admitted together with a diagnosis of ague. According to the attending physicians, the mother's fits seemingly corresponded to a quartan, the child suffered from a tertian type. Both claimed to have fallen sick three months earlier, after spending time in Stamford, Lincolnshire. Leslie was described as emaciated and with a sallow complexion, and her menstrual periods had not returned for nearly seven months following the weaning of her child. Fortunately, substantial doses of cinchona, administered orally to both Leslie and Margaret in the form of enemas, together with a good diet, turned things around and both patients survived their ordeal, leaving the Infirmary in better condition after a stay of ten weeks.[73] Progress notes placed in the Infirmary's clinical charts indicate that when physicians were able to administer larger amounts of Peruvian bark, the fever fits tended to cease. Although mixed with water, juices, or wine to make it more palatable, and administered to patients in divided doses, the cinchona powder remained a bitter draught for most patients to swallow and retain. Yet, the empirical findings of the bark's efficacy in the treatment of ague strengthened the hand of practitioners who argued for induction in the framing of scientific theory. 'Few medical theories have either truth or utility enough to enable us to predict', wrote James Mackintosh (1765–1832), a contemporary Edinburgh medical student, in his discussion of tertian fever. 'It is their highest praise if they can be reconciled to whatever empiricism or accident has discovered'.[74] While patient registers from both the Kelso Dispensary and the Edinburgh Infirmary suggested that ague in Scotland usually tended to be a benign and mostly curable disease, the cases extracted from student notebooks actually represented a special population of inmates. Indeed, more than two-thirds of them were admitted during the winter months following extended and stressful voyages from the endemic areas of south-east England where they had experienced the first debilitating paroxysms of ague. Precisely because of the severity of their symptoms, these patients were selected to the teaching ward because Edinburgh professors wanted their students to witness the medical management of typical and challenging cases.

Solving the puzzle:
ague in context

Based on the extensive historical information for Europe and especially south-west England,[75] one can convincingly assume that the bulk of eighteenth-century intermittent fevers or agues corresponded to what we now describe as being malaria, a characteristic parasitic disease that continues to prevail in many areas of the globe. Authors have established the probable presence of two agents, the *Plasmodium vivax* and *malariae*, in the blood stream of selected populations of eighteenth-century Europe, with occasional appearances of *Plasmodium falciparum*, more lethal and common in the tropics. In southeastern England the disease remained endemic until the early twentieth century.[76] Given the characteristics of its climate, this would not have been the case in Scotland. Cold winters and the brevity of warm weather would have made it very difficult for infected local mosquito populations to survive in significant numbers.[77] One must, therefore, conclude that ague in Scotland was mostly an import, a disease introduced by a steady stream of migrant workers and servants returning from England, traders from Holland and the rest of the Continent, and soldiers and mariners from tropical British colonies.[78] Once in Scotland, malaria temporarily spread into limited geographical areas, aided by local topography, microclimate, and availability of infected mosquito populations. Stagnant pools within marshes constituted ideal breeding grounds.

One can identify two types of people who brought ague to Scotland. First there were those individuals who experienced the initial episode while still at work during the late summer in the malaria-infested areas of south-west England. With the local workforce ravaged by malarial attacks and unable to cope with harvest work, seasonal imports were sought from surrounding regions. Among them were unemployed Scots, whose lack of immunity made them targets for malarial infection, following a normal incubation period of about two to three weeks for *Plasmodium vivax*. Most of these men and women experienced their first bout within the regions endemic for the disease. After the harvest, these sick labourers returned to Scotland, weakened by disease, poor diet, and strenuous travel. Here, many continued to suffer periodic and debilitating fits of fever well into the ensuing winter. Some malaria victims, already weakened by malnutrition – commonly anaemia and scurvy – were also prone to other ailments, including consumption and enteric conditions such as dysentery and typhus. Their subsequent fever paroxysms tended to become longer and more violent, accompanied by excruciating chest pains, weight loss, sometimes followed by death. Other malaria victims gradually recovered, going into spontaneous remission, only to experience further debilitating relapses of their disease during the following spring.[79]

A second group of ague sufferers actually had their first detectable febrile attacks in Scotland, nearly eight or nine months after returning from the English marshes. Here one can surmise that the responsible malarial parasite – *P. vivax* or *malariae* – had remained dormant in their bodies. As the evidence shows, a significant number of Scots suffered from the ague between February and May, a fact reflected in both the patient registers of the Kelso Dispensary and Edinburgh Infirmary as well as various parish reports. Since spring was always a critical period in the agricultural cycle, any disabling health problem, especially a high fever, received considerable attention. The economic implication of disabilities made ague a most unwelcome guest of the Scottish labourer. Some of victims usually had mild attacks and were expected to recover even without the employment of medicines.[80] There was, however, a third contingent of ague sufferers who periodically contracted the disease without leaving Scotland. There was no collective immunity to malaria in the Scottish population because the disease was never endemic in any particular area of the country. Yet, conditions for occasional direct infections with malarial parasites certainly existed. Local infected mosquitoes could easily infect an entire family who often lived in the same house with carriers or victims of malaria. The most common anopheline carriers – the *atroparvus* and *maculipennis* – were ideal culprits of infection because they bred in slightly saline water and easily entered human habitats.[81] Such contacts took place near marshes and during mild winters, when the dilapidated rural cottages became ideal hibernating spaces for infected vectors. This scenario could easily play itself out in circumscribed and protected coastal areas near the Firth of Tay as well as the Tweed estuary in Berwickshire.

Periodic forms of importation by a mobile population of Scottish farmhands working in south-west England, coupled with an occasional indigenous outbreak may have accounted for the rather sporadic presence of ague in Scotland throughout the eighteenth century. In view of what happened during the early 1780s in the Scottish Lowlands it is more difficult to explain the apparent epidemic episodes of this disease. How can the information gathered from the Kelso Dispensary and Edinburgh Infirmary registers be properly interpreted? Today we know that certain climatic, biological, and social conditions must be just right for epidemics of malaria to emerge. Often, even today, the exact causes of such events are difficult to determine, even though the problem is localised. Indeed, for malaria to become epidemic, a combination of factors must be in place. Firstly, the community must harbour a fair number of asymptomatic carriers with malarial parasites in their bloodstream; secondly, there should be a sudden increase in the number of mosquitoes capable of transmitting the plasmodium; and, finally, plenty of human bodies for the infected vectors to obtain their blood meals. The famous Kelso outbreak of 1781–2 in the Scottish Lowlands is congruous with such a confluence of factors.[82] The surviving evidence suggests that population growth and greater migration from the Highlands had created a veritable glut of seasonal workers in the region. As a hiring market for farm servants, Kelso sponsored a number of job fairs and certainly received more than its share of transient labourers, many of them previously exposed to malaria in the English fens. Those who stayed in farms surrounding the town lived in dark, confined, and filthy hovels not far from the swamps surrounding Kelso on the northern side of the Tweed River. Neighbouring parishes customarily provided separate cottages in the countryside to unmarried servants and working families who received board and cash wages. This practice brought a substantial number of young adults from different parts of the country into closer contact with each other. Also, dunghills, which created favourable conditions for the survival of infected anopheline hosts and their infective plasmodia often surrounded both townhouses and small rows of thatched, windowless cottages in the country.[83]

Another critical factor was the weather. According to extant meteorological records, the Scottish Lowlands were subjected to unusual climatic patterns between the years 1781 and 1787.[84] Most of this period experienced excessive rainfall during winter and spring, especially during the year 1782, when the area had one of the wettest months of May on record. This circumstance combined with an early snow created severe and extensive crop failures, triggering high unemployment among farm hands. Temperatures, on the other hand, were above normal from March to October with exceptionally warm and dry summers.[85] Strong easterly winds in the early 1780s may have possibly transported additional mosquito populations from the salt marshes in Berwickshire. Since the surrounding countryside around Kelso was still 'studded with swamps and morasses', stagnant pools of water created ideal conditions for breeding a larger population of malaria vectors.[86] Taken together, these circumstances help explain the sudden and unusual raise of malaria infections in the southern counties of Scotland.

Paradoxically, following the epidemics, ague appeared to decline in the late 1780s in south-west England and virtually disappeared from Scotland by the turn of the century. A contemporary explanation for its disappearance was the rise of agriculture.[87] Drainage of relatively impermeable clay soils in the Lowlands eliminated stagnant pools of water in many previously marshy areas, reducing mosquito populations. Struggling tenants were converted into prosperous farmers by growing tobacco and turnips; their living conditions, housing and diet improved.[88] Cultivation and drainage, while important, cannot however provide the whole answer for the decline of ague. Certainly, the anopheline vectors of malaria were robbed of their possible summer breeding grounds, but among Sinclair's parish reports, there were certainly a few that claimed a waning of ague while their marshlands still remained intact. As Adam Smith indicated in his *Wealth of Nations*, the increase in livestock and the improvement of land were parallel events.[89] Indeed, the new agriculture made it possible to usher in what was termed the 'turnip husbandry'. Land enclosure and abolition of infield and outfield systems of cultivation in favour of a rotation plan included root crops capable of feeding cattle, allowing herds to remain on the range during winters. Together with proper summer pastures, these changes allowed for the rapid multiplication of cattle and sheep.[90] After 1780, around Aberdeen, Angus, and the Scottish lowlands, it became profitable to bring cattle into these areas to be fed and fattened before export to England.[91] By 1800, for example, Berwickshire had 14,500 head of English shorthorn cattle; Roxburghshire, 16,400. There is no question that, given the partially zoophilic tendencies of the atroparvus and messeae mosquitoes, some of these insects began to detour from humans to cattle in search for their blood meals.

At the same time, the new demands of mixed farming, no longer seasonal, now precluded many farm hands from having to make yearly harvest migrations to the dangerous south-west English fens. Healthier local populations in those areas also lowered the demand for migrant labour. The reporter from Kirkbean parish in Galloway observed this trend. In the Lowlands, landless servants, often seasonally unemployed, could be hired for one year if married, six months if single. For those without farm jobs, urban employment at the growing textile industries nearby in Edinburgh or Berwick became attractive alternatives. Here, the incipient Industrial Revolution created new jobs, thereby indirectly helping to stop the exodus to England and the periodic importation of ague from the south and abroad.[92] Following the War of Independence, emigration to the former colonies in America was another attractive choice. Finally, changes in housing taking place in Scotland during this period proved less hospitable to mosquitoes. Gone were some of the dark and humid resting places for the irritating 'gnats'. As Sinclair rightly observed, 'since the houses of the tenantry and labourers were built of better materials, and rendered more convenient, warm, and cleanly, sickness is not so frequent'.[93] All these changes must have played an important role in the epidemiology of malaria.

Also not to be ignored were the increasingly effective medical treatments with sufficient doses of cinchona, self-administered or provided by physicians to suppress the febrile fits. Infusions and tinctures of the Jesuits' powder replaced the generous use of opium and alcohol, which had often led to addiction and poor health. Many sufferers were probably no longer infectious after receiving what would have amounted to near curative doses of the drug.[94] Thus, solving the riddle regarding the presence of ague in eighteenth-century Scotland must take into account the country's unique geography and climate, as well as the agricultural and industrial revolutions which took place on its soil late in that century. Diseases such as ague not only shaped Scottish history: their origins and evolution were expressions of an ecology that owed much to the particular biological, social, and economic forces that moulded Scotland in the late-eighteenth century.

Notes

1. W. Buchan, 'Intermitting Fevers or Agues', in *Domestic Medicine*, 9th edn (London: A. Strahan, 1786), 164.
2. G.E.R. Lloyd (ed.), 'Airs, Waters and Places', in *Hippocratic Writings*, trans. J. Chadwick and W.N. Mann (Harmonsworth: Penguin Books, 1978), 148–69.
3. The genre is fashionable. Among recent works see S. Watts, *Disease and Medicine in World History* (New York: Routledge, 2003), and K.F. Kiple (ed.), *The Cambridge World History of Human Disease* (New York: Cambridge University Press, 1993).
4. See K.F. Kiple, 'The Ecology of Disease', in W.F. Bynum and R. Porter (eds), *Companion Encyclopedia of the History of Medicine*, 2 vols (London: Routledge, 1993), Vol. 1, 357–81; also W.H. McNeill, *The Human Condition: An Ecological and Historical View* (Princeton: Princeton University Press, 1980).
5. W. Balée, 'Historical Ecology: Premises and Postulates', in W. Balée (ed.), *Advances in Historical Ecology* (New York: Columbia University Press, 1998), 13–29.
6. Background information is available in A. Learmonth, *Disease Ecology: An Introduction* (Oxford: Blackwell, 1988); see also N.F. Stanley and R.A. Joske (eds), *Changing Disease Patters and Human Behavior* (London: Academic Press, 1980).
7. For example, J. Riera Palmero and A. Rojo Vega, 'Spanish Agriculture and Malaria in the 18th Century', *History and Philosophy of the Life Sciences,* 10 (1988), 343–62; J. Riera Palmero, 'Work, Rice, and Malaria in Valencia in the Eighteenth-Century', *Physis,* 31 (1994), 771–85.
8. L.J. Bruce-Chwatt, 'Ague as Malaria: An Essay on the History of Two

Medical Terms', *Journal of Tropical Medicine and Hygiene,* 79 (1976), 168–76. Another hypothesis derives the word from the Gothic term 'agis', meaning trembling: H.A. Skinner, *The Origin of Medical Terms* (New York: Hafner, 1970), 12.

9. For malaria in Antiquity, consult M.D. Grmek, 'Porotic Hyperostosis, Hereditary Anemias and Malaria', in *Diseases in the Ancient World,* trans. M. Muellner and L. Muellner (Baltimore: Johns Hopkins University Press, 1989), 245–83.
10. M. Dobson, '"Marsh Fever": The Geography of Malaria in England', *Journal of Historical Geography,* 6 (1980), 357–89; and more recently by the same author 'Malaria in England: A Geographical and Historical Perspective', *Parassitologia,* 36 (1994), 35–60.
11. Consult S. Mason, *The Nature of an Intermittent Fever and Ague Consider'd* (London: J. Hodges, 1745). For a discussion of medical terminology, J.H. Dirckx, *The Language of Medicine: Its Evolution, Structure and Dynamics* (New York: Praeger, 1983).
12. W. Cullen, Clinical Lectures (Edinburgh: 1772–3), MSS Collection, Royal College of Physicians, Edinburgh, 127.
13. See comments by R. Porter in 'The Body and the Mind, the Doctor and the Patient: Negotiating Hysteria', in S. Gilman *et al., Hysteria Beyond Freud* (Berkeley: University of California Press, 1993), 225–6.
14. M.J. Dobson, 'Marshlands, Mosquitoes and Malaria', in *Contours of Death and Disease in Early Modern England* (Cambridge: Cambridge University Press, 1997), 306–27.
15. L.J. Bruce-Chwatt, 'The Anopheles Vector', in *Essential Malariology,* 2nd edn (New York: Wiley, 1985), 149–54; see also F.L. Dunn, 'Malaria', in Kiple, *op. cit.* (note 3), 855–62.
16. L.W. Hackett, *Malaria in Europe: An Ecological Study* (London: Oxford University Press, 1944); L.J. Bruce-Chwatt and J. de Zuleta, *The Rise and Fall of Malaria in Europe* (Oxford: Oxford University Press, 1980), 131–5.
17. See J. Ritchie, 'Ague in Scotland', in *The Influence of Man on Animal Life in Scotland: A Study in Faunal Evolution* (Cambridge: Cambridge University Press, 1920), 508–13.
18. For example, J.H. Brotherston, 'The Decline of Malaria', in *Observations on the Early Public Health Movement in Scotland* (London: H. K. Lewis & Co, 1952), 26–36.
19. The topic generated enough interest to spawn a dissertation by M.D.L. Finlay, 'An Enquiry into "the Ague" in Scotland', MD thesis, University of Edinburgh, 1978. See a summary 'Was Ague Malaria?', *Royal College of Physicians of Edinburgh Chronicle,* 9 (1979), 14–19. The author argues that ague was not malaria and could never have been endemic in Scotland.

20. One author, E.H. Ackerknecht, remarked that 'epidemiological and historical research embracing all aspects of the malaria problem rather confirm the thesis of the fundamentally social character of malaria'. See his *Malaria in the Upper Mississippi Valley, 1760–1900* (Baltimore: Johns Hopkins Press, 1945), 130. For background, H.M. Dutta and A.K. Dutt, 'Malarial Ecology: A Global Perspective', *Sociology, Science and Medicine,* 12 (1978), 69–84.
21. J. Sinclair, *Analysis of the Statistical Account of Scotland,* II parts (Edinburgh: A. Constable, 1825), reprint (New York: Johnson Reprint Corp., 1970), part I, 110.
22. *Ibid.*, 'On the diseases of Scotland', part I, section III, 135.
23. *Ibid.* For geographic orientation, consult T. Kitchin, *Geographia Scotiae* (London: S. Birt, 1749); G. Taylor, *Taylor and Skinner's Survey and Maps of the Roads of North Britain and Scotland* (London, 1776).
24. *Ibid.*
25. *Ibid.*
26. J. Sinclair, 'Parish of Peterhead', in *The Statistical Account of Scotland, Drawn up from Communications of the Ministers of the Different Parishes,* XXI vols (Edinburgh: W. Creech, 1791–9), Vol. XVI, 546. For a review of conditions in Scotland based on these parish reports, see J. Murray, *Life in Scotland a Hundred Years Ago as Reflected in the Old Statistical Account of Scotland, 1791–1799* (Paisley: A. Gardner, 1900).
27. *Ibid.*, 'Parish of Kirkden', Vol. II, 506; 'Parish of Careston', Vol. II, 483–4; 'Parish of Barrie', Vol. IV, 236–7; 'Parish of Tannadice', Vol. XIX, 372–83. More details in M. Steven, *Parish Life in Eighteenth-Century Scotland: A Review of the Old Statistical Account* (Aberdeen: Scottish Cultural Press, 1995).
28. *Ibid.*, 'Parish of Abernyte', Vol. IX, 140. Drainage of the Carse was described in J. Macculloch, *Malaria: An Essay on the Production and Propagation of this Poison* (London: Longman, Rees, Orme, Brown & Green, 1827), 38.
29. *Ibid.*, 'Parish of Eccles', Vol. XI, 230–42.
30. *Ibid.*, 'Parish of Roxburgh', Vol. XIX, 129.
31. *Ibid.*, 'Parish of Kelso', Vol. X, 588.
32. *Ibid.*, 'Parish of Kirkbean', Vol. XV, 121.
33. Anonymous, 'Causes of Insalubrity in Marshy Situations', in *The Edinburgh Practice of Physic, Surgery, and Midwifery,* 5 vols (London: G. Kearsley, 1803), Vol. I, 186; see also R. Robertson, *On Fevers which Arise from Marsh Miasmata and from Other Causes* (London, 1807). An essay delivered on November 1779 by R. Buck, a member of the Royal Medical Society of Edinburgh, was entitled 'What are the Qualities of Marsh Miasma Necessary to Produce Intermittent Fever?' It was transcribed in *Dissertations Read to the*

Royal Medical Society, Edinburgh (Diss. RMS), 95 vols. (Edinburgh: 1751–1833), MSS Collection, Edinburgh University Library, Vol. 11 (1778), 370–80.

34. W. Cullen, *First Lines of the Practice of Physic,* new edn, IV vols (Edinburgh: C. Elliot, 1788), Vol. I, 140–2.
35. A., *The Edinburgh Practice, op. cit.* (note 33), 141; see also the appendix on intermittent fevers in J. Lind, *Essay on the Diseases Incidental to Europeans in Hot Climates* (London: T. Becket, 1768).
36. *Ibid.*, 141. The remarks were attributed to a surgeon, Mr. Bradley, whose complete case of tertian fever was reprinted.
37. W. Cullen, Clinical Lectures delivered for John Gregory, February–April 1772 (Edinburgh, 1772), MSS Collection, Royal College of Physicians, Edinburgh, 281.
38. [J.C. Lettsom], *Reflections on the General Treatment and Cure of Fevers* (London: J.D. Cornish, 1772), 13. Even Cullen characterized East Lothian as 'aguish country'. See Cullen, *op. cit.* (note 12), 546–7.
39. James Gregory, Clinical Lectures (Edinburgh, 1783), in Medical Tracts II recorded by John Unthank, a student notebook in my possession.
40. Cullen, *op. cit.* (note 37), 282.
41. W. Hutchinson, 'Intermittent Fever', *Diss. RMS,* Vol. 18 (1785–7), 173–86. Several Edinburgh medical students wrote their dissertations on this important topic. See, for example, F. Buchanan, *De Febribus Intermttentibus Medendo* (Edinburgh: Balfour and Smellie, 1783); R.B. Spratt, *De Febre Intermittente* (Edinburgh: Balfour and Smellie, 1793); and A. Baron, *De Febre Intermittente* (Edinburgh: R, Allan, 1799).
42. F. Home, *Clinical Lectures Delivered in the Year 1769,* taken by John Goodsir (Edinburgh, 1769), MSS Collection, Royal College of Physicians, Edinburgh, 68.
43. The experience of managing labourers returning from the fens of Lincolnshire at St Thomas' Hospital in London is contained in G. Fordyce, *A Second Dissertation on Fever* (London: J. Johnson, 1795).
44. Cullen, *op. cit.* (note 12), 547.
45. W. Cullen, *Nosology or Systematic Arrangement of Diseases by Classes, Orders, Genera, and Species,* trans. from Latin (Edinburgh: W. Creech, 1800), 37. For the 'typhus' variety, see G.B. Risse, '"Typhus" Fever in Eighteenth-Century Hospitals: New Approaches to Medical Treatment', *Bulletin of the History of Medicine,* 59 (1985), 176–95.
46. For a complete summary of the nosological categories, see Anon., *op. cit.* (note 33), Vol. I, 123–95; and W. Cullen, 'Intermittents', in *Synopsis and Nosology,* trans. from Latin (Hartford: N. Patten, 1792), 1–5.
47. J. Mackintosh, 'Tertian Fever', *Diss. RMS,* Vol. 20 (1786–7), 204–22.

48. Cullen, Clinical Lectures for John Gregory, *op. cit.* (note 37), 281–2.
49. See W.F. Bynum, 'Cullen and the Study of Fever in Britain, 1760–1820', in W.F. Bynum and V. Nutton (eds), *Theories of Fever From Antiquity to the Enlightenment* (London: Wellcome Institute for the History of Medicine, 1981), 135–147.
50. S. Hinds, 'Has the Investigation of Proximate Causes Benefited the Practice of Medicine?', *Diss. RMS,* Vol. 19 (1785–6), 93–103.
51. Cullen, *op. cit.* (note 12), 127.
52. Widespread consumption among English farm workers is documented in V. Berridge, 'Fenland Opium Eating in the Nineteenth Century', *British Journal of Addiction,* 72 (1977), 275–84.
53. Hinds, *op. cit.* (note 50), 101.
54. Home, Clinical Lectures, *op. cit.* (note 42), 77.
55. To avoid the gastric side effects, a solution of bark was often administered by enema. See Cullen, *op. cit.* (note 12), 527–31. Decades earlier, Simon Mason – a Cambridge apothecary – had already employed the cinchona bark in Fenland patients with apparently great success. See Mason, *op. cit.* (note 11).
56. F. Home, 'Experiments with Regard to the Most Proper Time of Giving the Bark in Intermittents', in *Clinical Experiments, Histories, and Dissections,* 3rd edn (London: J. Murray, 1783), 1–13.
57. J. Lawson, 'What Are the Effects of Peruvian Bark?', *Diss. RMS,* Vol. 14 (1782–3), 384–5.
58. Anon., *op. cit.* (note 33), Vol. I, 132–3. For background, D.L. Cowen, 'The Edinburgh Pharmacopea', *Medical History,* 1, 2 (1957), 123-139.
59. W. Alexander, *Diss. RMS,* Vol. 19 (1785–6), 244.
60. *Ibid.*, 126–132. See also W. Saunders, *Observations on the Superior Efficacy of the Red Peruvian Bark in the Cure of Agues and Other Fevers,* 2nd edn (London: J. Johnson, 1782); S. James, *Observations on the Bark of a Particular Species of Willow Showing its Superiority to the Peruvian* (London: J. Johnson, 1792). For a summary M.J. Dobson, 'Bittersweet Solutions for Malaria: Exploring Natural Remedies from the Past', *Parassitologia,* 40 (1998), 69–81.
61. C. Wilson, 'Statistical Observations on the Health of the Labouring Population of the District of Kelso in Two Decennial Periods, From 1777 to 1787 and from 1829 to 1839', *Proceedings of the Border Medical Society,* (1841), 47–85. More details will be available my essay, 'Walk-in Physic in the Scottish Lowlands: The Kelso Dispensary, 1777–1802', in preparation.
62. *Ibid.*, 58–60. The statistics were also published in C. Creighton, 'The Epidemic Agues of 1780–1785', in *A History of Epidemics in Britain,* 2 vols (Cambridge: Cambridge University Press, 1894), Vol. 2, 366–70.

63. Table with the diseases of patients admitted to the Kelso Dispensary, printed in the annual reports *The State of Kelso Dispensary* (Kelso, 1780–81), Scottish Records Office, Edinburgh.
64. See lists of patients, giving age, diagnosis, and result of treatments, Kelso Dispensary documents, 1777–83, Scottish Records Office, Edinburgh.
65. G.B. Risse, 'Ague or Intermittent Fever', in *Hospital Life in Enlightenment Scotland: Care and Teaching at the Royal Infirmary of Edinburgh* (New York: Cambridge University Press, 1986), 133–35.
66. *Ibid.*, 82–89.
67. Edinburgh Infirmary, General Register of Patients, MSS Collection, Edinburgh University Library. Each volume contains between 500–600 pages. Because of the recording irregularities and omissions, twenty-five additional cases from 1794 to 1800 were omitted from the statistical analysis.
68. For patient destinations, see Risse, *op. cit.* (note 65), 89–108.
69. This occurred rather frequently. See *ibid.*, 172–6.
70. *Ibid.*, 228–38.
71. Case of Margaret McKay, in Thomas C. Hope, Clinical Casebook (Edinburgh, 1796–7), MSS Collection, Royal College of Physicians, Edinburgh. Such a therapeutic approach was often labeled 'Brunonian' – based on the theories and practices advocated by John Brown who was an extramural lecturer at the Edinburgh Medical Scholl between 1778 and 1782.
72 . Case of Kenneth Stewart, in John Hope, Cases of Patients in the Royal Infirmary Under the Cure of John Hope, MD, Edinburgh, 1781, MSS Collection, Edinburgh University. The entire patient record appears among selected clinical cases in Risse, *op. cit.* (note 65), 321–6.
73 . Cases of Leslie and Margaret Campbell, in Andrew Duncan, Sr, Clinical Reports and Commentaries, February–April 1795, presented by A.B. Morison (Edinburgh, 1795), MSS Collection, Royal College of Physicians, Edinburgh. For more details of Leslie's treatment see J.W. Estes, 'Drug Usage at the Infirmary: The Example of Dr Andrew Duncan, Sr', in Risse, *op. cit.* (note 65), 359–60.
74. Mackintosh, *op. cit.* (note 47), 214.
75. Dobson's extensive demographic study of the region during the seventeenth and eighteenth centuries includes maps, parish records and contemporary manuscript sources. See Dobson, *op. cit.* (note 14), 287–367.
76. G. Macdonald, 'Local Features of Malaria: North European and Asiatic Zone', in *The Epidemiology and Control of Malaria* (London: Oxford University Press, 1957), 71–3; and Bruce-Chwatt, 'Epidemiology of Malaria', in *op. cit.* (note 15), 166–209.

77. See, for example, P.F. Mattingly, 'Origin and Evolution of the Human Malarias: The Role of the Vector', *Parassitologia,* 15 (1973), 169–72; and his work *The Biology of Mosquito-Born Disease* (London: Allen & Unwin, 1969).
78. Among those afflicted by the disease in the 1750s were invalided soldiers from the Scots Brigade who had fought in Holland. See W. Grant, *An Enquiry into the Nature, Rise and Progress of the Fevers Most Common in London* (London: T. Cadell, 1771), 72.
79. Bruce-Chwatt, 'Vivax Malaria', in *op. cit.* (note 15), 57–9.
80. Unfortunately Scotland's old parish registers at the General Register Office tend to be rather cryptic in their entries and the majority omit causes of death until 1855. For information regarding Scotland's rural society and economy, R.A. Dodgshon, *Land and Society in Early Scotland* (Oxford: Clarendon Press, 1981).
81. One nineteenth-century author argued that Eastern winds brought malaria from Holland during spring. See J. Maccullough, *Malaria: An Essay on the Production and Propagation of this Poison* (Philadelphia: T. Kite, 1829), 149.
82. G.H.F. Nutall *et al.,* 'The Geographical Distribution of Anopheles in Relation to the Former Distribution of Ague in England', *Journal of Hygiene,* 1 (1901), 5–12, 23, 31; see also Bruce-Chwatt, 'Genesis of Malaria Epidemics', in *op. cit.* (note 15), 173–6.
83. For background information, M. Lochhead, *The Scots Household in the Eighteenth Century* (Edinburgh: Moray Press, 1948); and A.C. Chitnis, *The Scottish Enlightenment: A Social History* (London: Croom Helm, 1976).
84. 'Register of the Weather', in *Transactions of the Royal Society of Edinburgh,* 1 (1788), 206.
85. For Edinburgh, see R.C. Mossman's rainfall and temperature charts in *Transactions of the Royal Society of Edinburgh,* 39 (1896–9), 116 and 143.
86. K. Duncan, 'The Possible Influence of Climate on Historical Outbreaks of Malaria in Scotland', *Proceedings of the Royal College of Physicians, Edinburgh,* 23 (1993), 55–62.
87. Details in H. Hamilton, 'Agrarian Change', in *An Economic History of Scotland in the Eighteenth Century* (Oxford: Clarendon Press, 1963), 55–71. The author describes the effects of the Forfeited Estates Commissioners in Perthshire resulting in enclosures, drainage through the use of dykes and planting of moorland. Eviction of tenants in certain overcrowded estates was also mentioned. With increasing numbers of cattle being brought to the area to be fattened before export to England, those animals may have been ideal substitute targets of the remaining infected mosquito population.
88. See J.H. Bayliss, 'Epidemiological Considerations of the History of Indigenous Malaria in Britain', *Endeavour,* 9 (1985), 191–4. See also two works of J.E. Handley, *Scottish Farming in the Eighteenth Century* (London:

Faber & Faber, 1953), and *The Agricultural Revolution in Scotland* (Glasgow: Burns, 1963).

89. A. Smith, *An Inquiry Into the Nature and Causes of The Wealth of Nations*, III vols (London: A. Strahan and T. Cadell, 1796), Vol. I, 221–2.
90. For details, T.M. Devine, *The Transformation of Rural Scotland: Social Change and the Agrarian Economy, 1660–1815* (Edinburgh: Edinburgh University Press, 1994).
91. I.F. Grant, 'The Social Effects of Agricultural Reforms and Enclosure Movement in Aberdeenshire', *Economic History,* 1 (1926–9), 89–116. See also M. Gray, 'Migration in the Rural Lowlands of Scotland', in T.M. Devine and D. Dickson (eds), *Ireland and Scotland, 1600–1850: Parallels and Contrasts in Economic Development* (Edinburgh: J. Donald, 1983), 104–17.
92. T.M. Devine, 'Social Stability in the Eastern Lowlands of Scotland During the Agricultural Revolution, 1780–1840', in T.M. Devine (ed.), *Lairds and Improvement in the Scotland of the Enlightenment* (Dundee: University of Dundee, 1979), 65–6.
93. Sinclair, *op. cit.* (note 21), part 1, 135.
94. Anon., *op. cit.* (note 33), Vol. I, 128–33.

6

'Mill Reek' in Scotland: Construction and Management of Lead Poisoning

Since antiquity, the protean and often-elusive manifestations of lead poisoning were linked to a variety of agents. This study on lead mining and its health hazards in Scotland seeks to understand the social construction of 'mill reek'. The condition was linked to the rudimentary extraction and refinement techniques employed in the 'lead hillies' of Lanarkshire. As production became more profitable, the deteriorating health of miners came to the attention of physicians, prompting a number of medical studies to determine the causes of their sicknesses as well as design successful therapies to reverse them. In Scotland, new interest in chemistry stimulated a series of clinical and experimental studies concerning the toxic action of lead.

When we consider... how many human wants and human luxuries lead by its useful properties becomes subservient, it will readily be conceded that it may insinuate itself into the human body by means not obvious, unobserved and unsuspected.

Samuel Pett (1793)[1]

Background

The tradition of mining lead ore in Scotland can be traced back to Roman times. While never a large-scale activity with important economic implications, it nevertheless supplied metal to local and foreign markets. Spurred by reforms of the early Industrial Revolution, this industry employed several thousand workers by the late 1700s and supplied the metal to builders, paint manufacturers, and plumbers in Scotland, England, Holland, and Russia.[2] Most of the original mines were located along the western Scottish seaboard and further inland, southwest near the Lanarkshire and Dumfrieshire border. Since the sixteenth century, the latter location at high altitude attracted prospectors looking for gold and silver. In an isolated area known as the 'lead hillies' in south Lanarkshire, dozens of workmen toiled under extreme weather conditions. The winters, especially, were characterised by severe frosts and heavy snowfalls. The region provided the necessary natural resources to encourage the extraction of lead: surface water for washing-off the ore's impurities before smelting, working the pumps to drain mines, and turning the waterwheels that operated the smelt mills' bellows. Wood for timbering mine shafts and houses as well as the use of peat to fuel the furnaces were also plentiful in the hillsides near the mines. This was a great advantage after the adoption of peat and coal smelting in the 1690s.[3]

By the eighteenth century, two main locations could be identified for lead mining in Scotland: Wanlockhead in Dumfriesshire and Leadhills in Lanarkshire. Together they accounted for about eighty percent of the total Scottish lead production. Wanlockhead in the Lowther Hills operated since 1675 on land belonging to the Duke of Queensberry and its mines were rich in silver and yielded some gold.[4] Leadhills or 'Hopetoun' came into being in 1719 on a bleak hillside owned by the Earl of Hopetoun in the upper Clysdesdale, at the top of Glengonnar and on Friars Muir.[5] A visitor in 1796, described Leadhills as 'one of the highest spots – 2,200 feet above sea level – of ground in Great Britain which is cultivated'.[6] John Sinclair's *Statistical Account of Scotland* contains a brief report on the town written by the Reverend James Maconochie of the nearby parish of Crawford in Lanarkshire. It estimated the mining town's population in the 1780s to be around 970 people.[7]

By the 1720s, the Scottish lead mining industry employed around two hundred workers. During the American War of Independence, the British demand and price of lead soared, and the growing workforce reached nearly a thousand. By the 1790s, both Leadhills and Wanlockhead had become prosperous mining communities supplying smelted lead bars for fifteen to nineteen pounds sterling until the needs associated with the Napoleonic War in 1803 nearly doubled this price.[8] Given the modest size of this industry, investment in lead mining was initially difficult. Rich Scottish landowners such as the Earl of Hopetoun initiated some co-partnerships with Scottish merchants – often from Edinburgh and Leith – as well as English ones who leased the mining lands on a royalty basis and sold the product to overseas customers. Among these customers were the Scots Mines Company with its Royal Charter directed from London. Under the management of a Mr Stirling, the Leadhill mines were placed on an orderly and profitable footing. They employed about two hundred men in their heyday – around 1790 – and produced approximately 18,000 lead bars annually with an estimated profit of about 36,000 pounds sterling.[9] As his share, the Earl of Hopetoun received every sixth bar as rent. Thus, lead mines were regarded as potentially valuable assets, although most partners seemed less concerned with immediate profits given the volatility of lead demand and prices. In 1772, however, Joseph Black, then professor of chemistry at the University of Edinburgh and a key promoter of Scottish industry visited Leadhills. Reports circulated around this time regarding the finding of gold dust. Thus, the professor came as consultant to the Earl of Hopetoun on this 'question of gold'. But, alas, the precious metal remained elusive in the Lanarkshire hills.[10] Rather it was the exploitation of iron that contributed to Scotland's subsequent industrial development.[11]

Lead and mining life in Scotland[12]

Lead is usually available in the form of lead sulphide (galena) mixed with quartz, fluorite and calcite (spar). Ore fields containing lead generally present as complex systems of horizontal fissures or veins distributed quite irregularly, making it rather difficult to predict yields. Mining below ground traditionally began by sinking simple shafts or pits – also called 'grooves' – to discover a vein of ore. Once a vein was found, its productivity was determined and followed along its course by digging trenches and subsequent shafts.[13] At Leadhills, the lead ore vein ran from north to south, gradually dipping into the ground and reaching a total depth of 167 fathoms. Miners, called 'pickmen',[14] descended into the shafts using ropes and extracted the ore with hammers and pickaxes, trying always to separate the narrow vein of ore from the surrounding hard limestone. Carpenters and smiths joined them in constructing the shafts. Common labourers assisted by clearing away the rubbish. Rocks were moved into wheelbarrows and raised by ropes. The work was much more difficult, time-consuming and expensive than mining coal.

Gunpowder was employed to blast the shafts and trenches, creating a polluted environment full of smoke and dust composed of minute particles of rock and ore perceived to be poisonous. Proper shaft ventilation was necessary because of pockets of this 'foul air'. Moreover, existing shafts had to be cleared of water seeping through the rocks with the help of pumps. At Wanlockhead, hand pumps started to be employed in the 1720s, followed by more efficient steam pumping introduced after 1778 at both Leadhills and Wanlockhead. In fact, by 1782, Leadhills already had three Watts' steam engines employed as pumps or 'bab-gins'.[15] Their drawback was an increased consumption of coal and more pollution. These technical improvements in drainage allowed miners to work at even greater depth; to improve the odds for additional strikes.

Leadhills had a particularly 'fine brilliant, broad-foliated galena' containing about eighty percent lead.[16] However, once extracted, the lead ore or 'bouse' needed crushing, sorting, and washing to separate the lead sulphide from other parts of rock. Washers who used sieves, shovels and hammers, usually performed this sorting outdoors or in wooden sheds. Vats were filled with water to allow the fragments to be layered by specific gravity. Washing or dressing the ore was traditionally a chore performed by sons – mostly boys from the age of nine to nineteen – as well as by the miners' wives. By the eighteenth century, horses or water powered the crushing mills. These procedures were inefficient and discarded unnecessarily much of the lead. A better approach was to first 'roast' the powdered ore over a pit, 'ore-hearth' or small blast furnace, to expel some of the sulphur before proceeding to the actual smelting.

Melting the prepared ore was a twelve to fifteen hour process that took place in a shallow blast furnace using mostly peat instead of coal. A more expensive process used furnaces or smelting mills equipped with water-powered bellows that required skilled personnel. Other smelters employed a circulating air furnace that consumed eight times as much coal as a blast furnace, but needed less water to operate the bellows.[17] Here, the washed and partially separated lead ore was mixed with iron filings and salt, together with coal or peat. The red-hot fire melted the whole mass, dissipated the sulphur, and allowed the lead fragments to gradually coalesce into a paste that was placed on slabs or workstones. Lead monoxide (litharge) was skimmed like foam from the surface as the metal reacted with the air. It yielded two pigments, an orange-red lead oxide (minium) and another, white lead carbonate (ceruse). Finally the 'grey slag' was broken up into lumps while the liquid lead flowed into pots and was ladled to form pigs. While further smelting could make the lead softer and more pliable – as well as refine the liquid to extract silver – the process is called 'cupellation' – the additional costs were exorbitant for Scotland's small mining operations at this time. Leadhills yielded about five ounces of silver for every ton of lead ore. Both at Leadhills and Wanlockhead, the modest amounts of silver obtained during smelting were sold to Edinburgh goldsmiths.[18]

Both mining and smelting were preferably carried out at the same site. The location of smelters, however, was related to the availability of fuel – peat, coal, or wood – and places near water sources for power to blow the bellows of furnaces. Not surprisingly, the entire smelting process generated a host of poisonous fumes, prompting mine operators after 1800 to build long horizontal chimneys – up to half a mile – to dissipate such fumes and thus improve ventilation in the smelters. Smelters or 'refiners' were highly skilled workmen, placed at the top of the labour hierarchy. Many of the workers were English – fifty percent at the Scots Mines Company in 1750 – especially at the smelters, although the migration from the south waned by the 1770s. Scots apparently found mining unappealing in spite of the fact that it certainly trumped agricultural work. There was always a shortage of skilled and disciplined labour.[19] The more economic process of melting ore with peat in the 1690s replaced smelting with charcoal. This increased the proportion of ore smelted directly at the mines but diminished the earlier exports of lead ore during the seventeenth- and early-eighteenth centuries to foreign markets, especially Holland. Distribution of the lead made up a significant part of the costs of production. The bars of 'grey gold' were placed in bags and carted downhill fifty miles over a toll-free route all the way to Biggar because a shorter route to Dumfries was badly maintained. However, after the 1750s, when roads leading from the mines to Edinburgh and the port of Leith improved, transportation costs declined.

Mining life in Scotland's isolated and inhospitable mountain valleys was harsh. One traveller, Robert Heron, stressed the 'bleak, wild and lofty' features of the area and the 'austerity of the climate'.[20] Given the inclement weather and severe winters, most work was done during the summer by a cadre of skilled men. New arrivals nursed the hope of higher wages; or, burdened by debts, sought the solitude. The hours were irregular, although by the 1790s work was carried out around the clock in six or eight-hour shifts. Many miners were characterised as 'wicked', 'abandoned', 'thoughtless' and 'dissipated'. Drunken brawls were frequent enough to prompt licensing of ale sellers as a measure to control the access to alcohol. Offenders received corporal punishment. Both workers and supervisors shared the hardships of living in the high Scottish moorlands. Employers, like the Earl of Hopetoun, by adopting a somewhat paternalistic attitude towards the men's work and morals, prescribed a code of behaviour for each class of worker. Towards the end of the eighteenth century, resident managers achieved a degree of social bonding and solidarity among the miners by keeping them under close supervision and control.

Unlike the forced serfdom prevailing in British coal and salt mines, lead mining had a reputation of being managed in a somewhat more flexible and equitable way given the uncertainties surrounding its extraction. Most prevalent was the so-called 'bargain system', a form of partnership between small groups of miners and owners.[21] For a stipulated price, the miners committed themselves to raise a certain amount of ore or dig the ground for a particular distance. Another popular arrangement was the 'bing tale', wherein the miners were paid according to the number of 'bings' of ore extracted from the mine and washed by their family members for smelting. Miners could also dig in units of ground called 'meers'; each trench measuring twenty-nine yards of ore vein marked by wood sticks or 'stows'.[22] There was also the 'fathomtale' partnership in which the workers were paid according to the total number of fathoms driven through the ground. Unlike in England, miners never had the freedom of mining and selling ore independently. Under these conditions, their earnings fluctuated significantly depending on the success of exploration and ease of extraction. The average wage amounted to about eighteen to twenty pounds sterling per year.[23] Sporadic cash payments were often delayed. Most men needed frequent loans between payments, a practice that kept them perennially in debt to their employers although a number of subsistence allowances could often be negotiated. Credit was primarily extended by the company store. As Britain battled Napoleon during the 1790s, subsistence payments failed to keep pace with rapidly rising prices in spite of the fact that the price of lead had reached new heights.

Initially, most men lived in simple huts and tents, forming self-contained communities until the growing prosperity in the 1780s improved their lives and prompted the settlement of entire families and the construction of cottages. The presence of women and children tended to stabilise the Scottish mining communities. In sharp contrast to the previous lawlessness of a transient bachelor society, workers and managers developed a stronger sense of solidarity and community. Land was gradually reclaimed from the surrounding moors, and during leisure hours many miners developed private 'kitchen gardens' laid out for cultivating crops such as potatoes, corn, and other vegetables. Women engaged in spinning and sewing activities. Dwellers also built a chapel and established a circulating library, making contacts with schools and churches located in nearby villages and parishes such as Abington, Sanquhar and Crawfordjohn.[24] Merchants were encouraged to ply their business and provide supplies.[25] For its part, mining management set up a series of charity and special pension funds so if miners were injured at work, some owners awarded grants for medical expenses. However, following the peace of 1815, the war boom ended. When Spanish lead mines re-opened on the Continent, lead prices fell to sixteen pounds per ton and remained depressed in Britain well into the 1850s.

Miners spent the greatest portion of their wages on food and drink. Bread and other cereals constituted the everyday staples. Given the altitude of the lead mining dales, large-scale farming proved impossible, prompting the importation of most cereals and vegetables from lower arable lands. Oatmeal was cheaper than bread and easier to prepare. It could be eaten for breakfast as porridge with milk, at diners with broth and meat. Early on, much of this meat was salted. Home-grown potatoes were important together with fresh vegetables. Some families even kept their own herds of goats and some cows for milk, butter and cheese. In general, miners consumed more animal food than other workers of similar social status and eventually tea came to replace hard liquor as the general stimulant.

As a group, the Scottish lead miners remained fatalistic about their hazardous working conditions. The common wisdom that 'all mines are places where the air is bad' was taken for granted, a normal hazard that came with the job. Working in a dust-filled atmosphere with 'clouds of deleterious fumes' emanating from the busy smelters frequently caused a condition dubbed 'miner's complaint'. This included a series of respiratory ailments characterised by shortness of breath and wheezing, with 'black spit' – bluish-black mucus. Leadhills workers simply called it 'mill reek'. Other subtle or overt manifestations of sickness were gastro-intestinal and neurological disorders. As one eighteenth-century visitor reported, many miners and smelters came to suffer from the 'dry belly-ache', as well as 'palsies and sometimes madness' that could end in death.[26] By contrast, the Earl of Hopetoun boasted to the notable physician, Thomas Percival (1740–1804) that 'his miners are, in general, a very healthy set of men'.[27] The average life expectancy of a Scottish miner barely reached the late thirties, although one of them, John Taylor, published a brief narrative of his life and claimed to be a centenarian.[28]

During his travels through Scotland in 1776, William Gilpin (1724–1804) observed that the Leadhills mines 'as in all mineral countries, are destructive of health'. He added that 'you see an infirm frame and squalid looks in most of the inhabitants'. [29] The mines were blamed for the presence of pulmonary consumption and scurvy and only better ventilation of the smelt mills could improve the situation. The vapours or 'mill reek' drawn into the faces of the workers were obviously poisonous. They also destroyed the grass in surrounding areas and could kill grazing cattle and sheep affected by dry gripes. Shepherds were keen to keep their flocks at a safe distance. Many of the birds flying through the smoke perished. Dissections of dogs allegedly revealed fine lead particles in the stomach and inflamed intestines. The dangers prompted the removal of smelting mills from nearby settlements and the construction of tall flues or cupolas over the mills to amend ventilation. At Leadhill, the smelter was indeed moved from the village. Others at risk for chronic lead poisoning were men engaged in the manufacture of metal pots usually composed of equal parts of lead and copper, an amalgam achieved by fusing the metals together when subjected to heat. These workers were exposed to fumes emanating from the metallic mixture when poured into moulds. Moreover, individuals handling white lead powder were equally at risk. Traditionally, this product was frequently mixed with other ingredients to make enamel, a more durable and waterproof paint. Similar properties attracted potters who favoured the manufacture of lead-glazed ceramics as well as plumbers and manufacturers of pewter cooking utensils.

The multiple faces of lead poisoning: occupational and health aspects

During the Bronze Age, lead became one of the most popular metals obtained during the extraction of copper and silver. Over time, thousands of workers would have been involved in the mining of lead – it has been estimated that nearly 80,000 tons per year were produced during the peak years of the Roman Empire. While certainly affecting the slaves, prisoners, and lower-class workers directly involved in the metal's extraction, upper-class people were also exposed to lead contained in foodstuffs, water, wine, cosmetics and remedies. Lead was also a common ingredient in lotions, salves and ointments, as well as a preservative of fruit drinks and wines. To sweeten their dishes, Romans boiled down grape juice in leaded pots, producing a concentrate contaminated with the metal called 'sapa'.[30] As wine consumption soared during Imperial times, this syrup became a popular preservative for weak and sour wines since it would decidedly improve their taste. However, the grand hypothesis that chronic lead poisoning contributed to the decline of the Roman Empire by physically weakening its leadership has been since rejected as overly simplistic.[31]

Given this significant presence of lead in the ancient world, surprisingly little seems to have been known about its potentially toxic properties.[32] The effects of lead were often subtle and gradual, masked by the more dramatic actions of other metals such as arsenic and mercury that displayed immediate and often deadly toxicity. The paucity of medical reports has been explained as a function of the ancient physicians' professional standing. Practitioners moving in higher social circles with generously paid stipends, generally had little experience with the ailments afflicting lowly mine workers and slaves.[33] Nevertheless, some authors repeatedly associated lead exposure with disease, notably the appearance of severe abdominal spasms and paralysis of the extremities. In his work on antidotes for poisons, entitled *Theriaka and Alexipharmaca*, the Greek physician Nikander (185–135 BC) described a case of colic and paralysis following the ingestion of lead.[34] Dioscorides (fl. 54–68 AD) revealed a series of respiratory and paralytic manifestations associated with the vapours emanating from the manufacture of lead oxide.[35] The Roman architect Vitruvius, wrote about the dangers of drinking water from lead pipes.[36]

During the Middle Ages, lead was widely employed as a valuable building material for roofs, gutters, cisterns and pipes, as well as a component in the preparation of ornamental glass, glazes, weaponry, and pewter kitchen ware. Several authors seemed to have also focused on the connection between enamel – prepared with the addition of lead pigments – and symptoms of colic and paralysis experienced by manufacturers and the house painters who came in frequent contact with it. As German mining and manufacturing operations flourished in the fourteenth and fifteenth centuries, medical people began to pay greater attention to the deleterious effects of metals on human health. Arsenic, copper and mercury were among the early culprits. First Agricola's (1494–1555) *De Re Metalica* published in 1556,[37] and later Paracelsus' (1493–1541) monograph *Von der Bergsucht* of 1567,[38] contained information about the diseases and accidents of miners. These events proliferated in direct relation to the depth of the mines in which extraction took place.[39] For his part, Samuel Stockhausen (fl. 1619–56), a physician for miners working in the Hartz Mountains of the Duchy of Brunswick-Lüneburg, published a treatise in 1658 based on his own observations during visits to mines, smelters, potters and a number of experiments. By then, Stockhausen had become convinced that the metallic fumes inhaled around the furnaces were responsible for lead poisoning, a condition the Germans called 'Hütten Katze'.[40]

Since the Middle Ages, lead and other ingredients including spices, herbs, arsenic and sulphur, were routinely employed to adulterate sour native wines following poor grape growing seasons. Indeed, people employed ancient recipes, originally published by the author Columella, to prepare the Roman 'sapa'. After 1645, severe cold weather and poor harvests in the vineyards of France and southern Germany only accentuated the need for additives. The practice, however, triggered recurrent epidemics of a 'wine disease' in most wine-growing regions of Europe that involved gripping abdominal pains and paralysis of hands and feet. In 1572, one such episode afflicted the inhabitants of the province of Poitou, France, and was reported by Francois Citois (1572–1652), personal physician to Cardinal Richelieu in 1617. Citois' description and label of the syndrome as 'colic of Poitou' – latinised as '*colica pictonum*' or 'colic of the Pictons' (the people of Poitou) – was widely recognised by subsequent medical authors.[41] This 'bilious colic' and the paralytic complaints were said to be reversible following a prolonged regimen of cathartics and painkillers. Citois speculated about some astrological influences and attributed the colic to an excess of bile following older humoral views.

Eberhard Gockel (1636–1703) established a direct linkage between the manifestations of colica pictonum and the drinking of lead-adulterated wine in 1696. A prolific author and busy practitioner in the Imperial City of Ulm, a key wine-trading centre in southern Germany, Gockel attended to the health needs of monks living in two local monasteries when the 'wine disease' suddenly broke out in 1694. Working with two small population groups of people who contracted the ailment simultaneously, this physician was quickly able to discover the culprit: a wine found to be heavily laced with lead. Gockel's knowledge of old recipes allowed him to create an assay for testing all potentially adulterated wines for their lead content. In arriving at his conclusions about the potential toxicity of lead, he acknowledged the work of his near contemporary Stockhausen.[42] Citois' discovery triggered new laws that sought to ban the employment of litharge in wines, and prompted a wave of legislation against tainted wine throughout the Continent.

In England, Thomas Sydenham (1624–89) also commented on the appearance of colic and palsies following the liberal consumption of punch, a popular fruit drink mixed with rum. He revealed that colica pictonum was extremely common in the West Indies – notably Barbados and Jamaica – where it was known as the 'dry belly-ache' that 'destroys many persons'.[43] In a letter recalling his experiences with the 'bad effects of lead', Benjamin Franklin (1706–90) admitted that during his youth in Boston there were already complaints that New England rum was poisonous, causing abdominal cramps and 'loss of the use of limbs'. An examination of the local distilleries uncovered the fact that several of them employed a leaden condensation apparatus for their rum production believed to be the cause of the complaints. These findings prompted legislation in Massachusetts prohibiting the use of such equipment.[44] Franklin subsequently published, in 1745, an influential pamphlet written by the Philadelphia physician, Thomas Cadwalader (1708–79), on the 'West India Dry-Gripes' in which the author refuted the ideas espoused by Citois.[45] Having experienced similar instances in which the syndrome occurred following contact with lead fumes, Cadwalader pointed to this metal as the true culprit.[46]

Occurring mostly during the autumn, the so-called 'Devonshire colic' or 'cyder colic' had apparently been endemic for centuries in various regions of England. In the eighteenth century, following an expansion of Devon's orchards, increased cider consumption afflicted an ever-larger number of people with gastrointestinal and neurological symptoms, drawing increased medical attention. The English physician John Huxham (1692–1768) initially linked these manifestations to the consumption of this popular drink, suggesting in 1739 – like Citois before him – that it was caused by the tartar from fermenting apple juice capable of acidifying the body's bile.[47] However, more detailed studies carried out in the mid-1760s by another practitioner, George Baker (1722–1800) discovered that the presumptive culprit, cider, was heavily contaminated with lead because the presses employed in crushing the apples were traditionally lined with this metal.[48] Baker was influenced by Cadwalader's essay – provided to him by Franklin – in reaching his conclusions. Several subsequent presentations by Baker, including one before the Royal College of Physicians of London in 1771, reported similar experiences from other English practitioners, thereby confirming the link between colic and lead poisoning.

While the symptoms exhibited by ancient metallurgists who separated lead from silver were already well-known, occupational and social concerns for these workers lagged. In the first treatise published in 1700 and exclusively devoted to occupational diseases, Bernardino Ramazzini (1633–1714) quoted the authority of Agricola in saying that the mining of metals – essential for crafts and arts – was a regular form of torture and punishment because of its unhealthiness.[49] Ramazzini specifically focused on potters, who worked with calcinated lead for glazing their pots, linking their tremors and paralysis to this occupation. Not only did the workers inhale the metal while pounding and grinding the lead in marble vessels, they also drew its vapours as the potters melted it for coating the earthenware. According to Ramazzini, painters employing red and white lead pigment for greater durability of their paints also experienced milder forms of poisoning.[50]

Most authors agreed that just as harmful to painters and glaziers, who handled white lead, was exposure to 'mineral effluvia' of lead prevalent in mines and around smelters.[51] Observations reported in Vienna by Gerard van Swieten (1700–72) and Anton de Haen (1704–76), two students of Europe's leading physician, Herman Boerhaave (1668–1738), sought to categorically associate the term colica pictonum with lead poisoning.[52] De Haen's writings, including an accurate description of the clinical symptoms and underlying pathology, were widely quoted in eighteenth-century medical circles. His autopsies of several cases disclosed that the abdomen was the principal repository for the disease. The ileum and portions of the colon appeared indurate and severely constricted, surrounded by distended segments filled with gas. Many of the paralytic muscles displayed signs of atrophy and loss of tone and colour.[53]

In France, the physician, François Merat de Vaumartoise, informed his readers that between January and December 1766, 222 patients suffering from what he called the 'metallic colic' had been hospitalised at the Hôpital de la Charité in Paris. According to institutional statistics, 212 individuals (95.5%) were eventually cured and only ten had died (4.5%). Merat made a careful analysis of the patients' occupational status, identifying among the most common sufferers artisans, painters, plumbers and potters. His work re-affirmed the suspected link between exposure to lead and various respiratory, gastrointestinal and neurological symptoms. [54] Benjamin Franklin, for his part, recalled his visit to the same Parisian hospital 'particularly famous for the cure of that malady' in 1767 where he received a pamphlet highlighting Merat's findings. Other authors such as Theodore Tronchin (1709–81) pointed out a similar nexus. In 1757, Tronchin published an essay describing the poisonous qualities of the metal for miners, potters, and individuals being heavily medicated by quacks with lead acetate compounds. Tronchin also reported that affected miners would lose their balance and fall from ladders during their climb into the pits because of weakness in their hands and legs.[55]

In the last decades of the eighteenth century, there was growing medical concern about the effects of lead, especially the extremely painful lead-induced intestinal colic. By then, as noted in a previous essay, a much more health-conscious European society debated the effects of age and life-style and raised questions about the importance of an individual's constitution and occupation (Chapter 4). What groups in society were at risk of suffering such symptoms? How could these manifestations be distinguished from other ubiquitous gastric and intestinal cramps stemming from culinary over-indulgence or from spoiled food? In a letter written from Newcastle to Percival, a certain Dr Rotheram, who practised in the village of Hexham informed the Manchester physician around 1770 that he was being frequently consulted by workers from lead mines and smelting mills. Rotheram himself considered lead to be highly poisonous, especially when the particles were finely divided and, thus, capable of being absorbed into the stomach, lungs and pores of the skin. Although miners were usually quite healthy at the onset of their profession, the lack of airshafts to exhaust the volatile metal caused obstinate bouts of asthma, cough, and a bluish expectoration associated with severe constipation and muscular spasms. During smelting operations the lead fumes condensed in the cool air forming a white dust that blew into the faces of the miners.[56] The destructive nature of the lead vapours on the area surrounding smelting operations were described by Percival in a separate monograph on lead.[57]

Given the remoteness of the Scottish lead mines, self-reliance in health matters was essential: Wanlockhead's local library possessed copies of James Mackenzie's *The History of Health* (1758) and William Buchan's *Domestic Medicine* (1769).[58] If illnesses appeared more serious, nearby physicians could be summoned. At Wanlockhead in the early 1800s, the former navy surgeon James Martin worked for the Scots Mines Company. Fatal accidents were rare but men occasionally fell into shafts, others were injured in cave-ins following blasting. Small particles of stone could injure the eyes. The mining companies had employed some medical practitioners since the 1740s but their assistance had only a negligible impact. James Wilson, a surgeon from the village of Durrisdeer who attended Leadhill miners in the 1750s, promoted a number of measures designed to prevent lead poisoning. Miners were urged to breathe untainted air and take purgatives during the spring and autumn.[59] The customary diet rich in meat and fats among English mill men was believed to be useful as an antidote for poisoning effects. Sweet oil and a little aquavit were also considered preventatives. However, Scottish miners broiled mutton, beef and pork steaks on hot leaded grills so that the flesh would acquire an agreeable flavour. Percival pointed out that the deleterious effects of the fumes on the nervous system were compounded by the miners' practice of broiling their meat on newly cast, hot lead pigs. Workers were also encouraged never to begin mine work in fasting state. Poor diets and excessive consumption of alcoholic beverages weakened many workers. Cold was considered an important culprit and the men were advised to avoid going out into the cold air after labouring the entire day in hot smelters without wearing warm clothing. They were also told to drink warm soups or broth immediately after completing work in the shafts.

But there were other sources of poisoning. Following Paracelsus, physicians and especially quacks continued to prescribe high doses of 'sugar of lead' or lead acetate for inflammatory conditions, including fevers, phthisis and venereal diseases, a therapy that often triggered violent abdominal pain. Similar side-effects occurred in persons who frequently used white lead ointments for cosmetic reasons, often to disguise their pockmarked faces following recovery from smallpox. Confronted by these facts by the 1770s, some practitioners were now willing to abandon the internal use of lead, but felt that its external employment was still justified because of lesser toxicity.[60] One popular compound was the 'Saturnine Water of Goulard', a combination of lead acetate in brandy and water. It was widely used as an anti-inflammatory agent in plasters for tuberculous ulcers, superficial cancers and other swellings. The French surgeon Thomas Goulard of Montpellier developed the compound and enthusiastically proclaimed lead to be 'one of the most efficacious remedies in the cure of most diseases which require the assistance of surgery'.[61] However, writing in 1775, Percival reported several cases of fatal lead poisoning due to the employment of this remedy.[62]

In the end, both 'mill reek' and 'dry colic' appeared to be conditions with clear links to lead exposure. The colic was linked to lead-contaminated cider and rum produced by presses and distillation apparatus made from this metal.[63] The resulting syndrome featured painful abdominal cramps and progressive neurological features that began with muscular weakness and ended in irreversible paralysis and even death. Fumes from smelting lead and silver affected workers and refiners, the use of lead-pigmented enamel troubled painters, as well as glaziers, who handled earthenware vessels. For their part, 'austere' lead-adulterated German and French wines as well as Portuguese port slowly poisoned heavy drinkers, even causing what was then termed 'irregular gout'.[64] By the 1790s, most European and American medical men had concluded that lead was a potentially poisonous metal acting on the digestive and nervous systems of susceptible individuals.

Colica pictonum in Edinburgh: concept, symptoms, diagnosis and management

At Edinburgh University, in the meantime, the study of chemistry flourished under the leadership of William Cullen (1710–90) and Joseph Black (1728–99). Both academics were engaged in novel studies concerning the nature of air and combustion.[65] In Cullen's view, chemistry had an important role to play in the improvement of the practical arts. He envisioned chemistry as a bridge between natural philosophy and empirical activities such as agriculture, the bleaching of linens, and purification of salt employed by the fishing industry to preserve its products.[66] Economical goals were equally important as scientific achievements. The preparation of alkaline salts in Scotland was intended to free the country from importing them, a move 'of general benefit to the kingdom'.[67] In spite of his chemical interests, Cullen wrote surprisingly little about what he termed the 'peculiar' condition labelled colica pictonum in the corrected and enlarged edition of his *First Lines of the Practice of Physic* published in 1788. In fact, he omitted most references to lead and referred his readers to the work of George Baker who had written on the so-called 'Devonshire colic'.[68]

There were still debates about distinguishing between a *colica vegetabilis* which included the symptoms prevailing in cider country presumably caused by acid in fruits from *colica saturnica* and linked to the ingestion and inhalation of lead. Other labels continued to be employed, including the terms 'metallic', or 'painter's colic'. There was also a condition known as 'bellon', *rachialgia pictonum* or *metalica* producing sensory and motor impairments caused by the effects of lead and afflicting those living or working in the vicinity of smelting houses.[69] However, the traditional designation of colica pictonum or 'colic of the Poitou inhabitants' prevented practitioners from emphasising the linkage with lead poisoning and its occupational aspects. In his own classification of diseases, Cullen attempted to introduce some order into the nomenclature by including the genus 'colica' among the order of 'spasms'. 'Spasms', in turn, were placed in his second class of diseases, the so-called 'neuroses' or nerve-mediated ailments. Given the contemporary clinical confusion regarding the nature of intestinal cramps, Cullen distinguished seven distinct species including the *colica spasmodica, pictonum, stercoraria, meconialis* and others. He also recognised that poisoning with white lead could cause severe intestinal cramps as well as palsy of the hands, and that glaziers, plumbers and painters were primarily involved.[70] Reacting to the prevailing nosological confusion, the senior president of the Royal Medical Society's 1786–7 session, Edmund Goodwyn, refused to propose a specific name. He preferred to include colica pictonum 'amongst a numerous list of others that are daily met in practice to mock the pride of classification and teach us the imperfection of our art' (Chapters 2, 7).[71]

During the last decade of the century, two other Edinburgh academics with chemical interests, Thomas C. Hope (1766–1844) and Daniel Rutherford (1749–1819) showed an interest in lead poisoning. A professor of chemistry at Glasgow until 1795, Thomas Hope was considered a popular British scientist as well as the discoverer of a new mineral containing a metal called strontium – it was found in the parish of Strontian in Argyllshire. After 1795, Hope shared the Edinburgh chair of chemistry with Joseph Black. Similarly interested in chemistry, Daniel Rutherford, son of John Rutherford (1695–1779) former professor of practice of physic at Edinburgh, had been a student of Joseph Black. Rutherford followed Black's earlier discovery of 'fixed air' or carbon dioxide, writing his 1772 medical dissertation on the qualities of another 'noxious gas' later called nitrogen.

Promoted by its famous academics, chemistry developed into a popular subject of study at the University of Edinburgh, attracting a growing number of students.[72] Perhaps because of Hope and Rutherford, the so-called colica pictonum became an attractive subject for a series of clinical and experimental studies that combined both chemical and medical knowledge. Using the case of a 25-year-old glazier in a 1785 presentation to the Royal Medical Society of Edinburgh, a medical student named William Alexander admitted that colica pictonum constituted a formidable disease, alarming and dramatic in its progress and frequently fatal in its termination. Alexander, however, believed that this serious affliction had the potential of dramatically illustrating the great utility of medicine, since physicians, as true men of science, would eventually recognise the true nature of the disease and rescue their patients from its ravages.[73]

Speaking as a follower of John Brown's new pathogenesis – then the rage in Edinburgh – the student rejected lead as the sole cause for the intestinal and neurological symptoms, blaming instead prolonged and intense exposure to cold for the problems. 'Artificers who are employed in manufactures and exposed to the fumes arising from metals', Alexander explained, 'can scarcely be supposed to receive any considerable quantity into their stomachs'. He argued that paralysis of the upper extremities rather than colic was the first and frequently most dangerous manifestation of the disease. 'Miners who are obliged to work in water which holds a considerable quantity of lead in solution [can be] deprived of the use of their limbs without any symptom of colic occurring', insisted Alexander.[74] Replacing the contemporary nosological confusion, according to Brown's medical system, colica pictonum was simply characterised as 'asthenia', a universal condition of diminished bodily excitement (Chapter 3).[75]

Alexander and a group of Edinburgh students who were all members of the Royal Medical Society put the idea that lead compounds could debilitate the human body to the test. This student-run institution sponsored an Experimental Committee charged with the design and execution of animal trials to clarify a series of issues dealing with human physiology and physiopathology (Chapter 2). In this particular instance, Alexander and his schoolmates sought an experimental confirmation of their views about the action of lead by conducting a series of vivisections on rabbits. After exposing an animal's chest and opening the pericardium, the students applied drops of a lead acetate solution directly to the beating heart in one-minute intervals. In spite of bodily convulsions, the heart continued to contract with force and velocity, prompting experimenters to open the right ventricle and continue their lead drip. However, eighteen minutes into the test, the animal's heart ceased beating. Similar experiments were then conducted with cold water; death occurred after only eleven minutes. Alexander concluded that both acetate of lead – traditionally considered an astringent and sedative – as well as cold water had both exhausted the heart's excitement and caused it to stop. Thus, the proximate cause of colica pictonum was said to be a systemic bodily debility induced by the deficiency or removal of powers necessary to maintain a healthy excitement.[76] Alexander's subsequent experiments with other substances, including opium, alcohol, and arsenic established the notion that lead was really a stimulant power. Another medical student, Alexander P. Anderson, used these experimental conclusions to explain that muscular spasms, constipation and the paralysis from colica pictonum, were all symptoms of debility induced by lead as well as cold water. A stimulating plan of action was called to manage the condition. For example, opium and other stimulants such as musk and camphor might correct the debilitated, 'asthenic' condition of the body.[77]

Sponsored by the principals of Edinburgh University, William Robertson and George Baird, several contemporary medical dissertations also dealt with colica pictonum. In the 1780s, they included the theses of John Prendergast (1786), John Reid (1786) and Andreas Ponton (1787).[78] Other subsequent theses included those of John Beamish (1798), Joshua Dixon (1798), Morteus Moriarty (1804), David Hay (1809), and Matthew Kenny (1810).[79] The case of a 35-year-old male presumed to be a miner from Devonshire was initially presented by Samuel Pett in January 1793 to the Royal Medical Society, and later became the core of his 1793 medical dissertation.[80] Unlike some of his fellow students, Pett was emphatic in linking the disease exclusively to lead; rejecting all other hypotheses that included the action of other metals such as copper, antimony, mercury and arsenic. He cited numerous proofs pointing specifically to the epidemiology of the disease and its linkage to the occupational experiences of miners, plumbers, potters, glassmakers and painters. The cardinal complaints could be closely traced to the time and duration of exposure. Among additional causes of lead poisoning, Pett included the excessive internal and external administration of 'saturnine' compounds such as lead acetate still employed as an anti-inflammatory agent in cases of phthisis or mixed with opium and ipecac for analgesic pills.[81]

The multiple and sometimes subtle manifestations of lead poisoning continued to baffle physicians into modern times.[82] In late eighteenth-century Edinburgh, colica pictonum presented with a diverse set of symptoms, often imperceptible in their progress and occurring in no particular sequence. During his clinical rotation at the Edinburgh Infirmary's teaching ward from 1 November 1796 until 31 January 1797, Thomas Hope admitted and took care of four lead workers suffering from poisoning. Daniel Rutherford, in turn, managed two additional hospital patients during the summer session that extended from May to June 1799. For both clinicians, the cardinal symptom was a 'dry belly ache', a severe and gnawing pain, fixed and constant, radiating over the entire abdomen, especially the umbilical region and often increased during breathing. Violent pain in the stomach and abdominal cramps were often accompanied by obstinate constipation together with the sensation of a cord tightly tying down the intestines. Even a slight contact with bedclothes could trigger much pain.[83] Andrew T., a 32-year-old silver refiner 'exposed by his business to fumes of lead' was admitted to the Edinburgh Infirmary on 10 April 1795 by another university professor, Andrew Duncan Sr. The patient related successive one-hour bouts of violent abdominal pain, especially after dinner and at night, intense enough to render him unconscious.[84] If stools could be obtained through enemas, they were small hard knots like sheep's dung.

In the case of Alexander B., a 34-year-old worker admitted by Dr Hope on 27 December 1796, the story was also typical. The griping pains in the pit of his stomach and around the umbilical region accompanied by severe constipation had started seven weeks earlier, more than a year after he became employed in lead work.[85] Another 20-year-old patient, John L., was admitted to the hospital on 6 January 1797 complaining of similar symptoms. According to Hope, he 'was employed in lead works for two years but never felt the inconvenience from it.' An initial episode of colic was stopped following a brief absence from his employment.[86] During the initial

Figure 6.1

Edinburgh Infirmary Case

William F., aged 32, admitted 23 Aug 1781; discharged cured 17 Sep 1781. Total hospital stay twenty-five days. Attending physician John Hope.

History: He is by trade a painter and has been long subject to violent colic which begin with a sensation of weight and retraction of the umbilicus, and are accompanied with severe vomiting. He had an attack of this kind about a fortnight ago but by the use of different medicines passage of his belly was procured and the other symptoms alleviated in the course of two days. He has since, however, had a constant feeling of unusual heat, weakness and as it were emptiness in the abdomen accompanied, when greatest, with much anxiety. For some months, he has also had numbness and diminution of voluntary motions of the hands sometimes accompanied with swelling and redness of the knuckles.

Physical Examination: Pulse 100, tongue somewhat foul but moist; thirst natural, appetite very low, belly regular. The abdomen is soft and uniform, and he feels no uneasiness on pressure.

24 August: Take at bedtime 1 oz castor oil, 1 oz spirits of lavender with 4 ounces of water. 10 grains (antispasmodic) pills of asafoetida gum twice a day

25 August: Three stools obtained with immediate sensitive relief. Complains of want of sleep. Instead of broth to have a small bit of meat daily. Administer bolus at bedtime composed of Valerian powder and Canella alba.

26 August: A good night after the bolus. Took a morning dose of Glauber salts, which have operated well and with relief.

27 August: The operation of the salts continued till late last night.

28 August: A good night. Abdominal complaints greatly better. Complaining of flying pains across his shoulders. Patient to continue gum pills and take a tepid bath.

29 August: Sweated after the bath, is sensibly better.

30 August: To receive asafoetida julep.

31 August: [Patient] has discharged a good deal of wind by flatus and eructation since he began taking the julep and finds himself much easier.

1 September: To take 15 grains of Ipecac powders and 1 grain of tartar emetic in the evening (both emetics)

4 September: The flying pains are now his chief complaints. To receive a tepid bath.

5 September: Pain easier. [Patient] sweated profusely and has passed more flatus easily. To have 3 0z of ale four times a day.

6 September: Continues free of pain.

9 September: No change in the numbness and paralysis of his fingers. (Use of an electric machine) To have electric sparks taken daily from his hands and fingers for 8 days.
10 September: Infusion of chamomile.
17 September: More asafoetida julep. All complaints but weakness gone. Dismissed cured.

Source: J. Hope, *Cases of Patients in the Royal Infirmary Under the Care of John Hope, M.D.* (Edinburgh: 1781), MSS Collection, University of Edinburgh.

stages, many of the patients also complained of cold skin and clammy sweats, appetite loss and stomach unease, poor digestion, lassitude and weight loss. Duncan's patient, Andrew T., presented with a sallow face and was said to have had 'lost much flesh' in the previous five months. Another 25-year-old worker, John W., was admitted on 3 January 1797 and also placed under Hope's care with a similar diagnosis. He had only been employed in the mines for two months when symptoms started a fortnight ago and he was forced to leave his job. This patient also complained of heaviness in his chest and frequent vomiting after taking food.[87]

Rutherford's patients had more gastric complaints. William B., aged twenty-nine, another miner, was admitted on 11 May 1799 with symptoms that included violent burning pain at the pit of the stomach, nausea and vomiting of a dark purplish matter with a sweet taste. He was 'employed in lead work at Leith for about a month; attributes present symptoms to that', chronicled Rutherford.[88] The other labourer, 50-year-old Alexander G., came into the hospital on 8 July 1799. He provided a four-week history of nausea, pain and frequent vomiting, especially following meals, together with pain around the umbilicus and a tendency towards constipation following exposure to lead fumes and powder.[89] Some sufferers claimed to observe a bluish coloration of their skin, and a sweet taste in their mouths. On inspection, Alexander's tongue was covered with green or brownish matter, the breath offensive. This was followed by intense thirst, severe nausea and retching, with the vomiting only yielding some phlegm and bile.

Besides severe abdominal pains many sufferers of the disease also spoke of headaches and giddiness, followed by numbness and later outright paralytic symptoms affecting the muscles of hands and arms. Duncan's Andrew T. complained of numbness in all his limbs. When he was re-admitted two years later and seen by Hope on 15 November 1796, he could not even extend his right hand. Alexander B. experienced prickly sensations and slight numbness and displayed tremors in both his arms and legs. John L. appeared quite debilitated, with pain radiating into both arms and legs.

Because of muscular spasms, often the hands of all these patients were clenched in fists. After several weeks, debility lead to extensive dizziness, paralysis, and even convulsions, followed by insensibility and delirium, intermittent pulse, coma, apoplexy and death.[90] At times, the patients only voided small amounts of urine and seemed to experience painful abdominal episodes resembling those associated with kidney stones. Prognosis varied greatly depending on the length of the exposure to lead as well as the severity and duration of symptoms.

In dealing with this ailment, experience and skill were paramount in avoiding a protracted and unsatisfactory course of therapy. The approach of cleansing the 'prima via' was two-fold. Some practitioners employed both emetics to unburden the stomach and cathartics to empty the bowels from the hardened stools. Tartar emetic diluted in wine or other electuaries was prescribed together with mild cathartics such as infusions of senna with tamarinds, rhubarb or aloes. Because of its emetic power, a South Carolina practitioner, Lionel Chalmers, proposed specific treatment with ammoniated copper. Other purgatives like jalap and astringent alum (potassium aluminium sulphate) were employed to accomplish the same objective.[91] More common were laxative enemas using castor oil to bypass an already upset stomach. This was certainly part of Andrew Duncan Sr's management of the disease. For their part, patients were urged to drink warm broth or plenty of water. Small doses of opium continued to be administered while the pain was severe but practitioners often found themselves in a quandary. Prescribing opiates only accentuated the existing constipation. Strong purgatives and stimulants, in turn, increased the intestinal spasms and pain. The patients' sore bellies were also massaged. Bloodletting was usually banned because it would only contribute to the existing debility of the patient. Bland and nutritious food was recommended, including veal broth, jellies, and meat. Tonics composed of iron filings infused in wine with cinnamon were meant to stimulate the bodily systems and help restore weight.[92]

In addition to managing pain and the gastrointestinal symptoms, practitioners often also tried to ameliorate the neurological complaints. Numb arms and legs were rubbed with camphor oil and wrapped in flannel, paralytic limbs exposed to sparks generated by an electric machine with the expectation that some of the motion could be restored.[93] The Edinburgh Infirmary had possessed such an apparatus since 1750, and there were indications that by 1771 William Cullen had procured a portable machine to be carried to a patient's bedside. Towards the end of the century, most electric shocks administered to patients with paralytic symptoms were of moderate intensity. Ten to fifteen shocks were usually administered within a period of two to five minutes, the sessions repeated daily for a week, but the results were ambiguous at best.

At the Edinburgh Infirmary, Duncan's patient, Andrew T., received opium for his violent cramps and was discharged as 'cured' on 23 April 1795 after a twelve-day hospitalisation. His paralytic right hand had been subjected to electrical sparks but eventually he lost hope in getting better and demanded to leave the hospital. Rutherford's William B. was given both castor oil and a tincture of senna as well as a bolus containing laudanum. He spent nine days in the hospital and was also discharged as 'cured' on 20 May 1799. Alexander G. received a series of purgative enemas containing senna until the Infirmary's teaching ward closed at end of the academic year. His transfer to the ordinary ward for a final convalescence occurred on 26 July 1799. Hope's patient, Alexander B., was placed on oral castor oil, given opium tincture and ordered to receive abdominal fomentation. A week later, however, the cramps seemed to persist in spite of a successful evacuation of stools produced by laxatives. With only slight abdominal discomfort remaining, he was discharged as 'cured' on 10 January 1797 following a fourteen-day stay in the hospital. Subjected to a similar regime using calomel, a mercurial purgative, John W. left the institution 'cured' seven days after his admission while John L. required additional pain medication in the form of opium pills before departing as 'cured' on 17 January 1797.

In spite of the optimistic institutional discharge label, few patients were ever completely cured. Many sufferers of colica pictonum remained chronically ill and emaciated, afflicted with varying degrees of muscular atrophy, tremor and paralysis. Relapses of the painful colic were common, particularly if the men returned to their previous occupations. In Vienna, de Haen had suggested a long-term regimen of milk diet and electricity to build up strength and restore mobility but the results were inconclusive. Warm baths for relaxation and to alleviate pain were popular for short term relief. Bathing in mineral waters at prominent spas and gentle exercise at home were highly recommended. For those who could afford it, baths became an important component of the treatment. Many people suffering from paralytic symptoms went to Bath and were admitted for several months to the local General Hospital. Here, the patients were subjected to repeated warm baths and told to drink the famous mineral water. Institutional statistics reported eighty percent improvement among nearly a thousand patients previously admitted for a variety of ailments.[94] For miners and smelters, the ultimate prophylactic, of course, was to leave the lead mines for good and look for another line of work.

Conclusion

This discussion has highlighted an important shift in medical opinion regarding the importance and ubiquity of chronic lead poisoning in the second half of the eighteenth century.[95] Traditionally, miners were known to be frequently sick and have short lives. By the eighteenth century, however, lead mining had become a more prosperous business and the health and fitness of its skilled workers a greater concern for managers and owners exploiting their mines.[96] A better understanding of the multiple causes of toxicity and identification of key occupational factors helped practitioners institute a somewhat useful therapeutic regimen capable of reversing many of its early and disabling effects. Informed by the growing chemical revolution, Edinburgh academics in the 1790s welcomed the opportunity of treating a number of miners referred to the Infirmary's teaching ward and afflicted with symptoms of lead intoxication. Such an interest had perhaps been stimulated by the 1772 visit of Joseph Black to Leadhills and his relationship to the Earl of Hopetoun, an important patron of the Edinburgh Infirmary. The evidence suggests that some late-eighteenth-century physicians began framing an occupational relationship between lead exposure and a syndrome of crippling intestinal and neurological manifestations. Moreover, as reflected in the sample case history (Table 6.1), these practitioners were able to deal with some of the acute symptoms by resorting to their traditional evacuation measures. However, further studies about the occupational effects of lead on health were still needed to better define risks, detect patterns, and with the help of statistics, organise the findings.

Notes

1. S. Pett, 'De Colica Pictonum', in *Dissertations Read to the Royal Medical Society (Diss. RMS)*, 95 vols (Edinburgh, 1751–1833), MSS Collection, Edinburgh University Library, Vol. 30 (1792–9), 152.
2. See D.J. Rowe, *Lead Manufacturing in Britain. A History* (Beckenham: Croom Helm, 1983). The coverage of this publication ranges from 1778 to 1980. An older but still useful source of information is A.H. Stirling, *A Sketch of Scottish Industrial and Social History in the Eighteenth and Nineteenth Centuries* (London: Blackie, 1906). For England and Wales, consult R. Burt, *The British Lead Mining Industry* (Redruth: D. Truran, 1984).
3. A useful secondary source for this topic is W.S. Harvey, *Lead and Labour: The Miners of Leadhills*, a 2000 monograph dealing primarily with social issues, especially labour disputes during the nineteenth and twentieth centuries. It is solely available on the World Wide Web. See ch. 2,

'Early Days', ch. 3 'The Business of Mining', and ch. 4 'Wages and Conditions'.

4. T.C. Smout, 'The Lead Mines at Wanlockhead', *Transactions of the Dumfries and Galloway Natural History and Archaeology Society*, 39 (1962), 144–58. Mining history has become an independent and specialised field of study that includes social, political, economic, and technological aspects. However, most of the documentation and research is oriented toward nineteenth- and twentieth-century developments. For further research, consult R. Burt and P. Waite, *Bibliography of the History of British Metal Mining* (Exeter: University of Exeter Press, 1988). This publication and further updates are available through the Mining History Network on the Internet.
5. W.A.J. Provost, 'Lord Hopetoun's Mine at Leadhills: Illustrated by David Allan and Paul Sandby', *Transactions of the Dumfries and Galloway Natural History and Archaeology Society*, 54 (1979), 85–9.
6. C. Hatchett, *The Hatchett Diary: A Tour Through the Counties of England and Scotland in 1796 Visiting their Mines and Manufactories* (Truro: Barton, 1967), 101.
7. J. Sinclair, *The Statistical Account of Scotland*, XXI vols (Edinburgh: W. Creech, 1791–9), Vol. IX, 505–16.
8. For more information, see *A Select Bibliography Relating to the Mines at Leadhills and Wanlockhead* (Glasgow: Leadhills and Wanlockhead Mines Research Group, 1973).
9. W.S. Harvey, 'Lead Mining in 1768: Old Records of a Scottish Mining Company', *Industrial Archaeology*, 7 (1970), 310–18.
10. The best summary on this subject is T.C. Smout, 'Lead Mining in Scotland, 1650–1850', in P.L. Payne (ed.), *Studies in Scottish Business History* (London: Cass, 1967), 103–35.
11. A. Fleck, 'The Industrial Development of Scotland in the Cullen-Black Period', in A. Kent (ed.), *An Eighteenth-Century Lectureship in Chemistry* (Glasgow: Jackson, Son & Co, 1950), 107–25; see also H. Hamilton, *An Economic History of Scotland in the Eighteenth Century* (Oxford: Clarendon Press, 1963).
12. For an overview, C.E. Gregory, *A Concise History of Mining* (London: Pergamon, 1980); M. Lynch, *Mining in World History* (London: Reaktion, 2002). Also consult the British Mining Database on the Internet.
13. T. Houghton, *'Rara Avis in Terris' or The Compleat Miner*, 2nd corrected edn (London, 1738), 63.
14. For terms used by miners see W. Hooson, *The Miner's Dictionary* (Wrexham: W. Hooson and T. Payne, 1747).

15 . W.S. Harvey, 'Pumping Engines at the Leadmills Mines', *British Mining,* 19 (1982), 5–14.
16. Hatchett, *op. cit.* (note 6) 101.
17. G. Downs-Rose and W. S. Harvey, 'Lead Smelting Sites at Warlockhead, 1682–1934', *Transactions of the Dumfries and Galloway Natural History and Archeology Society,* 54 (1979), 75–84.
18. For details concerning the assaying of smelted lead ore, see W. Hardy, *The Miner's Guide or Compleat Miner* (Sheffield: F. Lister, 1748), 214–20.
19. For more details, see A. Campbell, *The Lanarkshire Miners: A History of Their Trade Unions, 1775–1974* (Edinburgh: J. Donald, 1979). Additional useful information can be obtained from nearby mines in North East England: C.J. Hunt, *Leadminers of the Northern Pennines, in the Eighteenth and Nineteenth Centuries* (New York: A.M. Kelley, 1970).
20. R. Heron, *Observations Made in a Journey Through Western Counties of Scotland in the Autumn of MDCCXCII,* 2 vols (Perth: W. Morison, 1799), Vol. I, 35–40.
21. W.S. Harvey, 'Miners' "Bargains" at Leadhills during the Eighteenth Century', *Glasgow Spelaeological Society Journal,* 2 (February 1970), 1–21.
22. Houghton, *op. cit.* (note 13), 64.
23. Sinclair, *op. cit.* (note 7), Vol. IV, 516.
24. See W.S. Harvey, 'A View of the Leadmines at Wanlockhead, 1775', in *Transactions of the Dumfries and Galloway Natural History and Archeology Society,* 54 (1979), 90–6.
25. J. Williams, 'The Day Book (1742–50) of William Hendry, a Wanlockhead and Leadmills Merchant', *Transactions of the Dumfries and Galloway Natural History and Archaeology Society,* 54 (1979), 167–72.
26. T. Pennant, *A Tour of Scotland MDCCLXIX* (London: B. White, 1772).
27. T. Percival, *Observations and Experiments on the Poison of Lead* (London: J. Johnson, 1774), 21.
28 . John Taylor died in 1770; he was supposedly 132 years old. See his autobiographical sketch in *Scots Magazine,* 33 (1771), 24–6.
29. W. Gilpin, *Observations, Relative Chiefly to Picturesque Beauty, Made in the Year 1776 on Several Parts of Great Britain, Particularly the High-Lands of Scotland,* 2 vols (London: R. Blamire, 1789), Vol. II, 176–7.
30. See R. Shepherd, *Ancient Mining* (London: Elsevier, 1993); and P.T. Craddock, *Early Metal Mining and Production* (Edinburgh: Edinburgh University Press, 1995). Significant amounts of lead were detected in wine experimentally prepared according to the directions provided by the Roman authors Pliny and Columella. See R. Kobert, 'Chronische Bleivergiftung im klassischen Altertume', in P. Diergart (ed.), *Beiträge aus der Geschichte der Chemie* (Leipzig: Franz Deuticke, 1909), 103–19. For an overview, H.A.

Waldron, 'Lead Poisoning in the Ancient World', *Medical History,* 17, 4 (1973), 391–9; A.C. Aufderheide, 'Lead Poisoning', in K.F. Kiple (ed.), *The Cambridge World History of Human Disease* (New York: Cambridge University Press, 1993), 820–7.

31 . There is an extensive literature on the presumed role of lead poisoning in the decline of the Roman Empire. The debate began by the publication of S.C. Gilfillan, 'Lead Poisoning and the Fall of Rome', *Journal of Occupational Medicine,* 7 (1965), 53–60; followed by J.O. Nriagu, 'Saturnine Gout Among Roman Aristocrats. Did Lead Poisoning Contribute to the Fall of the Empire?', *New England Journal of Medicine,* 308 (1983), 660–3; and L. Needleman and D. Needleman, 'Lead Poisoning and the Decline of the Roman Aristocracy', *Classical Views,* 4 (1985), 63–94. An informative rebuttal of this hypothesis can be found in J. Scarborough, 'The Myth of Lead Poisoning Among the Romans: An Essay Review', *Journal of the History of Medicine,* 39 (1984), 469–75.

32. J.O. Nriagu, 'Occupational Exposure to Lead in Ancient Times', *Science of Total Environment,* 31 (1983), 105–16; and more recently by the same author 'A History of Global Metal Pollution', *Science,* 272 (12 Apr 1996), 223–4; see also J.F. Healy, *Mining and Metallurgy in the Greek and Roman World* (London: Thames and Hudson, 1978).

33. This thesis was presented by L.G. Stevenson in 'A History of Lead Poisoning', PhD dissertation, Johns Hopkins University, 1949.

34. R.H. Major, 'Some landmarks in the history of lead poisoning', *Annals of Medical History,* 3 (1933), 218–19. A facsimile edition of Nikander's illustrated work from the Bibliothèque Nationale de France has been reprinted in 1997; see also A. S. F. Gow and A. F. Scholfield (eds), *Nicander: The Poems and Poetical Fragments* (Cambridge: Cambridge University Press, 1953).

35. This author's *De Materia Medica* was first printed in 1499. See R.T. Gunther (ed.), *The Greek Herbal of Dioscorides* (1655), trans. J. Goodyear (Oxford: Oxford University Press, 1934).

36. T.A. Hodge, 'Vitruvius, Lead Pipes and Lead Poisoning', *American Journal of Archeology,* 85 (1981), 486–91.

37. G. Agricola, *De Re Metallica,* trans. H.C. and L.H. Hoover (New York: Dover, 1950).

38. Paracelsus, 'On Miners' Sickness and Other Miners' Diseases', trans. G. Rosen, in H.E. Sigerist (ed.), *Four Treatises of Theophrastus von Hohenheim, called Paracelsus* (Baltimore: Johns Hopkins Press, 1941), 45–126.

39. G. Rosen, 'The Occupational Diseases of Miners During the Middle Ages and the Renaissance', in *The History of Miners' Diseases* (New York: Schuman, 1943), 39–88.

40. S. Stockhausen, *De Morbis Lithargiri* (On the Litharge Disease) (Goslar: 1658); see a later French translation: *Traite des Mauvais Effects de la Fumes de la Litharge* (Paris: Ruault, 1776).
41. Citois' original publication *De Novo et Populari Apud Pictones Dolore Colico Bilioso Diatriba* was published as *A Discussion of the New and Common Painful Bilious Colic among the Pictons* (Poitiers: Mesnier, 1626). An English translation of the first chapter of this book can be found in R.H. Major, *Classic Descriptions of Disease*, 3rd edn (Sprinfield: Thomas, 1945), 314–15.
42. J. Eisinger, 'Lead and Wine: Eberhard Gockel and the Colica Pictonum', *Medical History*, 26, 3 (1982), 279–302; and his more recent article 'Secret Poison: Episodic Outbreaks of Colic or "Wine Disease"', *Natural History*, 105 (1999), 48–53.
43. T. Sydenham, 'On Colica Pictonum', in *The Works of Thomas Sydenham, MD*, trans. R.G. Latham, new edn, 2 vols (London: Sydenham Society, 1850), Vol. II, 268.
44. 'The Famous Benjamin Franklin Letter on Lead Poisoning', dated 31 July 1786 and written by Franklin to Benjamin Vaughan. The letter is available on the Internet with its original capitalisation and spelling.
45. T. Cadwalader, *An Essay on the West-India Dry-Gripes* (Philadelphia: B. Franklin, 1745).
46. R.P. Wedeen, 'Punch Cures the Gout', *Journal of the Medical Society of New Jersey*, 78 (1981), 201–6. John Hunter experimentally confirmed Thomas Cadwalader's opinions in the early 1780s. See J. Hunter, 'Some Experiments Made upon Rum in Order to Ascertain the Cause of the Colic Frequent Among the Soldiers in the Island of Jamaica, in the years 1781 and 1782', *Medical Transactions of the College of Physicians, London,* 3 (1785), 227–49.
47. J. Huxham, 'A Small Treatise on the Devonshire Colic which was Very Epidemic in the Year 1724', translated and reprinted in *The Works of John Huxham* (London: W. Bent, 1788). For an informative secondary source H.A. Waldron, 'The Devonshire Colic', *Journal of the History of Medicine*, 25 (1970), 383–413.
48. G. Baker, *An Essay Concerning the Cause of the Endemial Colic of Devonshire* (London: J. Hughs, 1767), reprinted with some additions in the *Medical Transactions of the College of Physicians London* I (1768), 257–318, 319–63, 364–406 and second edition (1772), 257–315, 316–63, 364–406; see also H.A. Waldron, 'Sir George Baker and Lead Poisoning', *Proceedings XXIII International Congress History of Medicine* (London: Wellcome Institute of the History of Medicine, 1974), 1286–90.
49. B. Ramazzini, *Diseases of Tradesmen* (New York: Medical Lay Press, 1933), 17.
50. *Ibid.*, 53–5 and 67–71.

51. For an overview, C. Warren, *Brush With Death. A Social History of Lead Poisoning* (Baltimore: Johns Hopkins University Press, 2000).
52. G. van Swieten, 'On Colica Pictonum', in *Commentaries Upon the Aphorisms of Dr Hermann Boerhaave*, trans. from Latin, XVIII vols (Edinburgh: C. Eliot, 1776), Vol. X, 236–37.
53. See A. de Haen, *De Colica Pictonum Dissertatio* (Hagae: Comitum, 1745), trans. into French as 'Dissertation Sur la Colique de Poitou', *Journal de Medicine, Chirurgie, Pharmacie* X (1759), 508.
54. F. Merat de Vaumartoise, *Dissertation sur la Cholique Metallique* (Paris: Rigot, 1803); see also R. Christison, *A Treatise on Poisons in Relation to Medical Jurisprudence, Physiology and the Practice of Physic* (Edinburgh: A. Black, 1829), 421.
55. T. Tronchin, *A Treatise on the Colica Pictonum or the Dry Belly–Ach*[sic], trans. from Latin and ed. by R. Schomberg (London: W. Johnston, 1764). This work was originally published in Geneva in 1757 and also points out the dangers of drinking lead-contaminated water collected from leaden roofs in Amsterdam.
56. Percival, *op. cit.* (note 27), 92–110.
57. *Ibid.*, 23–5, 37–9.
58. J.C. Crawford, *Wanlockhead Miners Library* (Wanlockhead: Museum Trust, 1978). The Scottish Museum of Lead Mining located at Wanlockhead has a catalogue of this miners' library. See also W.S. Harvey and G. Downs-Rose, 'The Lead Mining Museum at Wanlockhead', *Industrial Archaeology*, 15 (1980), 11–29.
59. J. Wilson, surgeon at Durrisdeer, 'An Account of the Disease Called Mill Reek by the Miners at Leadhills', in a letter to Alexander Monro, *Essays and Observations, Physical and Literary*, I (1754), 459–66.
60. See W. White, 'Observations on the Medical Virtues of Lead', *Medical and Philosophical Commentaries*, 3 (1775), 72-80.
61. T. Goulard, *A Treatise on the Effects and Various Preparations of Lead*, trans. from French, new edn (London: P. Elmsly, 1775), 2.
62. See 'Extract of a Letter from Dr Percival to Dr Duncan on the External Use of Preparations of Lead', *Medical and Philosophical Commentaries*, 3 (1775), 199–205. This compound was created by the French surgeon Thomas Goulard in the 1760s.
63. Hunter later published his findings in a book: *Observations on the Diseases of the Army in Jamaica, and On the Best Means of Preserving the Health of Europeans in that Climate* (London: J. Johnson, 1796).
64 . The issue whether chronic lead poisoning was responsible for many of the symptoms included under the earlier label of 'gout' was advocated in J. Hardy, *A Candid Examination of What has been Advanced on the Colic of*

Poitou and Devonshire (London: T. Cadell, 1778); see R.P. Wedden, 'Irregular Gout: Humoral Fantasy or Saturnine Malady', *Bulletin of the New York Academy of Medicine,* 10 (1984), 969–79; and R. Porter and G.S. Rousseau, *Gout: The Patrician Malady* (New Haven: Yale University Press, 1998), especially 49–50. Analyses of eighteenth-century wines reveal a significant amount of lead and would support the notion of lead poisoning. Consult G.V. Ball, 'Two Epidemics of Gout', *Bulletin of the History of Medicine,* 45 (1971), 401–8.

65. J.R.R. Christie, 'William Cullen and the Practice of Chemistry', in A. Doig *et al.* (eds), *William Cullen and the Eighteenth-Century Medical World* (Edinburgh: Edinburgh University Press, 1993), 98–109; see also T. Hankins, *Science and the Enlightenment* (Cambridge: Cambridge University Press, 1985), 85–110.
66. For details, A.L. Donovan, *Philosophical Chemistry in the Scottish Enlightenment: The Doctrines and Discoveries of William Cullen and Joseph Black* (Edinburgh: Edinburgh University Press, 1975). A new survey of all contemporary scientific developments can be found in R. Porter (ed.), *Eighteenth-Century Science* (New York: Cambridge University Press, 2002). This is volume IV of a forthcoming eight-volume project, *The Cambridge History of Science,* edited by D.C. Lindberg and R.L. Numbers.
67. W. Cullen, 'Memorial to the Commissioners Managing the Annexed Estates', dated 19 March 1763, MSS Collection, National Library of Scotland. See Donovan, 'Moral Philosophy and Economic Improvement in Mid-Eighteenth-Century Scotland', *op. cit.* (note 66), 49–76.
68. W. Cullen, *First Lines of the Practice of Physic,* new ed., IV vols (Edinburgh: C. Elliot, 1785), Vol. III, 36–8.
69. B. Parr, *London Medical Dictionary,* II vols (Philadelphia: Mitchell, Ames and White, 1819), Vol. I, 462–5.
70. Cullen, *op. cit.* (note 68), Vol. IV, 18-38.
71. E. Goodwyn, 'Essay on Colica Pictonum', *Diss. RMS,* Vol. 18 (1785–7), 162.
72. S. Shapin, 'The Audience for Science in Eighteenth-Century Edinburgh', *History of Science,* 12 (1974), 95–121; and by the same author 'Property, Patronage and the Politics of Science', *British Journal of the History of Science,* 7 (1974), 1–41.
73. W. Alexander, *Diss. RMS,* Vol. 18 (1785–6), 410–25.
74. *Ibid.*, 416.
75. For information on John Brown's ideas, consult G.B. Risse, 'The Brownian System of Medicine: Its Theoretical and Practical Implications', *Clio Medica,* 5 (1970), 45–51.

76. H. Bowles, J. Jachman and W. Alexander, 'Experiments on Sugar of Lead to Determine Whether it be a Stimulus', *Diss. RMS,* Vol. 8 (1785), 85–121.
77. A.P. Anderson, *ibid.,* Vol. 24 (1789–90), 390–405. Anderson became a senior president of the Royal Medical Society for the 1790–1 session.
78. J. Prendergast, *De Colica Pictonum* (Edinburgh: Balfour and Smellie, 1786); J. Reid, *De Colica Pictonum* (Edinburgh: Balfour and Smellie, 1786); and A. Ponton, *De Colica Spasmodica* (Edinburgh: Balfour and Smellie, 1787).
79. J. Beamish, *De Colica Pictonum Complectens* (Edinburgh: C. Stewart, 1798); J. Dixon, *De Colica Pictonum* (Edinburgh: R. Allan, 1798); M. Moriarty, *De Colica Pictonum* (Edinburgh: R. Allan, 1804); D. Hay, *De Colica Pictonum* (Edinburgh: A. Smellie, 1809), and M. Kenny, *De Colica Pictonum* (Edinburgh: C. Stewart, 1810).
80. S. Pett's doctoral dissertation was *De Colica Pictonum* (Edinburgh: G. Creech, 1793).
81. Pett, *op. cit.* (note 1), 133–64.
82. J. Corn, 'Historical Perspective to a Current Controversy on the Clinical Spectrum of Plumbism', *Health and Society,* (winter 1975), 93–114.
83. This symptom was reported in a plumber; the case was presented by a medical student, Alexander P. Anderson, during the 1789–90 session of the Royal Medical Society. See *Diss. RMS,* Vol. 24 (1789–90), 390–405. For a modern interpretation, Y. Janin et al., 'The "Lead-induced Colic" Syndrome in Lead Intoxication', *Surgical Annual,* 17 (1985), 287–307.
84. A. Duncan Sr, *Clinical Reports and Commentaries, February–April 1795,* presented by A. Blackhall Morison (Edinburgh, 1795), MSS Collection, Royal College of Physicians, Edinburgh.
85. T.C. Hope, *Clinical Casebook* (Edinburgh, 1796–97), MSS Collection, Royal College of Physicians, Edinburgh.
86. *Ibid.*
87. *Ibid.*
88. D. Rutherford, *Clinical Cases* (Edinburgh: 1799), MSS Collection, Royal College of Physicians, Edinburgh.
89. *Ibid.*
90. Anonymous, 'Colica Pictonum', in *The Edinburgh Practice of Physic, Surgery, and Midwifery,* 5 vols (London: Kearsley, 1800-1803), Vol. 1, 435–6 and Vol. 2, 406–8.
91. T. Percival, *Essays, Medical and Experimental* (London), Vol. 2 (1767), 194; and Vol. 5, 172.
92. More details can be found in H. Clutterbuck, *An Account of a New and Successful Method of Treating those Affections which Arise from the Poison of Lead* (London: T. Boosey, 1794).

93. G.B. Risse, 'Electricity', in *Hospital Life in Enlightenment Scotland: Care and Teaching at the Royal Infirmary of Edinburgh* (New York: Cambridge University Press, 1986), 213–17.
94. Drinking and bathing in mineral waters at Bath and other European locations became quite fashionable. See R. Charleton, *An Inquiry into the Efficacy of Warm Bathing in Palsies* (Oxford: Clarendon Press, 1770). For an excellent secondary source consult A. Heywood, *A Trial of the Bath Waters: The Treatment of Lead Poisoning* (*Medical History*, Suppl. No. 10) (London: Wellcome Institute for the History of Medicine, 1990), 82–101, and by the same author 'Colica Pictonum: Taking the Cure in Bath', in R. Rolls *et al.* (eds), *A Pox on the Provinces* (Bath: Bath University Press, 1990), 101–10. Heywood and her colleagues at the Royal Infirmary of Bath conducted a series of studies regarding the physiological effects of these bathing practices and documented their success in removing lead compounds from the human body.
95. See recent aspects of this occupational hazard in C. Warren, *Brush With Death: A Social History of Lead Poisoning* (Baltimore: Johns Hopkins University Press, 2000); and P. Grandjean, *Widening Perspectives of Lead Toxicity* (Copenhagen: Fadl's Forlag, 1979).
96. For a broad perspective, R. Gillespie, 'Acounting for Lead Poisoning: The Medical Politics of Occupational Health', *Social History,* 15 (1990), 303–31.

PART III:
MEDICAL THEORY AND PRACTICE

7

Organising Medical Knowledge and Making Clinical Decisions: Phthisis and Student-Selected Case Histories

Clinical cases have traditionally been among the most important documents for understanding the representation, organisation, and transmission of medical information. In hospital practice, they provide a key form of medical discourse shaped by professional and social needs. Based on student casebooks and lecture notes, the essay analyses selected cases admitted to the Edinburgh Infirmary and labelled as 'phthisis' or 'pulmonary consumption', the most common and deadly ailment of the century. The intent was to employ a clinically complex disease and closely follow the words and actions of notable attending physicians exposing colleagues and students to the ambiguities of medical practice while attempting to save lives.

Introduction

> The best marked diseases, the most singular in nature, and the greatest variety of acute as well as chronic are chosen for [the clinical wards of the Royal Infirmary of Edinburgh]. Regular and circumstantial reports of every symptom belonging to the disease and every effect produced by the remedies exhibited are taken in the presence of students… There cannot therefore be a more useful addition to the medical college nor a more favourable institution for the improvement of the student, of the physician, or of medicine itself.
>
> Francis Home (1783)[1]

The practice of collecting memorable clinical cases has been a time-honoured tradition in medical practice.[2] As Foucault has noted, such texts are indeed valuable markers of epistemological activity.[3] In arranging their clinical experiences, practitioners engaged in a selection process based on prior knowledge and standards. For historians, such documents have long been among the most fruitful sources for grasping the representation, organisation, and transmission of clinical knowledge as well as understanding the actual management of past medical practices.[4] Newer approaches seek to interpret medical case histories as co-constructed narratives in which the sick and their healers collaborate to create unique stories of suffering examined within cultural contexts and from a rhetorical point of view. Indeed, these texts not only reflect practitioners' interviewing and organising skills, but also their ability to interpret the resulting information and make therapeutic choices. The clinical case history reveals much about the contemporary state of medical knowledge. It also provides valuable insights into decision-making and conditions governing professional authority and patient power.[5]

Individual records of clinical encounters were traditionally composed, collected, and preserved for purposes of future reference and study. Faced with difficult new cases, practitioners sought previous examples of bedside problem-solving and management in order to compare them with the situation at hand. From the seventeenth century on, when empirical information derived from the observation of patients became an increasingly respectable source of medical knowledge, casebooks began to proliferate.[6] Even authors writing for the fledgling medical journals of this period began to share particular case histories designed to either illustrate or, more importantly, to frame their clinical discoveries and conclusions.[7]

During the eighteenth century, the popularity of such documents soared with the medicalisation of hospital care and its potential to dramatically expand clinical knowledge.[8] Indeed, the social environment of hospitals came to play a central role in shaping new medical theories and sanctioning novel forms of patient management. Greater understanding of diseases came from patients on wards suffering acute, multiple, and often severe conditions. By abstracting salient disease manifestations – including anatomical lesions – sick persons became known merely for being carriers of particular dysfunctions. The fact that patients featured in institutional histories were recipients of charity, eliminated problems of medical confidentiality and etiquette associated with the care of private paying patients. In sum, the new modes of knowledge collected in hospital wards and casebooks became a new and important form of medical discourse elaborated within unique spaces and shaped by changing social and professional needs (Chapter 1).[9]

As noted elsewhere, the medicalising hospitals in Europe rapidly became a boon for eighteenth-century surgical and medical professionals.[10] As one local academic, Francis Home (1719–1813) observed, 'these charitable institutions [hospitals] amply repay the expense which the public bestows on them by promoting the study and practice of medicine'. Indeed, 'under one roof are collected a great variety of morbid cases to which students have an easy access and where a wide field is opened to physicians for the improvement of their science.'[11] To better organise bedside observations at the Edinburgh Infirmary, local university authorities reached agreement with hospital managers in 1750 to establish a separate teaching area at that institution. This ward was to be open only during the academic year from November to April and managed by university professors in three-month rotations.[12] Based on the model employed by Hermann Boerhaave (1668–1739) at Leyden's St Caecilia Gasthuis earlier in the century, Edinburgh's teaching ward opened with a capacity of twelve beds, six for males and six for females.[13] However, sustained student demand and the need for more hospital revenues encouraged the Infirmary's managers to expand this unit to thirty, and eventually fifty, beds during the 1780s. In a further move to accommodate the interests of the medical profession, university professors were authorised to choose their own patients from the pool of qualified applicants. Moreover, the professors could also request transfers of inmates from other parts of the institution who displayed unusual signs of disease, thereby ensuring a broader spectrum of clinical cases for their instruction. As a supplement to daily bedside instruction, the same professors organised a series of bi-weekly clinical lectures at the hospital to discuss selected cases.[14]

Hospitals like the Edinburgh Infirmary also provided opportunities to acquire anatomical and pathological knowledge. However, autopsies could not be routinely performed. The hospital managers only authorised a few dissections, usually conducted by surgical clerks employed by the institution who had never managed the deceased patients. Although the old tripartite division into physicians, surgeons and apothecaries was already crumbling under the weight of intense rivalry and professional competition, the ethics of a British physician–gentleman usually precluded his hands-on involvement with living bodies and corpses (Chapter 8). Lacking proper feedback from managing clinicians, the dissecting clerks simply composed brief and fragmentary reports that were dutifully filed with the rest of the clinical history.[15] Pathological anatomy continued to take a backseat to clinical findings. Under such circumstances, lesions were often misinterpreted, and the presumed causes responsible for death remained dubious. Despite the stigma attached to such examinations, surgeons were eager to perform human dissections on deceased inmates, especially those previously subjected to operations. Here the nature of incisions, the quality of sutures and postoperative infection could be eagerly checked.[16]

Journals, in each ward of the Edinburgh Infirmary, became the central repository of information concerning all ongoing patient developments and treatments. The registers were always available for professional perusal and required by statute to remain 'opened' on demand to every hospital donor – although in practice only the elected managers checked them carefully at their monthly meetings. A ward journal divided into seventeen separate columns allowed hospital practitioners to select and inscribe clinical details as well as organise the management of each patient under different rubrics that included basic data such as age and sex, symptoms and signs, diet and medications.[17] Some of the data concerning drugs and diets was additionally copied into a separate prescription book for the hospital apothecary in charge of compounding the drugs, as well as for the matron, cook, and nurses who arranged, prepared, and served the meals. Written in English, the ward journal acted as a medical filter, eliminating the voice and story of the patient in favour of the physician's summary account couched in terse, technical language. The large folio was kept on a desk with wheels so that it could be moved easily to the bedside when attending physicians and surgeons dictated their observations during daily rounds. Because the ledger was kept in a place of public access, all prescriptions and therapeutic indications entered in the journal were written in Latin to ensure confidentiality. The same approach was taken with intimate details linked to female menstrual status and the condition of sexual organs.[18]

Infirmary's clerks then modified and presumably abstracted the extensive documentation in the registers, and composed brief individual case histories for inclusion into another document, the ward ledger.[19] Like the journal, this ward ledger was to be updated frequently with the inclusion of progress notes and new prescriptions. On its last page, the ledger also had 'an index of the several patients and diseases mentioned in it'.[20] Some of this data was used to make entries in a general register of patients by recording name, ward, admission and discharge dates, diagnosis, and mode of hospital dismissal. Another perpetual register apparently contained an alphabetically arranged list of all the diseases seen in the hospital with cross references to particular ward ledgers and their respective patient histories.[21]

Student casebooks and lecture notes: a popular Edinburgh genre

Medical students, who wished to 'visit' with patients, 'hear' medical prescriptions or clinical lectures, attend operations and dissections, needed to purchase a 'licence'. With this admission ticket came a printed copy of regulations that needed to be 'cheerfully' observed. These rules were designed to ensure that the students were 'composed' and of 'decent carriage' while exercising their privilege of 'walking' the wards with the attending physicians and surgeons. Licence holders were told to keep their hats off and refrain from making noise while witnessing surgical operations in the amphitheatre. If found guilty of any 'indecent or irregular' behaviour that could be construed as 'hurtful to patients', the offending students forfeited their passes and were permanently excluded from entering the Infirmary.[22] Along with the ticket, students could use the hospital journals 'for taking copies of cases'. Clinical histories copied by Edinburgh students constitute key documents for an understanding of eighteenth-century medical practice. As already noted, the voice of the patient vanished after passing through the various stages of social and medical interpretation. Nevertheless, these records offer a unique window on contemporary clinical management in a charitable-institutional setting such as the Royal Infirmary of Edinburgh. From its inception, the hospital's elaborate registration system became an important factor for attracting medical students and surgical apprentices interested in clinical instruction. Indeed, a 1792 student guide boasted that,

> the Infirmary of Edinburgh is much superior to any similar institution in Britain for the purposes of medical education. The cases of patients are all regularly registered, and an account of their situation is daily given by the attending physicians.[23]

According to official regulations, on Saturday afternoons the 'clerk of the house' – a gentleman physician employed by the Infirmary – would 'read leisurely' – meaning slowly – from the teaching ward ledger in the operating amphitheatre. The assembled students who had paid for a ticket to participate in clinical instruction were encouraged to take 'notes of every cure they think worthwhile' pertaining to 'the whole of the practice' carried out in the Infirmary. For an additional fee, the clerk was even authorised to provide copies for students who, presumably, had better things to do than take dictation on their weekends.[24] By the year 1755, this practice had become popular enough to force an expansion in dictation. From the 1780s, as the clerks became overburdened with other duties, students were allowed to copy the information twice daily directly from the ward ledgers. New regulations approved in 1792 went even further, allowing students individually to borrow the books for such copying purposes at off-hours but precluding them from carrying the books out of the hospital.[25] Although authored by different individuals over a period of nearly thirty years, surviving student casebooks reveal an impressive homogeneity of structure, style, and content, suggesting that medical pupils closely followed an established protocol employed in the composition of the ledgers. Copying cases was, of course, only one aspect of acquiring clinical knowledge. Students were urged to interview the patients themselves before and after the rounds, questioning them or obtaining information from the nurses. Students 'ought to mark down regularly every day the situation of each patient by which means he will understand all the cases and become interested in the events,' proclaimed the 1792 manual.[26]

Not surprisingly, all surviving case histories appear to be direct products of dictation. The case histories often display a number of contemporary abbreviations and, hastily written in stages, frequently continue in later pages of a student's notebook to record subsequent developments.[27] Some students were more meticulous in their copying than others; they had their cases rewritten later in a legible and sometimes elegant fashion by an amanuensis.[28] A comparison among cases recorded in several contemporary student notebooks also reveals omissions and inaccuracies caused by the speedy transfer of information from ledgers to student notebooks. Some case histories have errors in dates, pulse readings, and the dosage of medications. More serious failures were oversights in listing symptoms and signs exhibited by certain patients, omitted diagnoses, and even neglected dietary instructions or daily progress notes.[29] Apparently, each student filtered the data according to his own interests and priorities.

One can also detect differences in the spelling of patients' names, dates of institutional admission and discharge between the ward journals, notebooks and the Infirmary's general patient register. Perhaps part of the problem was that several of the patients featured in these histories were originally admitted to other hospital wards before their transfer to the teaching unit. In turn, when the managing professor relinquished his rotation to another colleague, the remaining inmates were promptly discharged to the ordinary wards and no further details of their hospitalisation were therefore copied. Finally, given the increase in admissions and chronic lack of clerical assistance, periodic breakdowns occurred at all levels of this intricate registration system during the latter decades of the century. In this context, busy students copying clinical cases only added to the inconsistencies and omissions that already plagued all hospital records.[30]

Nevertheless, Edinburgh student case histories came to be fairly close copies of another constructed medical text, the ward ledger. Patients' voices, except for occasional terms, were, of course, omitted. As a result, they reveal very little personal information, except age, sex, – and sporadically – occupation (males) or married status (females). Some inmates were identified as soldiers and servants since the Edinburgh Infirmary had established special wards for their care. In exceptional cases there were references to previous hospital admissions, sick relatives, and place of residence. After listing name and age, as well as date of admission, all cases contained a brief history that enumerated the patient's key complaints. Instead of reproducing subjective experiences from the patient's own narrative, stereotypical combinations of symptoms and signs sought to convey specific medical meanings.[31] At times, symptoms were linked to environmental conditions, including cold weather, damp lodgings, and exposure to rain. Urban and rural accidents abounded. In one account, a ploughman came into the hospital with a paralysis of his left leg following a fall and collision with a large boulder.[32] Previous treatments were also recorded, revealing a multitude of popular practices such as bloodletting and the use of patented nostrums. If pertinent to the presenting condition, occupational relationships were revealed. For example, a mason who displayed an opaque speck on one of his eyes was recorded as having been busy hammering a stone fragment.[33] A glassmaker from Leith, in turn, complained of a chest ailment attributed to frequent temperature changes between his workshop and the outdoors.[34]

This so-called 'accession of symptoms' or 'discovery of disease' was sometimes followed by a number of diagnostic procedures.[35] Hospital physicians gave arriving patients brief physical inspections, determining pulse and respiration rates, skin colour, appearance of the tongue, and other obvious bodily signs.[36] Thus, at the time of admission, all new patients' pulses, their quality and rate, were determined and registered on the chart. These measurements were then repeated daily,[37] followed by reports about the condition of the inmates' skin, tongue, appetite, urine, and bowels. In the established structure of the Edinburgh case history a further component, if deemed useful, was the general appearance of the patient. Often, physicians were stumped by the clinical manifestations of their arriving patients, incapable of making a diagnosis or, in the language of the time, remaining 'under ambiguities'.

Following the patient's salient complaints and vital signs, the clinical records reproduced their first set of prescriptions written by the attending professors. Although all patients admitted to a hospital were supposed to receive similar routine treatments, the evidence obtained from the notebooks suggests the attending physicians individualised their therapies in response to particular patient needs and clinical situations. Progress notes, enumerating prominent symptoms and, when necessary, recording additional prescriptions, followed. Therapeutical actions were sometimes characterised as 'throwing' a preparation at the patient. Drug effects or 'exhibitions' were regularly noted, including the appearance of 'mischief' or side-effects. At times, the medicines were 'received with loathing' and comments were made about the patients actually 'bearing' individual doses. Physicians garnered success when the patient was said to be 'in the train', meaning on the road to recovery. Finally, the clinical record cited the patient's discharge status. Most left 'cured' or 'relieved', others 'by desire'. Allowing the dying to leave the institution was not unusual. For the managers it was a welcome strategy to reduce a hospital's mortality statistics.

It also served to meet the demands of some patients and their relatives to pass away at home surrounded by family and friends (Chapter 1).

Little is known about the criteria used by students to filter the information contained in hospital documents for their individual notebooks; however a major factor was the student's enrolment in the courses of clinical lectures. In some instances, the entries followed a strict chronological arrangement; in others, the students just show-cased a cluster of patients with similar ailments. Many had introductory indices listing the names and diagnoses of all selected patients. Some notebooks only contain female cases. One Edinburgh professor, James Gregory (1753–1821), boasted that many of the students, including himself, came to possess 'complete and regular journals of every prescription and symptom from the hour that the patient entered the ward till he was dismissed'.[38] Although the statement may have been rhetorical, there is no question that student casebooks from the Edinburgh Infirmary achieved a measure of popularity.

In addition to casebooks, medical students also collected notes or full transcripts from the clinical lectures given by their professors. First organised by John Rutherford (1695–1779) in the late 1740s, the clinical course had been intended to supplement the less formal instruction at the bedside. Three decades later, the lectures had officially become part of the medical curriculum and were delivered twice a week in the hospital's amphitheatre. During the academic year stretching from early November until the end of April, Edinburgh professors selected the topics and individual patients to be managed and discussed in the Infirmary's teaching ward. Whenever possible, groups of patients suffering from similar ailments were presented. This strategy allowed teachers to make comparisons as well as critical distinctions regarding disease evolution and treatment. Some students reproduced verbatim the teacher's remarks in shorthand and had them later re-copied in legible script by a professional copier. Thanks to their efforts, we can recover the candid voices of Edinburgh's most distinguished practitioners as they struggled at the bedside.[39]

In the special pedagogical setting of a teaching ward, some of Scotland's top medical practitioners freely shared their beliefs, experiences, and uncertainties as they engaged in clinical problem-solving. Professors like William Cullen (1710–90), James Gregory and Andrew Duncan Sr (1744–1828) were openly willing to express their clinical reasoning and justify particular therapeutic strategies. Pathological anatomy and certain clinico–pathological correlations were also attracting professional attention. As Cullen explained to his students, 'it is not improperly said that the earth hides the faults of physicians'. He concluded that 'if every patient that dies were opened, it would too often discover the frivolity of our conjectures and futility of our practice'.[40] Those speculations, and Cullen's penchant for theoretical explanations or 'great turn for system' regarding the underlying phenomena of health and disease, were often fanciful.[41] Delivered with much ingenuity, they both attracted and repelled students, making it at times necessary for the professor to back off and apologise. However, Cullen was also a bedside empiricist willing to reformulate his theories and classifications based on new clinical evidence. Moreover, he definitely remained a therapeutic sceptic: he believed it was his moral duty to make candid admissions and unvarnished comments on medical practice (Chapter 4). This prevented what Thomas Percival (1740–1804), in his medical ethics tract, called 'self-deception'.[42] At the end of Cullen's 1772 lecture series, he even felt compelled to apologise for exposing his audience to the ambiguities of eighteenth-century medicine and his own errors. 'I make no scruple in discovering my own mistakes', he allowed, and offered 'no apology for my own ignorance'. Moreover, Cullen conceded that 'I am imprudent in telling you my faults some of you will no doubt discover', but 'if you have taken as much pains to learn as I have taken to teach, you will not go without some instruction'.[43]

Carefully bound in leather folios – some labelled 'Medical Tracts' – both Infirmary casebooks and lecture notes constituted important reference works in physicians' libraries before more clinical information became available in printed sources. This fact ensured their survival long after much of the official hospital documents had vanished.[44] Most of this information was generated between the years 1760–1800, at the height of Edinburgh's popularity as Europe's most prominent medical school. The combination of individual patient histories and academic commentaries about their management offers a unique window into the world of eighteenth-century clinical decision-making. 'The manner in which I have proceeded is, I think, a good one', explained Cullen. 'First to give you in many cases a slight, at least some general view of your case, to let you know in what manner I view it and what plan of practice I chiefly intend.'[45]

Phthisis: a disease of consumption

Consumption is a bodily process popularly defined as the 'wearing away or consuming all the fleshy parts of the body'. It was considered to be the most common and deadly disease in eighteenth-century Britain. Foreigners dubbed it *morbus Anglicus* or the 'English Malady'. Often a term of derision and ridicule, the label covered a variety of so-called 'wasting' conditions, among them atrophy, cancer, scurvy, scrofula, venereal disease, dropsy, catarrhs, hysteria, and hypochondriasis (Chapter 9). Consumption was blamed, in part, on the country's peculiar 'coldness and dampness', as well as occupational factors and urban lifestyle.[46] Critics stressed the paradox of high living, with its excessive consumption of goods, for triggering physical wasting. Among the most prominently recognised forms was the consumption afflicting the lungs.[47] Eighteenth-century knowledge concerning pulmonary wasting, or *phthisis* was primarily based on the ground-breaking work of Richard Morton (1637–98) whose *Phthisiologia* (1689) was translated into English in 1694 and reprinted in 1720. Relying mostly on classical antecedents, Morton artfully linked a number of respiratory symptoms to the presence of small lumps or 'tubercles' in the lungs, which were discovered through dissections at the autopsy table. Although at this time pathological anatomy remained the faithful handmaiden of clinical medicine, the author constructed a hypothetical pathogenesis on the basis of contemporary humoral and chemical views of the body. Morton relied on ideas later expressed in more detail by the famous Dutch physician, Herman Boerhaave. He conceived the human body as a blend of solid organs, membranes and vessels, all composed of fibres, and less dense, fluid particles constantly flowing in particular mixtures among each other following the laws of hydrodynamics. The heart propelled blood through a network of vessels of decreasing size allowing individual organs to selectively trap its particles at various bodily locations to build tissues and produce secretions. When the normal interactions between circulating fluids and their conduits became disturbed, disease ensued. Fibres could become weaker, soft and lax, or too stiff, firm and rigid. When some vessels were relaxed or obstructed, blood particles could be forced into the wrong tissues and organs where they stagnated and produced inflammation.[48]

Morton's theory about the basic mechanism of tubercle formation was that 'crude' blood serum leaked into lung tissue. Even though such spills could potentially be dangerous, it was also possible they could be re-absorbed or converted into 'scars'. However, if the tissue fibres in the lungs lost their strength, circulation accelerated and blood acquired some toxic or 'sharp' particles, thereby inflaming the tubercles. Morton viewed the so-called 'ripening' of lung tubercles as a gradual inflammatory process that spread primarily through the lymphatic system and eventually became quite destructive, leading to the widespread formation of ulcers and cavities. The possibility of arresting these events in the lungs – confirmed by clinical and pathological studies – lent hope to sufferers and practitioners alike who were called to halt this progressive and eventually fatal path.[49] Boerhaave's contemporary, the German physician Friedrich Hoffman (1660–1742), took a further step by placing greater emphasis on the role of nerves in human physiology and pathogenesis. Hoffman came to subordinate Boerhaave's hydrodynamics to the integrative control of the nervous system.

Hoffman's view, based on Newtonian notions, was that nerves possessed ethereal particles flowing through them that provided all bodily fibres with degrees of tension necessary to carry out their normal functions. Moreover, through the actions of the nervous system, a certain 'sympathy' linked all bodily organs, ensuring the co-ordination of motions and the flow of fluids. Disease was the result of abnormal bodily movements triggered by changes in the nervous system. Increases in fibre tension or tone caused spasms, especially in blood vessels, while loss of tension resulted in fibre atony and paralysis. Hoffmann explained the formation of 'polypoid concretions' (tubercles) in the lungs as the result of nervous and circulatory disturbances that allowed the deposition of 'acrimonious' particles.[50]

Physicians had little to say regarding the possible causes of phthisis beyond merely enumerating the traditional constitutional liabilities, acquired through inheritance, which could interact with harmful environmental conditions. Most medical authors remained sceptical about the contagious nature of the disease. However, in 1722, a little-known English physician, Benjamin Marten (1704–82), advanced the idea that the 'original and essential' cause of this disease was certain species of minute living creatures. They were conveyed either through the air or the blood to the lungs where they nested and 'came to perfection'.[51] The idea was rejected due to the lack of empirical proof and the author's own admission that the theory was conjectural. Others, like Edward Jenner (1749–1823), of cowpox fame, speculated that tubercles were similar to insect-caused hydatid cysts he had observed in a variety of domestic animals during his rural practice in the 1790s.[52]

On the other hand, George Cheyne (1671-1743) took a broader approach, blaming Britain's contemporary affluent society's luxurious consumption patterns for the appearance of phthisis and other ubiquitous scourges.[53] Indeed, pulmonary consumption was considered a true disease of civilisation. Genteel, high living, including an over-indulgence of food and alcohol, lavish fashions and light dress, immoderate sexual activity and sedentary habits, all were believed to weaken the body, sending it into a gradual tail-spin of malaise and decay that ended in premature death.[54] Such a medical critique of irregular living habits was not surprising since physicians' clinical experiences were almost exclusively derived from affluent private patients. At the time, many were heavily invested in moral crusades that sought to fight the corruption of commercial society. Little attention was paid to their lowly and often sick domestic servants, who, living in close proximity, must surely have contributed to the rising incidence of lung diseases among their wealthy masters.

The prevalence of pulmonary phthisis among young, affluent women – their bodies naturally delicate and sensible – generated an extensive medical discourse. The notion that females lived in a perpetual state of constitutional and acquired weakness had a long history (Chapter 8).[55] Physicians believed that the very characteristics that made the female body pleasing to the eyes of men also made it susceptible to a myriad of frailties and inexplicable ailments. New cultural standards of bodily slimness, achieved through starvation diets laced with plenty of tea and coffee, were believed to further relax bodily fibres. With respect to pulmonary consumption, Francis Home pointed out that enfeebled females could easily become overheated when spending a great deal of time indoors, thus becoming more liable to the colder air as they moved outdoors. 'Effluvia' emanating from hot and crowded drawing rooms could be troublesome. Clothing that partially exposed women's upper bodies was thought to be dangerous to women's health. Because cold air seemed an important causal factor to consumption, an Edinburgh graduate, Thomas Beddoes (1760–1808), explained that the Scots had made themselves even more susceptible to the disease by exchanging their traditional thick and warm woollen plaids for lighter, more fashionable, cooler English linens. For Beddoes, consumption in women was obviously self-inflicted.[56]

In sharp contrast with medical reality, the prevalence of pulmonary consumption among the elite had a profound impact on late-eighteenth-century European culture. New and romantic representations of the disease clashed with the luxury model. Positive aesthetics of consumptive life emerged and focused primarily on young affluent persons suffering from the disease. These young people were portrayed as particularly fragile and delicate, sensitive and slender. They were considered to be victims of what Beddoes characterised as a 'devouring monster that stifles at his leisure the sons and daughters of the land'.[57] With their vitality seriously compromised, sufferers displayed a so-called 'hectic glow' created by pale skin, sparkling eyes, erotic red lips and rosy cheeks. Indeed, consumption became extolled as a process of ethereal transformation, a triumph of soul over flesh, heroically ending in premature death, represented as a final snuffing-out of the flickering, vital flame. The end was quite civilised: painless, slow and peaceful.[58]

Although much of the medical focus was on well-off consumptives, the labouring population was not completely ignored. In his account of diseases prevailing in Scotland, John Sinclair (1754–1835) admitted that consumption among the poor 'carries off the greatest number of persons about the middle period of life'.[59] Indeed, persons between the ages of fifteen and thirty were mostly affected, with females more liable to suffer from the scourge than males. Cullen and Beddoes pointed out the frequency of its respiratory form among individuals who were constantly exposed to dust such as stonecutters, millers, and clothing manufactures, including weavers, flax dressers, tailors and glovers. For their part, cotton workers were confined to crowded and overheated premises. Beddoes recognised the lack of 'good and comfortable accommodations among the poorer classes' as a factor contributing to consumption.[60] In Edinburgh's official mortality statistics, the category 'consumption' remained the most common cause of death in the late eighteenth century, accounting for almost a third of all recorded burials. Some observers linked the high prevalence of this disease to the city's severe air pollution created by fumes from coal burning during winters.[61]

Although its clinical course was fitful, phthisis displayed a progressive evolution that could be classified into several stages, based on particular bodily changes; each required a different prognosis and therapy.[62] Thanks to the findings of Giovanni B. Morgagni (1682–1771) and Joseph Lieutaud (1703–80), correlations between clinical events and pathological changes in the body were already in full swing.[63] The appearance of special lesions known as tubercles in the lungs had been widely observed and their variable evolution from clusters of pin-sized 'indurated' pocks to scars or larger pus-filled abscesses was duly noted at post-mortem examinations. Medical authors believed that these ulcers originated from infected lymphatic glands located in the lungs. As such they resembled the external buboes notorious in plague and syphilis. Still comparing tubercles to wound infections, physicians believed that such lesions often failed to heal because they were constantly contaminated by inspired air. The eventual disintegration and evacuation of tubercles destroyed the surrounding lung tissue and left behind extensive cavities, a process described by, among others, Matthew Baillie (1761–1823) at St George's Hospital in London.[64]

To establish a true anatomico–clinical synthesis, physicians needed to incorporate their correlations into a functional system in which clinical signs and pathological lesions could be interpreted within a mutually interacting physiopathology. The initial 'incipient' phase of pulmonary consumption featured a variety of respiratory symptoms: cough, mucous expectoration, and fever typical of the common cold or 'catarrh' – without signs of body wasting. However, asthma and the spitting of blood were a signal of concern to practitioners. Since Antiquity, coughing up blood – often a dramatic symptom – had suggested the presence of phthisis, but in the eighteenth century its occurrence was not exclusively linked to the presence of tuberculous ulcers.[65] Haemoptysis was seen as an independent phenomenon of vascular rupture, and like nosebleeds, often temporary and still capable of mending. Physicians speculated that the bronchial tubes and lungs were simply inflamed and thought these conditions were treatable with recovery likely.[66]

However, the persistence of haemoptysis, together with sharp chest pains, and an onset of a 'hectic fever' with a purulent expectoration definitely signalled the transition from an 'incipient' to an 'established' phthisis. The 'hectic' fever displayed a diurnal rhythm with spikes at noon and midnight, followed by profuse sweats. The fever was also responsible for the characteristic facial flushing and rosy cheeks. The symptoms of established phthisis strongly suggested an inflammatory condition: the presence of tubercles in the lungs. Medical authors speculated that the fully developed abscesses initially remained closed, containing an 'acrimony' or acrid matter. Except for providing ammunition for the fever, tubercles 'give little distress', declared Duncan Sr. However, as the disease continued to progress, these tumours broke open, and their contents were partially eliminated by expectoration, prompting sudden discharges of what was termed a 'vomica', a large amount of white or yellowish sputum said to have had a sweet taste.[67] Many practitioners, including Cullen, thought this sputum also entered the blood stream, poisoning the entire body. Physicians were similarly concerned about a potential stagnation and transformation of the effused blood into acrid pus in persons with haemoptysis because this process could further erode the lungs. In spite of increases in appetite, patients became debilitated and 'consumed', their flesh wasted.[68]

For eighteenth-century practitioners, colour, consistency, and taste of the expectorated sputum had important diagnostic implications. Here again, clinical and pathological observations converged to suggest a hypothetical progression of this fatal disease. Mucus was naturally transparent; pus always opaque. Still, a clear separation between purulent tuberculous phlegm and other material expelled during ordinary bouts of bronchitis and pneumonia remained elusive. 'Sink or swim' tests of the patient's sputum gave ambiguous results. Usually, the pus was supposed to break up and go down in a flask when sputum was immersed in water, while the mucus remained intact and floated.[69] Efforts to mix sputum with a solution of sulphuric acid or other salts apparently achieved a better separation. Cullen and other medical authorities often characterised the expelled tubercular matter as 'scrofulous', thus establishing a clear linkage between phthisis and a previously independent condition known as 'scrofula'.[70] For centuries, Britons had experienced the 'King's Evil', a disease of children and adolescents that affected the lymph nodes of the neck, producing hard but painless swellings that could turn into ulcers, draining a foul, whitish fluid often followed by spontaneous recovery.[71] By the eighteenth century, medical authorities considered scrofula another form of 'consumption' blamed on poor nutrition and damp climate. Seemingly widespread in southern Scotland, many of its sufferers and their offspring eventually also came to display pulmonary symptoms due to tubercular disease.

The third and final stage was an 'advanced' phthisis, in which the bodily conditions of its victims reached a critical level of deterioration. Debility and emaciation were extreme. A pale, emaciated countenance suggestive of the *facies Hippocratica* signalled the imminent demise. At this point, authors speculated that many tubercular lesions located in the lungs had finally ulcerated, spewing their purulent material into the bronchia while destroying the lung tissue and creating cavities. In this phase, previous symptoms – including frequent bouts of 'vomica' – were now severe. With the inhaled air presumably rendering the ulcerous matter even more acrid, its absorption into the body only accelerated the inflammatory status in the lungs. It likewise irritated the bowels. Legs and feet became swollen. Persistent coughing, purulent or bloody sputum, high fever, and the appearance of stubborn diarrhoea marked a gradual march towards death, with only periodic, short-lived remissions that falsely rekindled the patients' hope for a recovery. In fact, medical authors stressed the fact that most consumptives never relinquished their expectation for a final cure. Sufferers remained lucid until the very end – the mind alternated between euphoria and calmness – until ultimately delirium signalled the impending end.

Lung consumption at the Edinburgh Infirmary: decision-making at the bedside

Persons suffering from obvious pulmonary consumption – or its the medical term *phthisis pulmonaris* – were, in spite of its pervasive presence among members of the Scotland's lower working class, seldom admitted to the Edinburgh Infirmary.[72] Indeed, subjoined to the statutes governing that institution, was the statement that 'patients labouring under pulmonary consumptions, if the disease be advanced to the second or last stage, will suffer from the air of the hospital, however ventilated.'[73] At issue was the lack of what the surgeon John Aikin (1747–1822) branded as 'medicinally soft and pure' air. 'All diseases affecting the lungs, are, I fear, of that kind which can never receive benefit from even the sweetest and best contrived hospital', he remarked.[74] Eighteenth-century physicians were of the opinion that pulmonary consumption was 'absolutely incurable' in the long term and therefore 'improper' for treatment in hospitals. The exception to the rule suggested that 'in the beginning of the disease, while its nature is perhaps still equivocal, patients of this kind may be admitted.'[75] Thus, several 'incipient' cases were periodically admitted, especially to the Infirmary's teaching ward for pedagogical reasons.

Other respiratory conditions broadly defined as 'pectoral complaints' also eventually turned out to include a number of undiagnosed consumptives. Infirmary managers, for their part, considered the admission of phthisis cases an unwelcome event. At a time when official statistics were published and high cure rates important in attracting patrons, the potential of these patients for elevating institutional mortality figures could be potentially detrimental for raising funds (Chapter 1).[76] Moreover, the authorities were always fearful of admitting individuals who, in William Cullen's words, were true 'stick-fast' patients, defined as individuals whose multiple and chronic complaints would allow them to remain in the wards for long periods of time, preventing patient turnover.[77] Under such circumstances, the admission and management of consumptive patients demanded special caution and judicious clinical decisions from the academic physicians in charge.

An analysis of selected case histories taken from surviving student notebooks that recorded a total of 808 cases between 1771 and 1799 reveals the Infirmary's teaching ward managed twenty-four patients, thirteen males and eleven females, officially labelled as suffering from 'phthisis'. Two-thirds of the arrivals occurred on weekends, including Sundays, suggesting the gravity of the patients' complaints. There were significant age differences between the patients; the average age for the men was thirty, for women twenty–two. Included in the sample were individuals seen by John Gregory and William Cullen during the early 1770s, followed by patient clusters managed by James Gregory in the late 1770s and mid-1780s, and two additional groups in the 1790s supervised by Andrew Duncan Sr and Thomas C. Hope. In all instances, the student-copied case histories were matched with contemporary lecture notes and discussions from the respective Edinburgh professors who treated the patients. The words and actions of these practitioners at the bedside provide an intimate glimpse of eighteenth-century clinical practice, and especially of a clinically complex disease such as consumption. Of particular interest were the teachers' comments and rationale for justifying their clinical management.[78]

On 2 January 1772, John Gregory admitted James Murrain, an 8-year-old boy with a tentative diagnosis of intestinal worms. This was a rare event since the Infirmary seldom admitted children except when very young and in company of their mothers. The patient – or more likely his relatives – provided a straightforward account of abdominal pain, together with bouts of vomiting and diarrhoea, as well as fits of cough and fever. In addition, he seemed to be grinding his teeth and picking his nose. Murrain was said to be otherwise healthy and active until the last two years when he began to cough and lose strength. The abdominal complaints had started seven weeks earlier and had been treated with emetics and other medicines resulting in the expulsion of two or three worms. On inspection, the boy appeared wasted, and displayed several abscessed swellings on one side of his neck, suggestive of a common Scottish condition: 'scrofula'. When William Cullen assumed the clinical rotation in February 1772, the patient's great emaciation left no doubt about the underlying condition: pulmonary consumption. 'I formed a judgement of the disorder as soon as I had occasion to consider it', he told the students.[79] Almost a year later, Cullen admitted another patient, John Crookshanks, who failed to be included in a student casebook but probably arrived just before Christmas in December 1772. On admission, Crookshanks complained of cough and persistent chest pains. Together with his respiratory symptoms, this man appeared to have recently lost 'strength and flesh'. In this instance, Cullen seemed more hopeful, telling students that 'I thought it worthwhile to give you a well vouched instance of such a cure' since he presumed that the patient still had only a small number of tubercles in his lungs without ostensible suppuration.[80]

The next group of patients listed in the notebooks consisted of three male patients seen by James Gregory during his teaching rotation in the late autumn of 1779. The first was 20-year–old John Mathews, admitted on 9 November with chest pain and breathing difficulties. John complained of recurrent 'cough, pain of breast, and haemoptoe' from an exposure to cold twelve months earlier. The pain apparently shifted around the chest and the young man was fast becoming short of breath. Three days before admission, Mathews had been suddenly seized with persistent pain around the umbilical region of the abdomen, the complaint only temporarily diminished through massage. He was followed on 16 November by 30-year-old William Simpson. Simpson was quite hoarse and complained of a cough 'most troublesome when in bed'. For three months copious expectoration and hoarseness accompanied the cough, particularly during the night. He had difficulty breathing and his legs became periodically swollen. Next came a 37-year-old brewer, John White, who entered the institution on 7 December presenting with a history of coughing up blood.[81] When asked about this, he complained of repeated nosebleeds – he had been struck over his left eye months earlier – as well as blackish stools and progressive exhaustion.

James Gregory's second sample of presumed consumptive patients featured three females admitted to the Infirmary during the winter of 1787. All of them related similar respiratory symptoms. The first was 26-year-old Janet Hunter, a servant, admitted on 9 February complaining of violent bloody cough and frequent shivering fits. She also spoke of a lack of appetite, had lost strength and weight, and was unable to lie on her left side. Because of her persistent and violent coughing bouts she had been homebound for two months prior to being admitted. Hunter was followed by 19-year-old Ann Monro who arrived on 17 February complaining of chest pains and a short, 'tearing' cough, as well as suffering from headaches, cold clammy night sweats and a distended stomach. Finally, 31-year-old Jane Lindsay entered on 9 March with frequent cough and recurring vomiting of blood.[82] She was portrayed as being 'very much reduced and enfeebled' by her ailment, bedridden at home since the previous October because of her debility and lack of appetite.

Eight years later, during the late winter of 1795, another group of presumed consumptives arrived at the Infirmary's teaching ward then under the management of Andrew Duncan Sr. Among them was 34-year-old Daniel Robertson, a waiter, admitted on 3 February complaining of pains in his sternum. He also suffered from profuse night sweats and was quite emaciated. For at least six weeks, his severe cough had yielded a copious white expectoration streaked with blood but no purulent material, prompting a diagnosis of *phthisis catarrhalis* and hopes for a possible recovery. Daniel Robertson was followed by a 23-year old servant, Barbara Taylor, who came to the teaching ward on 11 March with acute pains in the left side of her abdomen as well as frequent cough. She seemed somewhat less compromised, had no bloody cough, but did experience regular night sweats. Four days later entered 29-year-old Daniel MacIntosh with chest pains and frequent cough 'attended by a very copious expectoration, sometimes of a gross, viscid matter, in general of a thin mucus'. Finally, on 22 March, Duncan admitted 30-year-old Margaret Dewer because of difficult breathing and sharp pains extending from the left shoulder to the sternum.[83] She also felt oppression in her chest and had difficulty breathing. This was amplified by a severe cough with copious expectoration of viscid, yellowish matter of a bad taste and odour that Duncan pronounced 'alarming'. Finally, a year later, Thomas C. Hope, then in charge of the teaching unit, admitted on 15 December 1796 15-year-old Kitty King. The patient complained of debility and depression. She had a violent cough attended with scanty expectoration tinged with a small amount of black blood.[84]

On the basis of their clinical histories, all patients except Kitty King were said to suffer from 'a fully formed hectic fever' characterised by alternating episodes of coldness and heat, followed by profuse sweat. Most had recurring and stabbing chest pains that prevented them from sleeping and forced them to lie on one side. As a result these individuals were quite exhausted, and several suffered from persistent diarrhoeas commonly associated with the end stage of phthisis. Indeed, many of them were said to have lost considerable weight – recorded in their charts as 'reduced in flesh and strength'. This was particularly true for the three women seen by Gregory in 1787 as well as Cullen's John Crookshanks and Duncan's Daniel MacIntosh. Most symptoms were blamed on the usual factors afflicting the lower class: hard labour, cold weather, damp lodgings, and exposure to rain. Barbara Taylor thought her 'frequent night watching' – keeping nightly vigils on a household member where she was working – was responsible for her sufferings.

Family histories were often sought to supplement the information provided by the patients about their own experiences. Perhaps as a diagnostic clue, the clinical history noted that both parents of Gregory's Jane Lindsay had previously perished from phthisis. In turn, Gregory's William Simpson claimed to have had a child who died of *tabes mesenterica*; another ailment frequently linked to early consumption. Among previous treatments patients took for their complaints prior to hospitalisation, were painkilling draughts. Gregory's patient John White had also been bled and Duncan's Daniel MacIntosh was blistered. As was usually the practice, the menstrual status of female patients was sought and reported. With the exception of Janet Hunter and Jane Lindsay, all the women claimed to be to be suffering from amenorrhoea since becoming ill. In Margaret Dewer's case, the menses had not resumed 'since her last lying-in, as she suckled her child till within these five weeks'.[85] The adolescent Kitty King had just experienced her menarche eight months earlier but reported no subsequent periods.

Physical data was usually restricted to general bodily inspections, pulse and respiration measurements and an examination of the tongue. Tall, thin and narrow-chested people endowed with lax and delicate fibres were more liable to become sick with pulmonary consumption. Towards the end of the century, Beddoes described a species of 'florid' consumption portrayed by an appearance of 'vivid' eyes, together with bright red cheeks, lips, tongue, and throat believed to arise from an excess of oxygen in the blood.[86] In several instances, the Edinburgh clinical histories contain similar remarks concerning the ruddy, plethoric complexion of certain phthisic patients. Gregory remarked that his patient, William Simpson, 'had the proper predisposing sanguineo–melancholic temperament'. Cullen focused on the association between 'scrofula' and phthisis; for example he remarked about the 'scrofulous habit' of John Crookshank. Both identifications represented a point of convergence between popular and professional notions that the body's surface disclosed significant signs of illness.[87] Additional testing of the sputum – if it could be obtained – were important for arriving at a realistic prognosis for each case. If patients continued to cough up fresh blood, the outcome was ominous. Before routine thermometry, the periodicity of a 'hectic' fever followed by profuse sweats could be simply detected by pulse measurements although 'inspections with the thermometer' were in use for other febrile conditions.[88] Observations of 'weak' pulses and 'fast' rates – over one hundred per minute – were common in patients' charts.[89] After taking John Crookshanks' pulse while he sat by the ward's fireplace in early February 1773, Cullen admitted to students that it was so fast 'as to pass my power of numbering'.[90] The man had an 'established' phthisis that would be extremely difficult to cure. But Cullen felt that there was still a small possibility the lung tubercles, currently engulfed in an inflammatory reaction, could be transformed into scar tissue. 'I thought it worthwhile to give you a well-vouched instance of such a cure', he explained. The fact that Crookshanks was allowed to be ambulatory and gather by the fire – a practice usually reserved for convalescents – suggested that Infirmary physicians had not yet given up on him. On the other hand, the patient's feeble pulse made Cullen fear that Crookshanks 'had not many days to live'. He remarked he had 'seen the same event of death take place merely from the debility'.[91]

Gregory was much more pessimistic, telling his student audience that anyone with a hectic fever, like that of William Simpson, had only one chance in a thousand of surviving the disease. Incipient cases, Gregory allowed, could perhaps be arrested, presumably under a regimen of proper diet, warm climate, and moderate exercise. Duncan was equally blunt in his prognoses. Referring to Daniel MacIntosh, Duncan was quoted in one student notebook as saying that this man was in a 'most debilitated state, and his disease was fatal…. Before the end of the course we shall see by dissection whether our opinion has been well founded.'[92] Yet, past clinical experience suggested that patients could linger for quite some time and that hospital stays, especially during the winter months, would actually protect them from acquiring other respiratory ailments, which usually hastened their demise. The notable exception was Kitty King, who, in spite of her chest pains and nocturnal cough was free of fever and appeared not be physically wasted, suggesting an incipient phthisis.

Playing for time: the treatments for phthisis

Contemporary medical authorities were keenly aware that in spite of advances in the understanding of the disease, the treatment of pulmonary phthisis remained ineffective. The clinical evidence regarding cases admitted to the Edinburgh Infirmary reveals some differences in therapeutic approach and emphasis among local academics managing the teaching ward. 'Incipient' cases like Hope's Kitty King were subjected to traditional 'antiphlogistic' measures that included rest, a light vegetarian or full diet supplemented by milk and fruit juices, bloodletting, gentle purgation, and perspiration. Vapour inhalations, expectorants and a blister over the sternum were prescribed for her dry cough. Tonics, often containing iron compounds such as ferrous sulphate were believed to strengthen the bodily systems. The professor also ordered a series of electric sparks to be administered over the lumbar and abdominal regions of this teenager in an attempt to restart her menstrual periods.[93]

All other patients featured in this sample suffered from established and advanced cases where physicians clearly had little to offer their patients except palliation for their most troublesome symptoms. The most important goal was the traditional Hippocratic stance to do no harm.[94] On one occasion, Cullen was emphatic in expressing this position. 'I have a rule in practice that I seldom push a remedy that may harm', he explained, 'as I would rather let a disease kill a patient than kill him by my medicine.'[95] Based on their prognoses of these advanced cases, it was obvious that treatments would hardly be successful. A third of the admissions had arrived during January in the dead of winter. Thus, the only therapeutic strategy was to bolster the general condition of the phthisic patients through rest, ample diet, and protection from cold weather until they could be discharged to 'pure country air' in the spring. In managing his patient John Crookshanks, shelter was precisely what William Cullen intended in 1772. He told his students:

> I allowed him to remain in the hospital since we were not pressed at the time for rooms and also because I thought that you might wish to have the opportunity of observing the progress of such a disease and especially the aftercourse of it.[96]

During clinical rounds and lectures, Cullen, Gregory and Duncan openly proclaimed their overall therapeutic strategy as merely palliative. A goat's milk and vegetable diet was meant to curb the general inflammatory process. Cooling and tonic draughts and juleps were believed to check the excessive effects of fever and strengthen the body. Opiates remained a double-edged sword. Their use was believed to increase inflammation but on the other hand, they also helped control the cough and facilitated rest and sleep while lifting the spirits. Emetics such as ipecac powder were administered in an effort to cleanse the lungs and stomach from the tuberculous matter being expelled by cough.[97] Blisters and issues were said to divert this harmful material from threatening vital organs such as the lungs to circumscribed areas of the skin. However, the pain created by these measures could further weaken an already debilitated patient.

Gregory was sceptical about all medical interventions. He was officially on record as being against subjecting hospital patients to clinical trials with new drugs until they had been tested in private practice.[98] Other professors, however, disagreed. In fact, Home openly published his conclusions regarding trials with various remedies in the treatment of phthisis pulmonaris.[99] Since he doubled for a time as both a hospital manager and attending professor, Gregory, fearing for the Infirmary's reputation, condemned Home's experiments.[100] Duncan's somewhat more aggressive approach in the 1790s seemed to follow Home's stance. In fact, the clinical records suggest that Duncan exploited the nearly hopeless prognosis of his phthisic patients by going well beyond palliation, and using a series of novel and untested treatments. Part of his strategy was born from new ideas about pulmonary physiology, which were based on an improved understanding about the nature and effects of atmospheric air. As noted earlier, this approach could be traced to Beddoes who in 1793 had published a work suggesting that consumption be caused by hyperoxygenated blood.[101] This conclusion stemmed from the clinical fact that the progression of pulmonary consumption appeared to slow or was even arrested during pregnancy. Several medical authors drew the inference that the additional oxygen requirements of the growing foetus were responsible for this phenomenon. In an attempt to correct the hypothetical imbalance, patients were experimentally treated for the disease through periodic inhalations of atmospheric air mixed with small amounts of carbon dioxide, nitrogen and hydrogen. Another contemporary authority, Erasmus Darwin (1731–1802), enthusiastically supported Beddoes' approach: 'Go on, dear Sir, save the young and the fair of the rising generation from premature death; and rescue the science of medicine from its greatest opprobrium'.[102] Home, for his part, claimed to have seen temporary improvements employing a 'mephitic' air, produced from pouring sulphuric acid on chalk as suggested by the chemist Joseph Priestley (1733–1804).[103] However, as reported to the student-run Royal Medical Society in 1795, individuals subjected to these therapies only experienced brief improvements of their symptoms. The treatments failed to stem the inexorable decline and subsequent death of these patients.[104]

While in the Infirmary, patients received a handful of medicines prescribed to provide relief for some of the most distressing complaints. In the case of James Murrain, the initial prescriptions included ipecac, a powerful emetic, and ten drops of laudanum at bedtime. His painful belly was rubbed three times a day with oil and kept warm through a flannel cloth cover. Placed on a regimen of purgatives that included rhubarb and calomel pills, the boy passed a number of worms. By the time Cullen took over Murain's management, the patient's general condition had significantly deteriorated. He appeared quite weak and further emaciated, and palliation seemed to be the only option, including the shift to a milk and gruel diet.

Cullen's other patient, John Crookshanks, was subjected to one venesection because of his difficult breathing and violent chest pain characteristic of pneumonia. He was already so weakened that he promptly fainted following the procedure, prompting Cullen to vow that he would not repeat the procedure. Cullen told students that decades earlier, practitioners had repeated such bleedings fifty to sixty times, thereby hastening the demise of their patients. Ipecac was Cullen's emetic of choice, 'throwing the stuff from the lungs'. He continued to emphasise that Crookshanks was probably riddled with 'scrofulous' pulmonary lesions, but still thought he was a candidate for drugs that might help restore strength as a last effort to avoid a fatal outcome. Therefore, Cullen experimented with a tonic, a decoction of indigo leaves recommended by Edinburgh's former professor of botany, Charles Alston (1738–61) for the successful treatment of 'scrofula'. From the progress reports during the first two weeks of January, the patient seemed to rally; his appetite returned and the cough and fever eased. In Cullen's opinion, the disease still remained within the reach of relief and it was important to bolster the patient's hopes for recovery.

Both Gregory and Duncan prescribed a stimulating regimen that consisted of a milk diet, supplemented in certain cases by meat dishes. White wine or porter beer was designed to improve the overall strength of the patients. In some cases, blisters were created on various parts of the chest. Other individuals received doses of a Peruvian bark infusion. The bark was considered to be a powerful restorative, although Home's experiments with this drug actually had found it to inhibit expectoration – which was believed to be the most effective mechanism for ridding the body of tuberculous matter.[105] All other medications were specifically meant to improve the symptoms of phthisis. They included the use of mucilaginous juleps, a bedtime draught usually containing an opiate to calm the cough and allow sleep; as well as, the ingestion of quantities of linseed infusions to soothe the throat and airways.[106] Only in the case of William Simpson did Gregory order a six-ounce venesection in response to an acute episode of laboured breathing.

Like Gregory, Duncan ordered the milk diet and routine symptomatic remedies including a mucilaginous mixture, opium diluted in sulphuric acid and spring water, as well as linseed infusion.[107] However, he also employed an experimental draught aimed at neutralising the alleged cause of the disease. Thus, all four of his patients received a powder composed of potassium sulphate and charcoal designed to chemically bind with the intestinal chyle and draw water, eventually to de-oxygenate the blood.

Thomas Garnett (1766–1802) had popularised this approach in his work on mineral waters.[108] Duncan meant to accomplish Beddoes goal by mouth because inhaling a mixture of gases was considered a more cumbersome and riskier procedure. Indeed, Duncan was quoted as saying to his students that 'besides using the proper remedies for these circumstances we may be induced to attempt an alleviation of [the patient's] calamities by producing a resolution of the tubercles before they arrive at suppuration.'[109] In spite of the addition of charcoal, however, both Barbara Taylor and Daniel MacIntosh reacted to the experimental medication with vomiting and diarrhoea. They both subsequently required additional doses of charcoal and opium to control these side effects.[110]

Daily progress notes, and new prescriptions illuminated the subsequent management of all consumptive patients. For example, because of his recurrent cough, John Mathews received from Gregory a useful emetic and expectorant: antimony potassium tartrate. For William Simpson, a blister was created on his chest in a last-ditch effort to improve his rapidly deteriorating condition. Duncan, in turn, also blistered Daniel Robertson and Barbara Taylor.[111] He allowed Margaret Dewer to sit near a fireplace located in the ward in order to aid her profuse perspiration – another traditional procedure designed to expel through the skin via sweat the harmful poisons thought to be trapped inside the body. Kitty King's cough persisted, prompting Hope to place another blister and leeches on her chest. A note in her chart on New Year's Eve indicated that 'the electrifying produced so much uneasiness as to cause her to faint'. No menstrual flow was observed.[112]

Ambulatory, tubercular patients were also encouraged to exercise their lungs and strengthen their pulses by walking through the ward or trying the Infirmary's swinging chair or wooden horse. Indeed, a week before her death, Gregory's Ann Monro was told to rock in the chair for half an hour every afternoon. Of course, what the Infirmary could not supply was the fresh country air everybody considered a key factor in any recovery. Cullen lamented both the patients' inability to escape those harsh Scottish winters for milder climates as well as engaging in 'long and assiduous exercise', or, especially, sailing (Chapter 4). 'None of these are applicable to our present patient', he admitted in reference to John Crookshanks' case, 'and all we can do is to employ a palliative course'.[113] 'Since the fatal event is probable', Cullen observed, 'it is of consequence to give temporary relief and to make this transition very easy and comfortable'. He was also emphatic in recommending that,

> in every period of the disease it is of the utmost importance to keep the mind calm, easy, and cheerful, for whenever anxious, corroding care, vexation, or

> uneasiness sits brooding on the imagination, medical assistance will be applied in vain.[114]

For his part, Gregory realistically predicted a downhill course for most of his phthisic hospital patients, preparing his students for that 'peculiar appearance of the face' they would be observing, namely the 'sharp features and circumscribed redness on the cheeks'.[115]

Whether such prognoses were communicated to the patients remains unknown. Most hospital patients were deliberately kept in the dark about the outcome of their treatments. 'In general you should never give the patient any hints with regards to the effects of the medicines they are taking', Cullen urged his students, 'the less medical knowledge they have so much the better.'[116] Contemporary medical ethics certainly supported the notion that in such situations truth-telling was not imperative. Neither was abandonment of the dying: physicians' visits and progress notes continued unabated until the end. According to Percival, disclosing the truth remained a 'painful conflict of obligations' in which the virtuous physician had to balance veracity and his professional duty to do no harm.[117] Cullen's decision stood in marked contrast with his candour in acknowledging errors in clinical judgement to students and colleagues as well conveying health-related knowledge to private clients (Chapter 4). Most phthisis patients, whether at home or on the teaching wards, clung desperately to life and forever hoped to recover. Infirmary patients suffering from 'phthisis' stayed for about forty days (males) and thirty-seven days (females).

Conclusion

Almost half of the patients suffering from phthisis in the Infirmary's teaching ward eventually demanded to be discharged when it became clear that their condition failed to improve. Others were dismissed as somewhat 'relieved' of their symptoms. A few sadly perished in the Infirmary. After a stay of fifty-two days, James Murrain, the young boy originally brought in because of intestinal worms, died on 23 February 1772. A complete post-mortem examination was duly authorised and probably carried out by one of the Infirmary's surgical clerks. On dissection, the lungs were observed to be a confused bundle of tubercular swellings, some the size of a pigeon's egg, others in advanced stages of suppuration. Both lungs also adhered to the pleura, another sign of previous inflammatory conditions. Moreover, the mesenteric glands were greatly enlarged, many the size of cherries and chestnuts. Finally, both kidneys seemed enlarged; the tissue riddled with similar tubercles and small abscesses. The final and official diagnosis was phthisis. Commenting extensively on this case in subsequent clinical lectures, Cullen discussed the frequency of worms in children but warned that not all manifestations should be automatically attributed to such an infestation. He summarised previous theories about the physiopathology of 'scrofula' and offered a possible linkage between bodily constitution, inflammation of the small intestine, and tuberculous mesenteric lymph nodes. Cullen commented that the findings 'now fully confirmed by dissection what I imagined was the case'. He urged that children exhibiting such 'scrofulous' lesions in their necks should always be suspected of having tubercles in other parts of their bodies, especially the lungs.

Cullen's other patient, John Crookshanks, died at the end of February 1773 after his condition had quickly deteriorated a month earlier. Once more, the professor was successful in securing permission for an autopsy and he blamed mistakes in pulse-counting for disguising the patient's true condition. The pathological findings were presented in great detail during a subsequent clinical lecture. Cullen used the opportunity to point out a number of correlations between the clinical progress of the disease and the pathological findings that conferred 'more certainty and clearness'.[118] He mentioned the deceased's smaller left chest cavity – probably a consequence of rickets – as being a common reason for greater susceptibility to tubercular lesions. The presence of numerous tubercles of various sizes in both lungs suggested the progressive nature of their appearance, a fact that made it very important for physicians to detect the disease in its incipient state. The lack of ulcerated lesions also prompted Cullen to caution his listeners that the lack of a purulent sputum or vomica should never rule out the diagnosis and that hectic fevers could be produced by internal absorption of pathological material from the tubercles.[119]

James Gregory discharged John Mathews on 28 November 1779, after a nineteen-day stay in the Infirmary. His discharge status was officially listed as 'relieved', but the available progress notes suggest the patient was still experiencing all the symptoms that had prompted him to enter the hospital in the first place. After just a week in the Infirmary, John White asked for his release and promptly left 'by desire' on 7 December of the same year. Not unexpectedly, another of Gregory's patients, William Simpson, had died just two days earlier, on 5 December, also after nineteen days of treatment. An earlier episode of difficult breathing had prompted Gregory to order a six-ounce bleeding. The final progress note read: 'was able to speak after the bleeding but died an hour after'.[120] Gregory returned to comment on this patient in a subsequent clinical lecture on 7 December, delivered on the topic of *phthisis pulmonaris*. Referring specifically to Simpson, Gregory was quoted as saying to the students that 'perhaps bleeding made his death at least easier'.[121] In this instance, an autopsy found that the 'lungs [were] most completely obstructed by tubercles, many of them suppurated'. Twenty-three ounces of fluid were extracted from the enlarged pericardial sac that occupied half of the thoracic cavity.[122] Additionally all three women hospitalised by Gregory in 1787 perished in the Infirmary. Janet Hunter died on 13 February, just four days after admission. The autopsy disclosed the presence of several tubercles and ulcers filled with purulent matter as well as fluid and adhesions in the left lobe of her lungs. Ann Monro lasted nine days but apparently her relatives granted no permission for a post-mortem examination. Jane Lindsay remained barely one week, her last days spent in a semi-comatose state. A limited dissection of her chest disclosed numerous lung tubercles in an ulcerated and 'scirrhous state' as well as multiple adhesions to the pleura and diaphragm.

Duncan's patients fared somewhat better. Daniel Robertson managed to leave the Edinburgh Infirmary on 21 April, nearly two and a half months after his admission. His cough was said to be better, and presumably his general condition improved to the point that Duncan optimistically assigned him the discharge category 'cured'. On 9 April, Daniel MacIntosh apparently asked Duncan to discharge him from the hospital after a stay of twenty-five days. The casebook reported the weakened patient was 'desirous of going into the country', so they 'let him be dismissed'.[123] The progress note for that final hospital day also indicates that this patient's cough continued undiminished, that he apparently was getting little sleep despite the medications, and that his limbs were much swollen. The note ends cryptically that 'he died in April', presumably shortly after his discharge from the Infirmary. Like many patients before and after him, MacIntosh perhaps did not wish to die in the hospital but in the company of family and friends, thus cheating Duncan out of a long-awaited autopsy that would confirm the clinical diagnosis. In summarising the case for students, Duncan was quoted as saying:

> We made trials of different remedies but without benefit....With a wish to breathe a purer air he was dismissed from our wards. Indeed I was disposed to think that his only chance for recovery was from country air and milk diet.[124]

Finally, Barbara Taylor and Margaret Dewer remained in the teaching ward until its closure at the end of the academic year in April. Both were 'dismissed with directions to retire to the country for the benefit of free air'. Taylor left following six weeks in the hospital, with her cough and chest pain somewhat improved. Her discharge was officially listed in the Infirmary's General Register of Patients as 'relieved'. Dewer left the Infirmary on the very same day after a thirty-four-day stay. Her discharge condition was recorded as 'nearly as before'. Unfortunately, the student copying the cases simply omitted Duncan's final summary. By 30 January 1797, Kitty King's strength had sufficiently improved and her cough abated somewhat. At this point, Hope, his academic rotation over, decided to transfer the patient to the regular medical ward for further convalescence. According to the patient register, she was discharged 'relieved' on 14 February 1797 after sixty-one days in the hospital.

For contemporaries, hospital care for pulmonary phthisis must have been a mixed blessing. The very fact that they were allowed to enter the Infirmary provided an opportunity for escaping their wretched abodes and the inclemency of Edinburgh's weather. Moreover, admission became a potent cause for hope since it suggested that, in the opinion of prominent attending physicians, their condition was still potentially curable. Such expectations, often dashed, prompted hospital patients to go along with the various treatments that legitimised their sufferings while appreciating the material 'comforts of the house'.[125] On the other hand, their compromised condition could hardly improve in an environment of potentially vitiated air and institutional contagion. For the Infirmary authorities, the high institutional mortality rates of hospital patients suffering from phthisis – fifty percent for this selected sample – was an unwelcome event. The managers were proud of the Infirmary's official statistics – especially the high cure rate (75%) with a low mortality rate (4%). Both statistics were extensively quoted, published and employed in attracting patrons. Everybody, of course, expected less favourable outcomes from the hospital's teaching ward. Because of their pedagogical needs for more complex and challenging cases, the professors in charge were probably resigned to lower cure rates. According to the data extracted from the student notebooks, the teaching ward's average mortality rate throughout the final decades of the eighteenth century actually fluctuated between eight and ten percent, still a far cry from the five-fold increase in deaths from those afflicted with phthisis. In his 1785 rotation, however, Duncan achieved his modest objective. Both Barbara Taylor and Margaret Dewer apparently did not lose further ground in the institution. Instead of dramatic therapies administered by Infirmary physician, the final outcome of phthisis hinged on the effects of pure air, better diet, and healthy living if the patients could only manage to leave the hospital for the countryside, a destination portrayed as wholesome and virtuous. Spring was about to arrive in Scotland, with its promise for a resumption of outdoor life.

At a time when both students and practitioners 'walked the wards' and observed large numbers of patients with a variety of illnesses during their daily clinical rounds, case-and notebooks provide a valuable record of contemporary clinical decision-making and therapeutic management at the bedside. Students employed them as invaluable memory aids of patient management. Despite their obvious limitations, these documents from the Edinburgh Infirmary constitute an invaluable source for historians interested in the construction, organisation, representation, and transmission of medical knowledge in eighteenth-century Britain. By providing a daily chronicle of clinical phenomena and medications designed to control them, these didactic records also constitute important documents for the history of therapeutics.[126] Certainly, the voices of actual patients virtually vanished from the documents, victims of professional interpretation and composition. Yet, the uniqueness of their sufferings and management survived in the medicalized narratives, recorded by hospital clerks and copied by students attending daily rounds. Each bedside event could merit a comment, while the treatments exposed particular therapeutic rationales and biases regarding the use of certain drugs and physical methods. Above all, Edinburgh professors attempted to instil a strong sense of therapeutical scepticism in their disciples. One former student, Edward Foster, strongly recommended 'to my countrymen' the Infirmary's clinical instruction, where 'lively description is painted, not only on the mind's eye, but on the eye of vision, by the labouring patients being stretched to view'. He indicated that the lectures were 'the only regular course of its kind anywhere given', promising that 'by a short attendance on them may be reaped all the advantages of a long experience.'[127]

Notes

1. F. Home, *Clinical Experiments, Histories and Dissections*, 3rd edn (London: J. Murray, 1783), vi-vii.
2. See, for example, the forty-two cases collected in the first and third books of a treatise called 'Epidemics' that belongs to the Hippocratic Corpus. Hippocrates, *Works*, trans. W.H.S. Jones, 4 vols (Cambridge, Mass.: Harvard University Press, 1972), Vol. 1, 187–287.
3. M. Foucault, *The Order of Things: An Archeology of the Human Sciences*, trans. from French (London: Tavistock Publications, 1970); see also A. Young, 'An Anthropological Perspective on Medical Knowledge', *Journal of Medicine and Philosophy*, 5 (1980), 102–16; and T. Osborne, 'Medicine and Epistemology: Michel Foucault and the Liberality of Clinical Reason', *History of Human Sciences*, 5 (1992), 63–93.
4. Later examples of medieval and Renaissance *consilia* can be found in N. Siraisi, T. Alderotti and His Pupils, *Two Generations of Italian Medical Learning* (Princeton, NJ: Princeton University Press, 1981), 269–302; see also L. Demaitre, 'Scholasticism in Compendia of Practical Medicine, 1250–1450', in N. Siraisi and L. Demaitre (eds), 'Science, Medicine, and the

University, 1250–1550: Essays in Honor of Pearl Kibre', *Manuscripta*, 20 (1976), 81–95.

5. The anthropological and medical literature on the topic is extensive. For further reading: A. Kleinman, *The Illness Narratives: Suffering, Healing, and the Human Condition* (New York: Basic Books, 1988); H. Brody, *Stories of Sickness* (New Haven: Yale University Press, 1988); E.C. Mishler, *The Discourse of Medicine: Dialectics of Medical Interviews* (Norwood, NJ: Ablex, 1984); and B.F. Sarf, 'Physician–Patient Communication as Interpersonal Rhetoric: A Narrative Approach', *Health Communication,* 2 (1990), 217–31.
6. S. Jarcho (ed. and trans.), *Clinical Consultations and Letters by Ipolito Francesco Albertini, Francesco Torti and Other Physicians* (Boston: F. A. Countway Library, 1989).
7. For example, the *London Medical Journal* published between 1781 and 1790, and *Medical Essays and Observations*, published by a Society in Edinburgh in 1732.
8. According to some authors, this coincided with the emergence of a new literary genre designed to generate compassion for the victims of disease and suffering. See T.W. Laqueur, 'Bodies, Details, and the Humanitarian Narrative,' in L. Hunt (ed.), *The New Cultural History* (Berkeley: University of California Press, 1989), 176–204. For details about the importance of a clinical history, S.J. Reiser, 'Examination of the Patient in the Seventeenth- and Eighteenth Centuries', in *Medicine and the Reign of Technology* (New York: Cambridge University Press, 1978), 1–22. The same author has recently published 'Creating Form Out of Mass: The Development of the Clinical Record', in E. Mendelsohn (ed.), *Transformation and Tradition in the Sciences: Essays in Honor of Bernard Cohen* (New York: Cambridge University Press, 1984), 303–16.
9. M.E. Fissell, 'The Disappearance of the Patient Narrative and the Invention of Hospital Medicine', in R. French and A. Wear (eds), *British Medicine in the Age of Reform* (London: Routledge, 1991), 92–109. For more details, see C. Rosenberg, 'Towards an Ecology of Knowledge: On Discipline, Context, and History', in A. Oleson and J. Voss (eds), *The Organization of Knowledge in Modern America, 1860–1920* (Baltimore: Johns Hopkins University Press, 1979), 440–55.
10. W. Blizard, *Suggestions for the Improvement of Hospitals and Other Charitable Organizations* (London: H. L. Galabin, 1796); see also G.B. Risse, *Hospital Life in Enlightenment Scotland, Care and Teaching at the Royal Infirmary of Edinburgh* (New York: Cambridge University Press, 1986); T. Gelfand, *Professionalizing Modern Medicine: Paris Surgeons and Medical Science and Institutions in the Eighteenth Century* (Westport, CT: Greenwood Press, 1980).

11. Home, *op. cit.* (note 1), V.
12. For details, C. Lawrence, 'Early Edinburgh Medicine: Theory and Practice', in R.G.W. Anderson and A.D.C. Simpson (eds), *The Early Years of the Edinburgh Medical School* (Edinburgh: Royal Scottish Museum, 1976), 81–94; see also Lawrence's essay 'Ornate Physicians and Learned Artisans: Edinburgh Medical Men, 1726–1776', in W.F. Bynum and R. Porter (eds), *William Hunter and the Eighteenth-Century Medical World* (Cambridge: Cambridge University Press, 1985), 153–76.
13. G.B. Risse, 'Clinical Instruction in Hospitals: The Boerhaavian Tradition in Leyden, Edinburgh, Vienna, and Pavia', *Clio Medica*, 21 (1987–8), 1–19.
14. For details, Risse, *op. cit.* (note 10), 240–78.
15. See, for example, James Gregory, *Clinical Reports*, 1 November 1795–1 February 1796 (Edinburgh: 1795-96), MSS Collection, Edinburgh University Library.
16. G.B. Risse, '"Before the Clinic was 'Born'": Methodological Perspectives in Hospital History', in N. Finzsch and R. Jütte (eds), *Institutions of Confinement: Hospitals, Asylums and Prisons in Western Europe and North America, 1500–1950* (New York: Cambridge University Press, 1996), 75–96.
17. This organisation follows in part recommendations contained in F. Clifton, *Tabular Observations, Recommended as the Plainest and Surest Way of Practicing and Improving Physick* (London: J. Brindley, 1731).
18. I have been unable to locate examples of such a ward journal. A description of this document is found in W. Maitland, *The History of Edinburgh* (Edinburgh: Longman & Cadell, 1779), 460.
19. Surviving fragments of a ledger have been found and briefly analysed in Risse, *op. cit.* (note 10), 96–7. The document summarizes cases hospitalised in a male ward largely filled with soldiers for the years 1773–6. See 'Ward Journal, 1773–6', MSS Collection, Edinburgh University Library.
20. Maitland, *op. cit.* (note 18), 460.
21 I am indebted to Michael Barfoot at Edinburgh University for more detailed references to the Edinburgh registration system contained in two documents not included in my 1986 book: *Medical Essays and Observations,* 1 (1752), V-XXII – this is the 4th edition; the original article was published in 1732. See also Royal Infirmary of Edinburgh 'Minutes of Managers', MSS Collection, Edinburgh University Library, Vol. 1, (1728–41), 239–43.
22. [R.I.E.], 'Minutes of Managers', Vol. 6, 1 October 1792, 157–8.
23. [J. Johnson], *A Guide for Gentlemen Studying Medicine at the University of Edinburgh* (London: Robinson, 1792), 45.
24. J. Stedman, *The History and Statutes of the Royal Infirmary of Edinburgh* (Edinburgh: Balfour & Smellie, 1778), 47–89.
25. [Johnson], *op. cit.* (note 23), 38–9.

26. *Ibid.*, 47.
27. Details in Risse, *op. cit.* (note 10), 296–301.
28. *Ibid.*, 45–56.
29. This is particularly true for the following casebook: A. Duncan, Sr, Clinical Reports and Commentaries, February–April 1795, presented by A. Blackhall Morison (Edinburgh, 1795), MSS Collection, Royal College of Physicians, Edinburgh.
30. Risse, *op. cit.* (note 10), 45–9.
31. *Ibid.*, 110–12. In a few instances the histories speak of whistling air pipes, stitches or darting chest pains, but it is not clear whether these complaints actually represent the patient's voice.
32. Case of William F., in Duncan, *op. cit.* (note 29).
33. Case of Thomas S., in James Gregory, 'Clinical Notes and Lectures' (Edinburgh, 1779–80), MSS Collection, Royal College of Physicians, Edinburgh.
34. Case of Duncan M. in *ibid.*
35. Risse, *op. cit.* (note 10), 108–18.
36. R. Porter, 'The Rise of Physical Examination', in W.F. Bynum and R. Porter (eds), *Medicine and the Five Senses* (Cambridge: Cambridge University Press, 1993, 179–97.
37. In the case of John Crookshanks, one of his patients suffering from phthisis, Cullen commented that 'today he was sitting by the fire in an erect posture. I felt his pulse and it was so feeble and frequent as to pass my powers of numbering, and from the feel that I had of it then, I would say that he has not many days to live.' in W. Cullen, 'Clinical Lectures' (Edinburgh, 1772–3), MSS Collection, Royal College of Physicians, Edinburgh, 277.
38. James Gregory, *Additional Memorial to the Managers of the Royal Infirmary* (Edinburgh: Murray & Cochrane, 1803), 431.
39. An English practitioner employing shorthand claimed to have collected 5,000 cases from the Stafford Infirmary over a period of ten years 'for his public and private practice'. T. Fowler, *Medical Reports on the Effects of Bloodletting, Sudorifics and Blistering in the Cure of the Acute and Chronic Rheumatism* (London: J. Johnson, 1795), VI.
40. See Cullen's clinical lecture delivered on 21 April 1772, dealing with the case of Elizabeth MacInnis, in Thomson/Cullen Papers, MSS Collection, University of Glasgow Library. A slightly different version is contained in the following student notebook: W. Cullen, 'Clinical Lectures, delivered for John Gregory, February–April 1772' (Edinburgh, 1772), MSS Collection, Royal College of Physicians, Edinburgh, 290–1.
41. M. Barfoot, 'Philosophy and the Method of Cullen's Medical Teaching', in A. Doig *et al.* (eds), *William Cullen and the Eighteenth-Century Medical*

World (Edinburgh: Edinburgh University Press, 1993), 110–32.

42. C.D. Leake (ed.), *Percival's Medical Ethics* (Baltimore: Williams & Wilkins, 1927), 107. For an analysis of contemporary medical ethics, L. Haakonssen, *Medicine and Morals in the Enlightenment: John Gregory, Thomas Percival and Benjamin Rush* (Amsterdam: Rodopi, 1997), 1–45.
43. Cullen, Clinical Lectures for John Gregory, *op. cit.* (note 40), 339.
44. A volume entitled 'Medical Tracts II' contains an abridged version of William Cullen's clinical lectures delivered for John Gregory between February and April 1772, together with other notes from James Gregory's presentations. According to an inscription, these lecture notes were apparently taken by John Unthank, who became professor of botany at the Royal College of Surgeons of Ireland. This manuscript is in my personal possession.
45. Cullen, Clinical Lectures for John Gregory, *op. cit.* (note 40), 339.
46. G. Cheyne, *The English Malady, or A Treatise of Nervous Diseases* (London: 1733).
47. R. Blackmore, *A Treatise of Consumptions and Other Distempers Belonging to the Breast and Lungs* (London: J. Pemberton, 1725).
48. For details, L.S. King, 'Hermann Boerhaave, Systematist', in *The Medical World of the Eighteenth Century* (Chicago: University of Chicago Press, 1958), 59–93.
49. R. Morton, *Phthisiologia: Or A Treatise of Consumption* (London: W. and J. Innys, 1720). For a modern summary, W.D. Johnston, 'Tuberculosis', in K.F. Kiple (ed.), *The Cambridge World History of Disease* (New York: Cambridge University Press, 1993, 1059–68.
50. L.S. King, 'Hoffmann' in *The Road to Medical Enlightenment, 1650–1695* (London: Macdonald, 1970), 181–204.
51. B. Marten, *A New Theory of Consumption: More Especially of a Phthisis or Consumption of the Lungs* (London: Knaplock, Bell, Hooke and King, 1722). See especially chap II, 'An Inquiry Concerning the Prime, Essential and Hitherto Accounted Inexplicable Cause of Consumption', 31–74.
52. For details, R.Y. Keers, *Pulmonary Tuberculosis: A Journey Down the Centuries* (London: Baillière Tindall, 1978), 20–35.
53. R. Porter, 'Consumption: Disease of the Consumer Society?', in J. Brewer and R. Porter (eds), *Consumption and the World of Goods* (London: Routledge, 1993), 58–81.
54. For details, T. Beddoes, *Essay on the Causes, Early Signs, and Prevention of Pulmonary Consumption for the Use of Parents and Preceptors* (Bristol: Biggs and Cottle, 1799).
55. In William Cullen's medical system, proof for the fragile nature of humans – notably females – was similarly couched in speculative notions of lax fibres,

soft nerves, and greater systemic excitability within their bodies. At the centre of most complaints were losses of bodily tone and vigour that directly affected all organs and vessels. The best source for this information is W. Cullen, *First Lines of the Practice of Physic*, new. edn, IV vols (Edinburgh: C. Elliot, 1788). See also W.F. Bynum, 'Health, Disease and Medical Care', in G.S. Rousseau and R. Porter (eds), *The Ferment of Knowledge: Studies in the Historiography of Eighteenth-Century Science* (Cambridge: Cambridge University Press, 1980), 211–53.

56. Details in R. Porter, 'Civilization and Disease: Medical Ideology in the Enlightenment', in J. Black and J. Gregory (eds), *Culture, Politics, and Society in Britain, 1660–1800* (Manchester: Manchester University Press, 1991), 154–83.
57. Beddoes, *op. cit.* (note 54), 11–2.
58. C. Lawlor and A. Suzuki, 'The Disease of the Self: Representing Consumption, 1700–1830', *Bulletin of the History of Medicine,* 74 (2000), 458–94.
59. J. Sinclair, 'On the Diseases of Scotland', in *Analysis of the Statistical Account of Scotland* (Edinburgh: A. Constable & Co., 1825), part I, 138.
60. R. Porter, *Doctor of Society: Thomas Beddoes and the Sick Trade in Late Enlightenment England* (London: Routledge, 1992), especially 99–107.
61. Edinburgh's Bills of Mortality were periodically published in *Scots Magazine.*
62. See 'Of the Phthisis Pulmonaris or Consumption of the Lungs', in Cullen, *op. cit.* (note 55), Vol. II, 356–423.
63. G.B. Risse, 'La Synthèse entre L'Anatomie et la Clinique', in M.D. Grmek (ed.), *Histoire de la Pensée Médicale en Occident*, 3 vols (Paris: Éditions du Seuil, 1997), Vol. 2, 177–97; see also L.S. King, 'The Rise of Modern Pathology', in *The Medical World of the Eighteenth Century* (Chicago: University of Chicago Press, 1958), 263–96.
64. M. Baillie, *The Morbid Anatomy of Some of the Most Important Parts of the Body* (London: J. Johnson and G. Nicol. 1793). A secondary source for this author is A.E. Rodin, *The Influence of Matthew Baillie's Morbid Pathology* (Springfield: C.C. Thomas, 1973).
65. W. Pagel, 'Humoral Pathology: A Lingering Anachronism in the History of Tuberculosis' *Bulletin of the History of Medicine*, 29 (1955), 299–308.
66. 'Of the Haematemesis or Vomiting of Blood', in Cullen, *op. cit.* (note 55), Vol. III, 51–60.
67. Duncan, Sr, *op. cit.* (note 29).
68. For details, T. Reid, *An Essay on the Nature and Cure of Phthisis Pulmonaris*, 3rd edn (London: T. Cadell & W. Davies, 1798).
69. Gregory, *op. cit.* (note 33). Cullen also commented on this subject in his lectures: Cullen, *op. cit.* (note 37), 110.

70. 'Of Scrophula or the King's Evil', in Cullen, *op. cit.* (note 55), Vol. IV, 359–81; consult also R.K. French, 'Scrofula (Scrophula)', in Kiple, *op. cit.* (note 49), 998–1000.
71. M. Bloch, *The Royal Touch: Sacred Monarchy and Scrofula in England and France*, trans. J.E. Anderson (London: Routledge and Kegan Paul, 1973).
72. A randomised sample of 3,047 diagnostic entries obtained from surviving folios between the years 1770 and 1800 from the Edinburgh Infirmary's General Register of Patients only lists thirty-four cases of phthisis or consumption. A third of them entered during the month of January and sixty-one percent were males. See Risse, *op. cit.* (note 10), 141–5.
73. Anonymous, *The History and Statutes of the Royal Infirmary of Edinburgh* (Edinburgh: Balfour and Smellie, 1778), 88.
74. J. Aikin, *Thoughts on Hospitals* (London: J. Johnson, 1771), 51.
75. Anon., *op. cit.* (note 73), 88.
76. For early efforts at quantification and statistical analysis see U. Tröhler, '"To Improve the Evidence of Medicine": Arithmetic Observation in Clinical Medicine in Eighteenth and Early Nineteenth Centuries', *History and Philosophy of the Life Sciences*, 10 (1988), 31–40.
77. Cullen, Clinical Lectures for John Gregory, *op. cit.* (note 40), 1.
78. This examination has been possible through a comparison of cases and lecture notes including those taken from Cullen, *op. cit.* (note 37); Cullen, Clinical Lectures, for John Gregory, *op. cit.* (note 40); James Gregory, *op. cit.* (note 33); Duncan Sr, *op. cit.* (note 29); James Gregory, 'Clinical Lectures and Cases' (Edinburgh, 1787), MSS Collection, National Library of Medicine, Bethesda, Maryland.
79. James Murain's case was extensively discussed by William Cullen during two clinical lectures in February 1772. It gave the professor a chance to express his views and treatment of phthisis, as well as discussing the autopsy findings. A full copy of his remarks exist in the manuscript Medical Tracts II, *op. cit.* (note 44), 30–64.
80. Cullen, *op. cit.* (note 37), 115.
81. Cases of John Mathews, William Simpson, and John White in James Gregory, *op. cit.* (note 33).
82. Cases of Janet Hunter, Ann Monro, and Jane Lindsay, in James Gregory, *op. cit.* (note 78).
83. Cases of Daniel Robertson, Barbara Taylor, Daniel MacIntosh, and Margaret Dewer, in Duncan Sr, *op. cit.* (note 29).
84. Case of Kitty King, in T. C. Hope, Clinical Casebook (Edinburgh: 1796–7), MSS Collection, Royal College of Physicians, Edinburgh.
85. Case of Margaret Dewer, in Duncan Sr, *op. cit.* (note 29).

86. See T. Beddoes, *A Letter to Erasmus Darwin, MD on a New Method of Treating Pulmonary Consumption* (Bristol: B. Rosser, 1793). The document was dated 30 June 1793.
87. Such apparent parity in reading the sick human body allowed patients to retain considerable interpretative control over their illness and engage in vigorous self-therapy. See M.E. Fissell, *Patients, Power, and the Poor in Eighteenth-Century Bristol* (Cambridge: Cambridge University Press, 1991).
88. W. Falconer, *Observations Respecting the Pulse* (London: T. Cadell Jr and W. Davies, 1796); G. Martine, *Essays and Observations on the Construction and Graduation of Thermometers, and on the Heating and Cooling of Bodies*, 3rd edn (Edinburgh, 1780); Cullen, *op. cit.* (note 37), 122–3.
89. James Gregory, *op. cit.* (note 33). According to the anonymous note taker, the lecture on phthisis was delivered on 7 December 1779, two days after the death of William Simpson.
90. Cullen, *op. cit.* (note 37) 277.
91. *Ibid.*
92. Duncan, Sr, *op. cit.* (note 29).
93. Hope, *op. cit.* (note 84).
94. See, for example, C. Packe, *An Explanation of that Part of Dr Boerhaave's Aphorisms, Which Treats of the Phthisis Pulmonalis* (London: M. Cooper, 1754).
95. Cullen, *op. cit.* (note 37), 541. For details, G.B. Risse, 'Cullen, the Seasoned Clinician: Organization and Strategies of a Successful Medical Practice in the Eighteenth Century', in Doig *et al.*, *op. cit.* (note 41), 133–51.
96 . Cullen, *op. cit.* (note 37), 273. An extensive discussion of the patient's autopsy findings by Cullen is reproduced in Risse, *op. cit.* (note 10), 344–5.
97. For example, see M. Griffith, *Practical Observations on the Cure of Hectic and Slow Fevers and the Pulmonary Consumption* (London: B. White, 1776).
98. James Gregory, *op. cit.* (note 38), 479.
99. *Ibid.*, 112–27.
100. For a detailed discussion of the therapeutic options, consult Risse, *op. cit.* (note 10), 177–202.
101. Additional information on Beddoes can be obtained from D.A. Stansfield, *Thomas Beddoes MD, 1760–1808, Chemist, Physician, Democrat* (Dordrecht: D. Reidel, 1984).
102. The letter from Darwin to Beddoes was dated 17 January 1793. It is included in Beddoes, *op. cit.* (note 86), 67.
103. Home, *op. cit.* (note 1), 122–5.
104. W.C. Darling, 'Phthisis Pulmonaris', *Diss. RMS,* Vol. 33 (1795), 18–34.
105. Home, *op. cit.* (note 1), 119–20.
106. For most eighteenth-century drugs, consult W. Lewis (ed.), *The*

Pharmacopoeia of the Royal College of Physicians at Edinburgh (London: J. Nourse, 1748). It also contains an appendix titled 'The Dispensatory for the Use of the Poor in the Royal Hospital at Edinburgh,' 338–62, that lists many of the in-house preparations prescribed by Infirmary physicians.

107. Duncan's therapeutics were examined in some detail. See J.W. Estes, 'Drug Usage At The Infirmary: The Example Of Dr. Andrew Duncan, Sr.', in Risse, *op. cit.* (note 10), 351–84.
108. T. Garnett, *A Treatise on the Mineral Waters of Harrogate*, 2nd edn (Leeds: T. Gill, 1794).
109. Duncan Sr., *op. cit.* (note 29).
110. Risse, *op. cit.* (note 10), 372. J.W. Estes also lists eighteenth-century medications in his *Dictionary of Protopharmacology, Therapeutic Practices, 1700–1850* (Canton, MA: Science History Publications, USA, 1990).
111. For more details of Robertson's treatment, *ibid.*, 358–9.
112. Hope, *op. cit.* (note 84). The entire case is reproduced in Risse, *op. cit.* (note 10), 318–21.
113. Cullen, *op. cit.* (note 37), 115. For the therapeutic effects of exercise, J.C. Smyth, *An Account of the Effects of Swinging Employed as a Remedy in the Pulmonary Consumption and Hectic Fever* (London: J. Johnson, 1787).
114. Medical Tracts II, *op. cit.* (note 44), 509.
115. James Gregory, *op. cit.* (note 33).
116. Cullen, *op. cit.* (note 37), 51.
117. Leake, *op. cit.* (note 42), 195; Haakonssen, *op. cit.* (note 42), 167–73.
118. The epistemological issues regarding clinico–pathological correlations are discussed in G.B. Risse, 'A Shift in Medical Epistemology: Clinical Diagnosis, 1770–1828', in Y. Kawakita (ed.), *History of Diagnostics, Proceedings of the 9th International Symposium on the Comparative History of Medicine – East and West* (Osaka: Tanaguchi Foundation, 1987), 115–47.
119. Risse, *op. cit.* (note 10), 344–5.
120. James Gregory, *op. cit.* (note 33).
121. *Ibid.*
122. *Ibid.*
123. Duncan Sr, *op. cit.* (note 29).
124. *Ibid.*
125. These issues are discussed in S. van der Geest *et al.*, 'The Anthropology of Pharmaceuticals: A Biographical Approach', *Annual Review of Anthropology*, 25 (1996), 153–78.
126. G.B. Risse and J.H. Warner, 'Reconstructing Clinical Activities: Patient Records in Medical History', *Social History of Medicine*, 5 (1992), 183–205.
127. E. Foster, *An Essay on Hospitals* (Dublin: W. G. Jones, 1768), 52.

8

Framing Gynaecology in Edinburgh: The Perplexing Nature of Women's Bodies

Eighteenth-century gynaecological views and practices have remained virtually unexamined. This paper focuses on 'female troubles' and their admission and treatment at the Edinburgh Infirmary based on medical publications, hospital registers, casebooks and student notes. Such activities took place amid serious battles between gentlemen physicians and surgeon–midwives wishing to expand the range of their practices. After reviewing fanciful explanations of menstruation and the purported fragility of female bodies since Antiquity, the analysis describes the actual medical management of menstrual irregularities and other related conditions. Most of the treatments were rooted in traditional domestic and folk approaches, exposing the contradictions and paradoxes surrounding explanations of women's pathology.

Introduction

> Wretched surely and unequal seems the condition of the female sex, that they who are by Nature destined to be the Preservers of the human race, should at the same time be made liable to so many diseases.
>
> John Friend (1729)[1]

On Sunday, 10 November 1785, Euphemia McKay, a 26-year-old married woman, sought admission to the Edinburgh Infirmary. Unfortunately, the voice of eighteenth-century hospitalised patients is no longer available. According to the surviving clinical chart, she appeared 'pale and languid in her looks' and told the admitting medical clerks that for the past three days she had experienced dizziness and headaches, 'dimness of sight', oppression in the chest and an occasional sensation of having a lump in her throat. To relieve her suffering, she had taken some purgatives. Euphemia indicated that her monthly menstrual flow had not resumed for the past three years. According to the patient, this predicament stemmed from a difficult pregnancy with periodic vaginal bleeding that eventually culminated in prolonged labour and stillbirth.[2] The story and nature of her complaints persuaded the clerks to admit Euphemia and send her upstairs to the teaching ward with a working diagnosis of *amenorrhoea.* James Gregory (1753–1821), then professor of the theory of medicine, was currently in charge of that ward. Like other university professors sharing the clinical rotation, Gregory always seemed interested in collecting challenging cases for teaching his students. 'Female complaints' were deemed particularly difficult to manage.[3]

While this analysis focuses primarily on the biomedical views of female bodies, it also seeks to understand the socio–cultural context of eighteenth-century clinical encounters between middle-class male practitioners and deserving poor, urban females.[4] While considerable information exists concerning views of female physiology and pathology during the preceding century,[5] eighteenth-century gynaecological practices have remained virtually unexamined and the topic is usually subsumed under the broader subject of midwifery.[6] By contrast, historians have probed Victorian views of women and how medical theories and practices played a crucial role in justifying and reinforcing traditional images of female fragility and inferiority.[7] However, it is possible to learn about eighteenth-century gynaecological theories and practices by reviewing clinical case histories from the Royal Infirmary of Edinburgh, recorded by contemporary students in the years 1770–1800.[8] This information provides an unparalleled source for examining the context, meaning, and treatment of various female conditions as mediated by competing medical systems and professionals. Moreover, it reveals the importance of social class in assessing the nature and pathology of female bodies.

Eve's nature explained: women's bodies since Antiquity

Before probing events in eighteenth-century Edinburgh, it is necessary to summarise earlier entrenched views concerning female bodies. Throughout history, medicine played a prominent role in defining feminine qualities and attributes. It participated in the establishment of gender myths, differences, and stereotypes. Views of female bodies were shaped as much by culture as biology. Such multiple discourses primarily originated from male voices strongly influenced by contemporary sexual roles and divisions of labour.[9] But gender also played a fundamental role in shaping these ideas. Healers can only be truly successful if they manage to understand and empathise with the sufferings of their patients through comparison with their own experiences. Much has been written about the virtues of 'wounded' healers. Because of their experiences and perceptions, male physicians were not only prone to misread female bodies but also to misrepresent their manifestations.[10]

In several treatises of the Hippocratic Corpus, *gyneikeia* or 'women's things' already represented a peculiar body of knowledge and practice. Derived from folk wisdom and transmitted from mothers to daughters,[11] many of these ancient ideas were developed from assumptions based on a limited range of anatomical and physiological observations.[12] Central to these ideas was the distinctiveness of the female body within prevailing mechanistic and humoral frameworks. In contrast to men, women were believed to be softer by nature, endowed with spongy flesh capable of absorbing and retaining fluids. A central conduit providing air and nourishment ran from the nostrils and throat to the anus and vagina with lateral passageways to special female organs like the breasts and womb. The womb was conceived as a hot, two-chambered jar or wineskin, capable of absorbing the male seed and cooking it properly to create another human being. Because the uterus displayed a certain visible mobility in pregnancy and birthing, as well as protruding into the vagina, the ancient Greeks believed that it could also wander around the abdomen. Indeed, the womb was believed to roam upwards towards the liver in search of humidity, pushing against the diaphragm, obstructing the central channel and creating a sensation of suffocation. Most of these physiological assumptions were based on external observations and analogies with animal anatomy. Within this biological construction, the ancient Greeks viewed women's bodies as fundamentally different and inferior to that of males. Subsequent refinements stressed the cold and moist quality of the female constitution which was thought to be responsible for its flaws, vulnerability and need of monthly purges. Later, Alexandrian anatomy, based on human dissections, de-emphasised the differences between males and females – their sex organs were believed to be merely transposed – as well as placed some constraints on the notion of a wandering womb. Galen used a social reason for bestowing his ubiquitous concept of humoral 'plethora' on women who kept indoors, neither engaging in strenuous labour nor exposing themselves to direct sunlight.[13]

Cultural and environmental contexts may have been critically important in shaping such ideas. Was the ideology of the fertile female with regular menstrual periods based on the Hippocratic practitioners' limited exposure to a more affluent clientele of women? On average these women must have been better nourished and less physically burdened with hard work. Specific historical and cultural shifts in menstrual patterns were indeed related to changes in diet and physical activity.[14] Because of frequent pregnancies and long periods of lactation, continuous menstrual cycles may not necessarily have been considered a 'natural' occurrence during the fertile period of a woman's life. Early physicians used ancient biological and cultural constructions of femininity to justify gender roles in Graeco-Roman society. Their tone was strongly misogynist and pronatalist. They used Aristotelian notions of generation to stress the primacy of the male seed over the passive female seed. All potential movements of the womb made women unbalanced and unpredictable, in need of male control and domestication. It also made them unfit for pursuits outside the home. The main determinant of women's wellbeing and fertility was correct reproductive functioning. Marriage and pregnancy were considered natural health preservatives, capable of forestalling the appearance of many ailments.

During the Middle Ages, classical views of female nature based on anatomical and physiological differences persisted, including the purported tendency towards vascular plethora and need for regular monthly discharges. By the mid-sixteenth century, the physician Caspar Wolff (1525–1601), published a collection of texts about women and fertility issues. This work revealed the gradual establishment of a legitimate and specialised area of study and practice for male physicians.[15] Physicians began to theorise that because of women's smaller skin pores and vessels, they possessed a traditional inability to deal with bodily fluids. During mature age, this deficiency resulted in monthly accumulations of excess blood and the need for monthly discharges to restore balance. Associations between menses and moon cycles reinforced notions of physical and mental mutability. The coldness and humidity of a woman were responsible for bodily characteristics such as broader hips, narrower shoulders, and decreased strength. To top it off, this humoral mix also affected women's control of their emotions and rationality.[16] However, the conflicting views about the womb – its potential movements and capacity to affect behaviour and generate local diseases – continued to be vigorously debated.

Another anonymous compilation, known in English as *Aristotle's Master Piece*, continued to promote classical views and prejudices. First published in 1684, the text was reprinted throughout the eighteenth century. Among its multiple topics were sections discussing the periodic 'weeping' of the womb, retention or overflowing of the courses, false menses or the 'whites', as well as dropsy, inflammation and tumours of the womb.[17] Endowed with these purported physical – and mental – deficits, women were considered unsuited for exposure to the affairs of the outside world. In fact, they were often considered potential threats to the social order in need of restraint and control from stable and rational men.[18]

During the seventeenth century, however, new ideas regarding the importance of both circulatory and nervous systems in human physiology finally modified the ancient views. Sexual differences were reassessed on the basis of new anatomical discoveries regarding the structure of the ovaries and uterus. This knowledge led to dramatic shifts in the perception of the female body.[19] Indeed, the publication of Thomas Willis' (1621–75) highly influential *Anatomy of the Brain* in 1664, accomplished a veritable paradigmatic change by placing all physiological and mental actions under the direction of the brain and nerves. His student, John Locke (1632–1704), and Lockean ideas regarding the mind's reception of sensations and capacity for creating ideas and feelings enhanced the shift.[20] In this new nerve-centred world, the solid bodily components trumped traditional humours. Encouraged by Newtonian optics, the transmission of sensations through the nerves was believed to operate according to iatromechanical principles.[21] Subtle, ethereal particles pulsed through solid bundles of nerve fibres. Both the quality and speed of such communications relied on the quality and state of its fibres. Expanding on previous studies, the Swiss physician Albrecht von Haller (1708–77), announced in 1752 the existence of two properties, irritability and sensitivity, located in the fibres of nerves and muscles.

New theories of human physiology were based on these experimental findings. William Cullen (1710–90), the most prominent eighteenth-century representative of the Edinburgh School, also placed greater emphasis on the role the neuromuscular system played in the phenomena of health and disease. He believed the presence of a nervous power was responsible for the transmission of sensations to the brain as well as the execution of voluntary and involuntary motions.[22] A proper degree of 'excitement' in the nerves assured the normal transmission of impulses for blood circulation, chemical combinations, secretions and muscular activity. The unsexed brain became the chief mover and governor of rationality and emotions, displacing the traditional influences exerted by the powerful womb. In theory, at least, this 'neurocentric' body could be equally shared by men and women. To accommodate previous notions of physical female inferiority, however, eighteenth-century medical authors, including George Cheyne (1671–1734), posited the notion that women naturally possessed 'weaker' nerves composed of delicate, slender, and less compact fibres. The gendered anatomical differences allowed for quicker sensations and conferred on women a higher degree of 'sensibility'.[23] Operating within a more flexible and delicate nervous system, medical authorities linked this ambiguous quality to women's identity, emotions and behaviour. Moral superiority, sociability, passion and vivacity of spirit were considered expressions of a heightened state of female sensibility. Sensibility, defined as the ability to perceive and respond to sensory impressions, became a key bodily attribute linked to the quality of women's bodily fibres and fluid imbalances.[24] In the words of the English physician John Friend (1675–1728), those toiling in the field of women's diseases were 'being led away by their fantasies' in the formulation of the 'most abstruse and hidden principles'. By doing so, they became 'interpreters of their own dreams'.[25]

Based on these assumptions, a chorus of male voices characterised females as being naturally fragile, weak, and irritable. 'We naturally associate the idea of female softness and delicacy with the correspondent delicacy of constitution', observed John Gregory (1724–73), another Edinburgh professor.[26] Women's spongy flesh was said to possess a peculiar 'laxity of body fibres', and their nerves were endowed with soft and thin outer membranes capable of receiving the smallest impressions. The weaker sex was naturally disposed to perceive greater pain sensations and be more receptive to the impact of emotions such as fear, anxiety and grief, which created a heightened state of nervous irritability.[27] Such qualities were great liabilities to women since they created a proclivity for refined living and fashionable consumption in Britain's new commercial society.

Scientific ideas of female nature and health reflected the social conditions in which they were constructed. Indeed, class remained a fundamental category for exploring the medical views and treatment of women.[28] Ambiguities about female physiology and pathology stemmed in great part from the physicians' meagre empirical basis for this knowledge obtained from brief clinical exposures to two fundamentally different groups of women. Generalisations, popularised in the print media, were primarily based on experiences with the affluent class of women. Patients seen in private practice were married, socially secure and protected, and tended to household chores. Most were reasonably nourished, experiencing earlier menarche and later menopause. They also tended to have fewer pregnancies, abortions and stillbirths, and their periods were more regular and substantial. In a gambit designed to appeal to prospective female patrons, eighteenth-century practitioners stressed the delicacy and sensitivity of women's bodies. In fact, they transformed such apparently flawed physiological qualities into fashionable assets, making them part of upper-class identity. However, the purported greater sensibility was also a replay of previous notions of the weaker sex's emotional instability, which required male control and discipline.

In the end, such fanciful conclusions about women's bodies merely revealed the physicians' determination in claiming an important role in the treatment of 'female troubles'. The basic Hippocratic notions and subsequent stereotypes about females continued throughout the eighteenth century, including the idea that women were naturally destined to be procreators and homemakers. Emphasis on fertility and pregnancy – to the exclusion of other issues – reflected widespread fears of a demographic decline.[29] In his popular publication *Domestic Medicine*, William Buchan

(1729–1805) insisted that women were well adapted and fit for their life as mothers and homebodies which 'did not require much strength'.[30] Reproductive imperatives also explained the renewed focus on the uterus – now an irritable organ in 'sympathy' with others – as the key source of 'female trouble'. Since women's health revolved around their capacity to reproduce, the excesses of a refined lifestyle came to be perceived as important risk factors. Luxury and indolence, gluttony and generous alcohol consumption, as well as frequent sex were believed to generate plethora, disease, and a shorter life span. Other practices bound to affect the delicate female frame included excessive socialising and reading. Even the perusal of romantic novels could produce a nefarious sexual arousal. 'Late hours and lying in bed in the morning are very hurtful to weak nerves', determined Cullen in 1782.[31] The very embodiments of femininity – structural fragility and laxity – paradoxically created a fateful predisposition to disease. Most eighteenth-century physicians were convinced that plethora triggered serious ailments, from fevers to arthritis, phthisis to dyspepsia, skin troubles to cancer.[32] Even a contemporary self-help manual emphasised this quality of the female body, explaining that what 'renders her the most amiable object in the universe' also subjected her to 'an infinite number of maladies to which every man is an utter stranger'.[33]

Poor women were often single, socially marginal and vulnerable. Those living in urban environments often sought medical assistance in hospitals and dispensaries. Many joined the new labour force created by the budding Industrial Revolution. Romantic notions claimed that country people and workers lived longer than the rich because of their robust constitution, frugal diet and vigorous physical activity. Most, however, were chronically malnourished because of their poverty and traditional deference to male family members in the distribution of limited food rations. They admitted experiencing a late menarche and early menopause, with infrequent, scanty and irregular menstrual periods. When married, these women usually had more pregnancies, abortions and stillbirths, and were prone to many other illnesses.

Given the frequency and temporary nature of many female disorders, most women, rich and poor, first dealt with their infirmities by employing home remedies or consulting family members and irregular healers. Professional advice was only sought if symptoms persisted and the affected women began to fear for their reproductive capacity and future health. Physicians, for their part, simply blamed most conditions on constitutional weakness. The limited clinical experience and diagnostic methods as well as contemporary mores hampered practitioners, dominated by their paying customers. Complete reliance on the clinical history and inadequate opportunities for follow-up distinguished most private practice in eighteenth-century Britain.[34] Gentlemen practitioners who made sporadic house calls to examine sick females risked offending their patient's virtue. For elite physicians who dared to make such an examination, the potential penalty for offence was loss of reputation and income. Because of an absence of clinical information gleaned from physical exams, gynaecology, in essence, remained a mysterious branch of healing, based on the rhythmic appearance and disappearance of bodily fluids.

In an effort to medicalise women's complaints and lend them legitimacy, menstrual irregularities together with vaginal, uterine and ovarian conditions were readily included in eighteenth-century nosologies or classification of diseases. Even critics suggested that it was of greater importance to patients that practitioners 'should be competent to class' the complaint 'under its proper head' rather than attempt to remove or cure a disorder.[35] In his own 1769 *Nosology*, Cullen included the most important feminine afflictions among one of his classes of diseases: 'neuroses' The label applied to generalised nerve-caused ailments affecting sense and motion. 'Amenorrhoea' or menstrual suppression came to be defined as a local pelvic problem. In turn, 'menorrhagia' or excessive menstrual flow, and 'leucorrhoea', a non-specific vaginal discharge, were classified as inflammatory conditions. Cullen's scheme became a popular heuristic and didactic device useful to physicians and students. His classification was entirely based on clinical distinctions and justified by bedside clues that tended to confirm previous assumptions. Nosology was also believed to be essential for the improvement of therapeutics. Remedies needed to be 'adapted not only to every genus, but to every species, and variety of disease'.[36]

'Female troubles' increasingly came under the jurisdiction of surgeons who began devoting their practices to childbirth. Establishing a theoretical framework for midwifery to achieve greater professional status was consonant with the strategies guiding general medicine. Among their most prominent members were the surgeons William Smellie (1675–1728), John Leake (1720–92), Thomas Young (1726–83), Alexander Hamilton (1739–1802) and William Hunter. Their writings relied on traditional views of female physiology, couched in humoral and iatromechanical terms. Most of these men elected to follow the eclectic medical systems elaborated by the Dutch physician Herman Boerhaave (1668–1739), and his contemporary, the German physician Friedrich Hoffmann (1660–1742). Boerhaave and Hoffmann had both skilfully integrated key physical and chemical insights to build a comprehensive human physiology and pathology that came to influence contemporary perceptions of the female body. Male midwifery's ascendancy, particularly in Britain, occurred against the backdrop of a demographic reality: the significant rise in birth rates between 1750–1800. With their superior understanding regarding the anatomy of reproductive organs, male midwives aggressively began to carve out their own surgical speciality by medicalising childbirth, and by extension, all related female diseases. Indeed, according to William Hunter (1718–83), women became 'more acquainted with people of our profession', shedding some of their traditional modesty and reticence regarding disclosure and management of gynaecological disorders.[37] Nevertheless, the spectre of the male midwife as sexual predator persisted.[38]

Menstruation: a 'local female peculiarity'?

Perhaps the most important factor in establishing gender differences and linking all feminine disorders was the formulation of a comprehensive theory of menstruation. Menstruation was unique to women and had always been a bodily as well as cultural phenomenon subject to competing interpretations, taboos, and ambiguous interventions. Throughout history, explanations of this occurrence remained central to the understanding of female physiology. On the positive side, this phenomenon was a mysterious cosmic event, linked to the tides, seasons and moon cycles. Menstrual blood seemed to play a role in the formation of new life because of its magical fertilising quality. At the same time, it was interpreted as a threat to males and a challenge to the social order. As such it often led to the social and sexual isolation of menstruating women.[39] Since Biblical times – 'curse of Eve' – menstrual blood has also had a negative connotation. Within certain cultures it was considered to be a polluted, possibly poisonous and toxic substance.

In classical times, menstruation was seen as an untidy, often painful – albeit necessary – occurrence, periodically weakening the female body and temporarily exposing it to humoral imbalances. Authors emphasised the normality of women's regular menstrual flow as a sign of good health and fertility, with all irregularities considered pathological and in need of medical treatment. In Hippocratic treatises, the phenomenon was viewed as a regular cleansing necessary for preserving good health. A woman's regular purge or *catharsis* was interpreted as shedding potentially decaying blood originally earmarked for the growth of a foetus. Deprived of its natural outlet, menstrual blood could also search for another exit, including the nose, mouth, nipples, and the anus in the form of haemorrhoids. Employed throughout history, remedies called emmenagogues were expected to 'draw down' the blood. Many also had a reputation as abortifacients. Menstrual retention, in turn, was considered to be the principal culprit for a host of women's troubles. Trapped in the body because of a clogged uterus, the surplus blood was believed to be liable to corruption, causing infertility, pain and numerous other diseases.[40] Authors such as Galen advocated stimulating measures to rid the female body of dangerous congestion due to internal obstructions. This would restore the necessary humoral balance.

During the Middle Ages, the toxic quality of the 'flowers' – a metaphorical term for menstrual blood implying the promise of a fruit – gave rise to literature concerning the mythical dangers of the 'venomous virgin'.[41] In this view, the menses were associated with uncleanness and transmission of malignant diseases. For their part, leading Renaissance authors similarly supported the Hippocratic notion of menstruation as a beneficial catharsis of superfluous blood subject to dangerous decay. Physicians such as Jean Fernel (1497–1558) re-affirmed the poisonous effects of menstrual blood on plants and animals as well as its capacity to produce potentially fatal diseases such as cancer, epilepsy and consumption.[42] Others stressed the Galenic idea of vascular plethora with displacement of excess blood into other bodily organs including the brain.

In early modern Europe, biases congruent with newer commercial goals of population growth encouraged the medical norm of regular menses. Periodic menstrual discharges were essential, not merely as reflections of female health, but for reproduction.[43] Shifting paradigms of the female body in the seventeenth century affected the explanation of menstruation but both the mechanical and iatrochemical explanations failed to challenge the core of ancient notions.[44] In fact, William Harvey's (1578–1657) blood circulation scheme placed new emphasis on the importance of blood and its dynamics within the body. Menstrual bleeding acquired even greater significance and management of the cyclical phenomenon was placed in the hands of learned physicians as part of an emerging rational and scientific medicine.[45] Chemical models posited a particular fermentation of blood in the uterus that increased vascular pressure. Since the blood was thought to turn poisonous, it periodically eroded the uterine vessels, forcing a discharge. Competing views pitted the traditional humoral paradigm against more novel assumptions based on the action of the nervous system. In this version, the flow occurred because of uterine irritability and leakage of engorged uterine arteries.[46] All theories converged on the ideal of menstrual regularity.[47]

Europe's leading eighteenth-century expert on menstruation, John Friend, also believed in the notion of vascular plethora. Originally published in 1703, his *Emmenologia* was translated into English in 1729. The older humoral view still postulated that the mature female constitution was capable of preparing supplemental amounts of blood intended for the nourishment of a foetus inside the womb and for milk following birth. If neither of these events took place, a compensatory mechanism or 'local peculiarity' provided for the periodic release of these excessive fluids.[48] Even before menarche, adolescent girls were considered to be in special jeopardy. Their delicate constitution and excessive nervous sensibility frequently led to eating disorders, triggering the 'green sickness' or chlorosis already described by the ancients. If young women starved themselves in an effort to acquire the fashionable and erotic pale complexion, their blood would thicken and fail to circulate through the uterus. If they consumed excessive amounts of food, excess blood and vascular plethora resulted. Following this rationale, the catamenia acted as a regular safety valve designed to remove the 'redundancy of blood' produced in the system. Pre-menstrual symptoms such as headaches, nausea, back pains, and swollen, tender breasts expressed this congestive state.[49] So did painful menstrual periods.[50] The symptoms were widely acknowledged to be more frequent in 'women of fashion and a delicate nervous constitution' than their 'lower rank' sisters who were 'strangers to those refinements and inured to exercise and labour'.[51] Gone was the notion that menstrual blood was venomous, but the flow was still defined as 'morbid flux' placing women at risk.

By the later eighteenth century, menarche was expected around the age of fifteen.[52] Reflecting both physical and mental conditions, the precise timing was a result of a number of speculative causes. According to Cullen and his followers, as soon as the compact pubescent uterus expanded through the addition of blood vessels, menstruation could begin.[53] In warmer climates sexual maturation and menarche occurred at an earlier age. Early menarche was linked with immorality and the young women suspected of reading erotic literature or engaging in masturbation.[54] By contrast, physicians practising in hospitals were aware that 'girls of the poorer sort' had a delayed onset of their menses.[55] In his clinical lectures, Cullen explained the considerable variations in the onset of menarche, indicating that 'no time can be precisely assigned as proper to the sex in general'.[56] He blamed late menarche on women's 'lean and dry habit', poor nutrition and hard work.[57]

Entrenched in traditional views, eighteenth-century practitioners and their female clients viewed menarche in unfavourable terms because it introduced a cycle of dangerous congestion and increased susceptibility to disease, not to mention the hazards of pregnancy and childbirth. When some women failed to experience menarche well into their twenties, the delay was considered pathological, an affection of immature ovaries and systemic body debility labelled by Cullen *amenorrhoea emansionis* and subject to medical treatment.[58] Virginity was another medical concern: the cleansing and decongesting menstrual flow could be obstructed by narrow uterine vessels and the hymen, thereby forcing a diversion of the blood to other parts of the body. In cases of an imperforated hymen, Andrew Duncan Sr and others recommended an incision with a lancet or trocar to facilitate the periodic expulsion. To lower their risk of dangerous pelvic congestion and disease, young women were urged to get married early, have frequent sex and get pregnant.[59] The ideal cure that would regularise and expedite the monthly flow was childbirth, since it promoted the full maturation and expansion of the uterine vessels.

Whether rich or poor, practitioners recognised that after menarche young women went through a two or three year period of irregular menstrual cycles and infertility. This fact was viewed as part of the 'natural tendencies of the system' impervious to medical treatment. More recent theories of human physiology subordinated all vascular changes to the tension or degree of irritability prevailing in the human nervous system. In women, following the maturation of the uterus and ovaries, local stimuli from the genitals as well as mental impulses in the form of sexual desire, created enough excitement in the uterine vessels to allow for the periodic discharges. However, no periodic flow could be established until the diameter of the uterine vessels was large enough to allow the blood to escape.

Medical men observed that 'women of quality' seemed to normalise their periods sooner and began discharging greater amounts of menstrual blood than their poorer sisters.[60] This traditional medical emphasis on menstrual regularity has been interpreted as a component of strategies designed to restrict, repress and reform women's bodies and minds; and thus, secure social and moral order. Beyond that, regularity was closely associated with proper muscular tone in the women's vessels. Cullen's disciple, John Brown, further associated regular menstruation with a healthy sex life. The stimulus Brown called 'venereal emotion' or 'power of love' was capable of exciting the uterus to periodically shed its blood: 'The more they give way to that passion, the more freely do they experience this discharge within certain boundaries', he asserted. Privation of sexual intercourse not only produced menstrual irregularities but was also said to have a debilitating effect on the body. Excessive systemic irritability tended to close the organ's arteries through vascular spasms that halted discharge. Defined by Cullen as *amenorrhoea suppresionis,* this was a disease in which adult women with a previous history of cyclic flows, who were not pregnant, experienced a cessation of menses.[61]

The opposite but less frequent gynaecological disorder was excessive menstrual bleeding or *menorraghia,* included in Cullen's class of 'haemorrhages' and popularly known as an 'immoderate flow of the menses'.

For Cullen, this label represented painful menstrual periods or *dysmenorrhoea*,[62] a condition of general debility leading to excessive arterial relaxation and consequently profuse and irregular bleeding.[63] Locally, the ailment resulted from vascular congestion capable of irritating the uterus. Instead of causing spasms, the womb's vessels became excessively relaxed.[64] Medical authors cited frequent miscarriages, botched abortions and difficult deliveries causing the uterus to 'overstrain' as possible causes of irregular bleeding. Frequent straining from chronic constipation could cause a similar state as the abdominal contents were thrust into the pelvis, resulting in both haemorrhoid and vaginal bleeding. Some of the women suffering from this condition were older, obese, or nearing menopause. As women aged, became weaker, and had less sex, vascular responses and excitability in the uterus lagged.[65] Many of the factors believed to trigger menorrhagia were also linked to an unhealthy lifestyle. Women suffering from this condition were blamed for lingering too long in warm chambers, spending too much time in bed having sex, eating rich foods and drinking excessive amounts of alcohol, tea and coffee. Excessive exertion and dancing could also be harmful.[66]

Each month, the normal menstrual discharge consisted of six to twelve ounces, evacuated over a period of three to five days.[67] Physicians professed to be amazed by the fact that such minor and slow blood withdrawals could effectively reverse the postulated systemic congestion. Following menstruation, even women's external appearance often improved. Skin and eyes regained lustre and bodies recovered strength. Paradoxically, greater blood withdrawal in the form of nosebleeds, discharges from haemorrhoids and therapeutic bloodletting never achieved similar results. Like other critical stages of human development such as teething, puberty and old age, 'out of order' menstruating women were considered to be particularly vulnerable to disease. Because of 'sympathies' between the uterus and several vital organs, other bodily systems were equally at risk.[68] Women needed to learn all the facts concerning their monthly 'weakness' without 'false modesty' in order to ward off serious consequences. Physicians recommended pubescent girls receive early instruction so that they would later be able to manage 'the most critical period of their lives'. Failure to know and practice such precepts could easily ruin a woman's health and most importantly, impair her powers of procreation.[69] Physicians frequently linked menstrual irregularities without pregnancy to two specific diseases: 'dropsy' and 'phthisis.' The former label represented a number of cardiovascular conditions while the latter suggested a lung problem, notably tuberculosis associated with the spitting of fresh blood (Chapter 7). Both were chronic, wasting ailments that eventually would prove fatal.[70]

When the menses began, women were urged to take great care and avoid anything that could possibly interrupt the flow and create a dangerous obstruction. Risk factors included a lack of fresh air, insufficient exercise, and fashionable straightlacing. With regard to diet, excessive ingestion of fish or other heavy meals would not only hurt the stomach but also negatively impact the uterus and impair the needed discharge. 'At the approach of a period you must take care to keep the bowels regular', admonished Cullen in a letter to one of his patients.[71] Every cold and acid food or drink that soured the stomach needed to be omitted. This included milk products and fruits. Moreover, tea drinking was dangerous because of its alleged weakening effects (Chapter 4). Lastly, medical authorities were also quite aware that emotional distress could play havoc with women's menstrual cycles. As one author admitted, 'nothing hurts more the nervous system and particularly the concoctive powers than fear, grief and anxiety'.[72] A lack of menses was attributed to a 'frightening episode'.[73] To avoid irregularity, physicians recommended 'sprightly amusements' or 'innocent festivity'. They also praised the power of poetry and painting as 'perpetual sources' for pleasing the female mind.[74]

All determinants of menstrual regularity seemed to ultimately rest on the conduct of women who experienced them. Violations courted disaster. Females received a precise blueprint for proper physical, emotional and social behaviour officially sanctioned by society. Issued in the name of health preservation, such maxims not only tried to justify and support the prevailing social and cultural views about women, but also tended to perpetuate their roles as breeders and homemakers. Because of their wide diffusion, these causal relationships seem to have been widely accepted by the women themselves, regardless of social position and income. At best, the rules stressed individual responsibility and provided confidence that a careful life-style would be rewarded with health, promote fertility, and shield oneself from dreaded diseases. At worst, the medical notions served to shift causality to social and behavioural recommendations that only privileged women could possibly follow.

Finally, women experienced another dramatic event, the 'cessation of menses' – now termed menopause – which generally occurred between the ages of forty-five and fifty. Prior to this event, many women experienced menstrual irregularities; a condition called 'dodging'. However, medical authors were uncertain about the proper timing of this cessation, generally placing it within the decade after the age of forty. One prominent English physician, John Fothergill (1712–80), admitted that the onset of menopause was 'a period in the life of females to which they are taught to look with some degree of anxiety'.[75] In a consultation with one of his aristocratic clients, Cullen tried to reassure his patient that the timing of menopause depended on her constitution, and that 'a formal stoppage may take place in a manner that will do no harm'.[76] Nevertheless, the popular notion that menstruation was a natural channel for the discharge of 'whatever had a tendency to produce diseases' fostered great concern and apprehension when the flow decreased and eventually stopped completely. Accepting the ancient tenets of 'catharsis', some women became terrified at the approach of menopause, believing that their bodies would fill up with noxious fluids. The excess blood was believed to accumulate throughout the body, especially in the brain and abdomen, genitalia and legs. Other complications were fibrous tumours in the uterus, or worse yet, fatal corroding cancers of the breast and uterine cervix.

Eighteenth-century authors directed their new nerve-centred theories to describe this 'change of life'. In doing so, they resorted to the same vascular uterine physiology that explained menarche and menstrual flow. As women approached menopause, a permanent arterial blockage resulted from the advancing rigidity of the vessels. First the condition was local but it soon triggered a general state of increased nervous debility with hot flushes, breathing difficulties, numbness and paralysis, as well as swelling and stiffness of the joints. Virtually any other discomfort was blamed on this weakness. Commenting on a female patient's soft and irritable fibres, Cullen spoke of a 'weakened system giving a tendency to paralysis and liable to the most violent spasmodic affections'.[77] Once again, authors pointed to the excesses of a 'refined' existence. Life-style and body weight became influential factors. More importantly, sterile women who had failed to perform their reproductive duties were identified as 'most apt to suffer at the decline of life'.[78]

Although a majority of women transitioned through their changes of life without professional assistance, the ideas expressed by medical authorities regarding their inherent fragility lingered and were consonant with contemporary life-spans and disease burdens. In fact, the concern about health risks linked to menarche and menopause was prompted by changes in the age structure of the population in Georgian Britain and higher death rates among adolescents and menopausal women.[79] Since menopause became such an important health concern, a few women even demanded to be bled in a futile attempt to simulate the lagging, periodical discharges. These women were encouraged by physicians who agreed with the notion that a failure to drain the accumulated blood would lay 'the foundation for an irrecoverable bad state of health during the remaining part of life'.[80]

'Female troubles' at the Edinburgh Infirmary

Why would lower-class women like Euphemia McKay, suffering from a non-life-threatening condition, seek admission to a hospital on a Sunday morning? To be sure, both rich and poor adult women accepted the notions stressing their natural inferiority and the importance of regular menses as a barometer for their physical health. Following the debilitating stillbirth episode, it was either Euphemia or, more likely her husband that was fearful of her future childbearing potential. Or could Euphemia's lack of menstrual periods be masking a welcomed or dreaded pregnancy? If the latter circumstance were true, was she hoping that an aggressive medical approach would help her abort? Perhaps her previous experiences with illness played a role in the decision to seek help. Who persuaded her to abandon the traditional domestic measures popular at the time to deal with her symptoms? Self-help manuals and oral traditions suggested a host of traditional herbal remedies to act as cathartics, emmenologues, and abortifacients. In Euphemia's case, the purgatives she took had not been helpful and maybe it was time to try something else. Perhaps her sponsor, a financial supporter of the Infirmary and owner of admission letters, suggested hospitalisation. Females identified as the 'poorer sort who live in towns' composed more than half of the inmate population. 'Condemned to sedentary employment', they were often judged to be potentially 'bad breeders', an important concern in an era when the working population was a key factor in achieving national power and prosperity (Chapter 1). No matter the motive, posing as an invalid at the Infirmary's Admissions Room during the winter months was bound to draw attention, especially among university professors scouting for challenging cases.

Eighteenth-century Edinburgh hosted a large population of young adults from vulnerable social and occupational positions. Servants and apprentices of both sexes usually lived in the master's house where they could obtain food and clothing. Single women in service were not free to marry. While waiting for the economic independence of their mates, some couples engaged in 'irregular' marriages without religious blessing – the Church of Scotland after the 1770s had been forced to relax its previously tight social control. Late marriage and illegitimate births increased. However, lack of privacy and sharing of beds in extremely cramped conditions placed strains on their servants' virtue and reports of rape by masters and other male attendants were not uncommon. If pregnancy occurred, maidservants were always considered guilty and dismissed from service.[81] Women frequently denied their pregnancies; midwives were summoned by the church to examine suspected cases. Lying about venereal disease was also prevalent. Employers who wished to rule out pregnancy or treat suspected venereal disease of their female servants sent them to the hospital, ridding themselves of sick workers and avoiding any further responsibility. Whether dispatched to the hospital by their sponsors or on their own volition, the relative institutional anonymity of the Infirmary and the opportunity to rest, be fed and cared for could seem attractive to these women.[82]

By the second half of the eighteenth century the rituals of pregnancy and childbirth as well as associated 'female troubles' were no longer exclusively staged and controlled by women. The traditional solidarity and bonding with regard to childbirth, lying-in and dying were beginning to dissolve, creating additional options for potential patients. Gynaecology was not viewed as a separate and special concern of any group of healers. Britain's competitive marketplace forced all practitioners – regulars and irregular – to make claims regarding their curing abilities with respect to a broad spectrum of diseases. Boundaries remained fluid between midwives, female and male irregulars, surgeons, male midwives, and gentlemen–physicians in private and hospital practice. All these healers sought to expand their marketability by claiming expertise in managing menstrual disorders and uterine diseases.

In Edinburgh, the Town Council established the first chair of midwifery in 1726, and Thomas Young became the first university professor there in 1756. In fact, members of the city's Incorporation of Surgeons had already attempted to create a school of midwifery in the 1730s. Male midwives acquired considerable prestige and power in spite of the fact that as surgeons they were usually not considered to be gentlemen. There was also growing support in Edinburgh for teaching midwifery as an elective to students. Later in the century, every practising physician was encouraged to learn its techniques. Young, who also possessed a medical degree, was the first to provide clinical training at the Infirmary. He also helped establish a small lying-in ward for such an instruction.[83] Conversely, aspiring men-midwives were told to attend medical courses, thus attempting to further blur the somewhat fuzzy borders between physicians and surgeons practising gynaecology.[84] John Gregory (1724–73), professor of the practice of medicine, discussed the problem in 1772, stating that 'if a surgeon or apothecary has had the education and acquired the knowledge of a physician, he is a physician to all intents and purposes ..and ought to be respected and treated accordingly.'[85]

However, turf battles between them were inevitable. With a generous supply of physicians and surgeons, Edinburgh was an extremely competitive medical marketplace after 1750. At the turn of the century, James Gregory estimated that seventy-five to ninety percent of the city's medical practice was carried out by surgeon–apothecaries functioning as 'ordinary physicians in every family'.[86] His very public war-of-words with John Bell (1762–1820), a young surgeon who was part of the rotation attending the Infirmary, highlighted the differing professional visions of elite medical practitioners and surgeons (Chapter 1).[87] In his 1784 publication, Young's successor, Alexander Hamilton, insisted that midwifery was not merely empirical but derived from a systematic theory. He dedicated his book, *Outlines of the Theory and Practice of Midwifery*, to William Cullen 'a gentleman conspicuous for extensive knowledge in every department of science', as a gesture of deference to a gentrified, former naval surgeon.[88] To frame his explanations, Hamilton borrowed extensively from Cullen's nerve-dominated female body, subscribing to the concept of delicate nerves and constitutions weakened by sedentary life. He also retained the ancient plethora theory of menstruation. Hamilton was instrumental in the creation of another separate public charity, the Edinburgh Lying-in Hospital, which opened its doors at the recommendation of the University's Academic Senate in 1791.

A 1792 guide published for prospective students prominently advertised the academic midwifery courses. This led to a personal and literary confrontation between James Gregory and Hamilton's son and eventual successor James.[89] By that time, Hamilton's new book on the management of female complaints also included diseases which occurred 'in the unimpregnated state' and 'medical subjects for the use of families', including young infants.[90] 'Nothing more strongly stamps the character of *Gentlemen* than a quick sensibility and delicate attention' to the 'weaker and softer sex', wrote the surgeon John Aikin (1747–1822).[91] For their part, physicians intent on medicalising these areas of practice emphasised the importance of female physiology and pathology, arguing that they were uniquely qualified to treat women. Indeed, physicians in charge of the Edinburgh Infirmary's teaching ward were rotating professors and also Fellows of the local Royal College of Physicians. These men were determined to preserve 'medical' gynaecology within the purview of gentlemen practitioners. Women constituted a large segment of their private practices. In fact, nearly a third of Cullen's medical consultations through the mails dealt with so-called 'female troubles'.[92] There was concern that a certain reticence to deal with reproductive matters based on notions of gentility was no longer appropriate in an era of medicalisation and increased professional competition. Physicians, for their part, insisted that they alone were in possession of knowledge necessary to place female complaints within a broader framework of physiology and pathology. Because menstrual irregularities and menopause were linked to a host of other non-surgical diseases, it was imperative that they be considered and managed by medical practitioners.

The decorum surrounding private practice provided limited clinical exposure to female complaints. As a result, medical students and their teachers were circumscribed in their ability to gain knowledge regarding 'female troubles'. However, hospital practice offered new opportunities. Indeed, the Edinburgh Infirmary periodically admitted gynaecological cases, especially to the teaching ward as late-eighteenth-century education gradually evolved towards the formation of general practitioners.[93] Professors definitely wanted students to become acquainted with the clinical nature and management of 'female troubles'. The medical elite obviously expected that some of these problems would be instructive to students and medical intervention might benefit the patients. Thus, teachers and students made strenuous efforts to subsume female sexual functioning within the prevailing general medical theories while at the same time borrowing additional knowledge for their diagnoses and therapies from contemporary anatomists and man-midwives. Attending physicians occasionally posed, at least rhetorically, as reluctant participants, but they were actually keenly interested in advancing their own knowledge and reputation as benevolent and charitable healers. Like true gentlemen, they offered protection and assistance to 'weak' and 'delicate' poor women seeking help.[94]

Voluntary hospitals, such as the Edinburgh Infirmary with its separate wards for female patients, provided more sympathetic space for housing such cases. However, the relative paucity of these admissions and the charitable nature of the institution hindered the pedagogical objectives.[95] In fact, these limited hospital experiences tended to perpetuate the universal stereotype of female fragility and propensity for chronic disease.[96]

In accordance with contemporary mores and notions of benevolence, Edinburgh Infirmary patients came under the protection of the managers (Chapter 1). Hospital physicians and students were cautioned 'not to shock the delicacy of tender females'. In fact, both groups were urged to act with great discretion, mostly relying on the information furnished by patients on admission and subsequent encounters during ward rounds. Based on extant student casebooks, a total of 619 women can be identified as patients admitted to the teaching ward between the years 1770–1800. Their average age was twenty-three years, the youngest being fourteen; the oldest sixty-two. One patient out of four was listed in the casebooks as being a servant. When treating a wide spectrum of women's complaints, elite physicians were keenly interested in determining the menstrual status of such patients. Such information was recorded for 341 of these women in their prime reproductive years, revealing that more than sixty percent of them reported irregular or missed periods. Since these hospital populations were arbitrarily selected on the basis of medical and social criteria (Chapter 1), it remains unclear whether such a high proportion of menstrual problems was similarly present among affluent women or the population at large.

With the influx of 'deserving' poor women into dispensaries and hospitals, institutional physicians were compelled to seek new causal relationships between life-style and menses. The usual linkages between affluent living and menstrual disorders were not always applicable to 'common females'.[97] But how could so many poor women suffer from such irregularities when conventional wisdom depicted them as strong and hardy? In his *Medical Instructions,* John Leake insisted that 'the poor female cottager who uses exercise in the open air, eats the coarse but wholesome bread of industry and drinks from the cooling stream is seldom troubled with those maladies which afflict the rich and indolent'.[98] Never at a loss for explanations, eighteenth-century physicians responded by expanding the range of possible causes. They now stressed the danger of excessive exposure to cold air, overexertion, damp linen clothing, cold water bathing as well as walking with wet feet while menstruating. Cold drinks were considered especially dangerous.[99] One patient's history read: 'Menses suppressed for the last six weeks from drinking a draught of cold milk while profusely perspiring'.[100] Malnutrition also seemed to be prevalent among those that earned low wages. Cullen claimed that among the lower-class patients seen at the Edinburgh Infirmary, the menses virtually ceased during the winter months, only to return with 'the advancing warmth of spring'.[101] The menses also set up a similar predisposition to several diseases, from catarrhs to fevers, rheumatism to ascites. 'More of the [female] sex date their diseases from cold caught while they are out of order than from all other causes', observed Buchan.[102]

What could women anticipate from physicians who openly professed their puzzlement about female physiology and pathology, and seemingly had little to offer beyond a number of familiar domestic and few aggressive but equally ineffective treatments? Most 'deserving' poor who experienced 'female complaints' and made their way to the Edinburgh Infirmary probably had modest expectations. As with men, sickness was an important source of physical and emotional distress, especially for those living alone away from their families. Housed in cramped quarters, they often found it impossible to rest. They were also reluctant to impose their health burdens on relatives and friends.[103] Instead, they sought reassurance through medical opinion. Diagnosis and treatments from some of the most famous and powerful physicians in all of Europe was considered perhaps a last resort that fuelled hope.

Infirmary physicians labelled and managed patients, guided primarily by oral reports from the inmates themselves, nurses, and at times from consulting midwives. It was a tedious, frustrating and unreliable method, which encouraged fraud and outright malingering, and easily led to misinterpretations and errors. Deception was often a necessary tool for patient admission; suspicions of 'female duplicity' abounded.[104] Nurses and most inmates – bound by gender, class and occupation – may have conspired with each other and withheld crucial details about their illnesses. As a result, the information gleaned from patients was often considered incomplete or untrustworthy. Patients who eventually admitted being pregnant were promptly expelled.[105] Gender, traditional taboos, and professional decorum dictated the nature and limits of physical examination.[106] Like true gentlemen, Cullen and other elite physicians limited their search for physical signs to visual inspections and pulse-taking. They eschewed the use of hands and avoided touching the female body internally to prevent damage to their own reputations. Investigations of the *naturalia* could be interpreted as sexually offensive. The procedure was still an important source of female embarrassment prompting occasional accusations of sexual assault and rape.[107] Only when absolutely necessary, were surrogate midwives called in to perform them. The lack of such an examination – a requisite among man-midwives – could have been another encouragement for prudish women to seek a medical admission.

Discretion and secrecy were essential in gaining women's trust and respecting their 'natural delicacy'. To preserve a degree of patient confidentiality, menstrual status and prescriptions were exclusively recorded in Latin in the patient registers.[108] Nurses assigned to the ward functioned as informants to confirm the veracity of complaints and rule out malingering. Notes such as 'this discharge is perceived as coming from the vagina' appeared on some clinical charts. Menstruation, however, could never be completely standardised. Every woman possessed her own periodicity, which was shaped by constitutional and environmental factors. Medical authorities emphasised the critical nature of the menses and their potential for creating windows of vulnerability. As a result, poor women who began menstruating during their hospital stay emphatically refused to take remedies prescribed for them, notably emetics and purgatives. Others used the opportunity to vigorously resist bloodletting.[109] If complications ensued or the patient's condition deteriorated at a later date, practitioners feared they would be blamed. 'The consideration of the presence of catamenia has thrown every practitioner upon occasion into a very doubtful and hesitating practice', complained Cullen, adding that 'I do not know that the subject has been fully canvassed or considered.'[110]

This refusal to follow medical orders on account of their menstrual status remained a key challenge to the professional authority of eighteenth-century physicians regarding 'female matters'. Like local church authorities, attending physicians probably called in midwives to perform pelvic examinations in cases of suspected pregnancy. Size of the uterus and conditions of the cervix remained for medical eyes only, inscribed in the ward journal using Latin terms. '*Os uteri ad tactum clausum*' – the mouth of the uterus remains closed – read the progress note in a casebook, suggesting that some of the patients were subjected to internal examinations for the purpose of ascertaining pregnancy through the status of the womb.[111]

Many attending professors remained sceptical about their diagnoses. Male physicians often failed to grasp the meaning and significance of female complaints since they had no way to gauge them in relation to their own bodily representations. Such doubt and confusion prompted brief therapeutical trials for diagnostic purposes – a traditional approach to cope with uncertainty. Failure of treatment was blamed on insufficient or misleading information or the lack of efficacy attributed to most traditional drugs and other methods of treatment. For hospital physicians the medical art was already quite conjectural, but managing women was even more perplexing. Most gynaecological problems were seldom fatal. Thus, the professional staff was deprived of opportunities to conduct postmorten examinations and their ability to link symptoms with pathological changes discovered in the reproductive organs.[112]

The most common gynaecological condition seen at the Edinburgh Infirmary was *amenorrhoea*. In most instances, this menstrual stoppage was of considerable duration, followed by the appearance of other symptoms of systemic debility. According to another Edinburgh professor, Francis Home (1719–1813), 'there is no disease which appears more frequently in the clinical ward than the amenorrhoea either in a simple or complicated state as a cause of a multitude of disorders.'[113] This presumptive diagnosis was always fraught with ambiguity for both the women who exhibited it and the practitioners called upon to restore the periods. First pregnancy had to be ruled out, especially if patients provided fragmentary histories or their 'reckoning' of menstrual periods proved confusing or inaccurate.[114] According to Duncan, an apparent menstrual obstruction could be due to pregnancy 'but the view of the female may be to obtain an abortion'.[115] Much was at stake. James Gregory admitted that 'we are frequently deceived by women with child who wishing to get rid of their burden, produce a miscarriage', adding that 'many cunning patients gave incorrect menstrual histories to hide their pregnancies'.[116]

Discussing Euphemia McKay's case, an Edinburgh medical student reiterated that pregnancy was not easy to diagnose and those physicians who misdiagnosed it 'may forfeit their reputation', particularly if their regimen of drugs resulted in miscarriage.[117] Patient narratives that suggested they were suffering from morning sickness were not helpful; physicians were urged to carry out careful inspections of the skin and palpate the abdomen to detect possible foetal movements after the fourth month of gestation. In doubtful cases, a midwife was called in to ascertain the condition of the cervix and furnish a report of her findings. Such vigilance often paid off, with pregnancy confirmed in several instances, some in unmarried servants. The findings were translated into Latin and recorded in the ward's journal. Other common reasons for *amenorrhoea* were recent miscarriages, traumatic births, and prolonged breastfeeding. It was not uncommon for poor women to continue without periods six to eight months after weaning their children. In most cases, however, no obvious cause could be blamed for the menstrual suppression except perhaps the weather and season of the year. Women suffering from the disease often complained of headaches, vertigo, difficult breathing, stomach cramps and back pain. Their median age was twenty-five, average for all female hospital admissions, and they usually remained in the institution for about three weeks. Since clinical teaching in Edinburgh followed the academic calendar from November until April, most admissions occurred during the winter months, a time when *amenorrhoea* was believed to be the most obstinate.

Managing 'female troubles'

Treatment for menstrual disorders was admittedly on a 'precarious footing'. According to Cullen, such management was 'a tedious process unfit for a clinical [teaching] ward' since a rapid turnover of cases was desirable to provide students with greater opportunities to observe interesting cases.[118] Nevertheless, Cullen admitted that 'I well know that the public will expect attempts from us in most cases'.[119] Brief institutional stays and a restricted in-house formulary discouraged therapeutic innovation. To protect its charitable image, moreover, Infirmary rules discouraged clinical trials (Chapter 1). The traditional therapeutic rationale based on humoralism was recast in language consistent with the new nerve-mediated theories. However, the actual treatments followed very much in the footsteps of the ancients.[120] Many treatments were rooted in domestic and folk approaches widely collected for centuries in self-help receipt books. While lecturing to medical students in 1772, Cullen acknowledged that:

> I don't know of any ready certain effectual means for exciting the menstrual flux and for my comfort, I have found some of the most eminent practitioners of these days joining me in this.[121]

The overall goal of treatment for *amenorrhoea* was ostensibly to restore the tone and strength of all bodily systems, especially the nerves, muscles and blood vessels. This approach demanded a plentiful diet and use of the traditional depleting procedures together with tonic remedies and stimulating exercise 'within and without doors'.[122] Instructions for carriage, horseback riding and 'violent leaping', appropriate for wealthier private patients, were expected to jar loose the retained blood. In addition, hospital physicians also attempted to relieve the obstruction through the administration of herbal and chemical compounds acting as antispasmodics and emmenagogues. These included the madder root (*rubia tinctorum*), a traditional remedy containing a powerful dye that tinged the urine a deep red colour. The original rationale for administering this emmenagogue was its presumed sympathetic magical action on the uterus that would hopefully lead to a resumption of the menses. Popular on the Continent, the remedy was administered by Francis Home to nineteen Infirmary patients during the 1770s with seemingly good results. Of those given the root powder dissolved in water, two-thirds soon claimed to have resumed their menses but the hospital physician was unclear about its mode of action. Sabine, a tincture made from juniper berries, castor and myrrh, was also reported to be a potent emmenagogue. However, the use was problematic because of its potential as an abortifacient.[123] Trials with other drugs were occasionally attempted, such as the administration of mercury, considered a universal stimulant and cure-all.[124] Opium was also given with the expectation that its action would relax the stubborn arteries in the uterus while taking care of other complaints such as headaches and cramps.

The goal was to stimulate the uterine arteries since they seemed to be constricted by severe spasms. They needed sufficient relaxation for discharging the collected blood. For this purpose blood had to be shunted towards the pelvic area. Among the standard strategies, physicians insisted in cleansing the bowels with purgatives and emetics. They also prescribed hot footbaths, enemas and even vaginal irrigation.[125] Rubbing the lower abdomen and legs with a flannel or flesh-brush was common. Two flannel cloths dipped in hot water were alternately placed on the skin and left there until the warming effect wore off. Performed by nurses, the entire procedure usually lasted about half an hour and was repeated once or twice a day. Warm water-bottles could also be placed over the genitals. Some patients were asked to sit up near the ward's fireplace so that the debilitating effects of coldness could be neutralised. If the menstrual obstruction was longstanding, the resulting systemic plethora or vascular congestion demanded the removal of blood from the body by other means. Artificial bloodletting in the form of venesection was meant to imitate the patient's ability to naturally discharge the noxious excess. It was usually prescribed if the patients displayed other symptoms of systemic congestion such as headaches, dizziness, a flushed face, and laboured breathing. At the Edinburgh Infirmary, nearly half of the patients suffering from amenorrhoea were bled; the average amount withdrawn was slightly over eight ounces. The lower extremities of the body, preferably the saphaenous veins located in the legs, were the preferred sites for such bleedings, although it was difficult to extract required amounts of blood from smaller vessels.[126]

More drastic was the use of 'gentle' electric sparks applied to the pelvic area and the back at intervals of two to three minutes for half an hour daily. On average, this electrification would continue for about a week unless the patient showed signs of menstruating. Although the sparks could be frightening, the effects were described as pleasant: they produced local warmth and a certain feeling of exhilaration. By contrast, the occasional compression of the femoral arteries first advocated by Alexander Hamilton was quite traumatic. This treatment was prescribed for periods of forty minutes or until the patients 'complained of pain and weight in the region of the uterus'.[127] The purpose was to produce greater congestion in the uterus and pressure in the obstructed vessels, forcing them to open up. Home observed that 'young ladies' – presumably private patients – 'would never submit to this operation', prompting him to try it 'among the commonalty'. Between 1769 and 1778, he reported a series of six Infirmary cases and claimed only one dubious success.[128] Both electrification and arterial compression were scheduled during evenings and administered by surgical assistants. Not surprisingly, several Infirmary patients refused these procedures and promptly sought permission to leave the hospital. Other female patients under active treatment for menstrual complaints also requested their discharge. Those who endured the various treatments without success were given palliatives and told to wait for warmer weather so that nature could take care of their troubles. All treatment failures were blamed on the physiological inconsistencies of the female body. If nothing seemed to work, Edinburgh physicians fell back on the presumed Hippocratic link between sexual intercourse and normal menstrual function. Cullen spoke hopefully about the favourable effects attributed to 'the exercise of lawful venery'.[129] Brown emphatically recommended the 'gratification of love'. Sex was believed to provide just the right 'gentle stimulus' to all organs involved in generation. Another pleasurable activity designed to stimulate pelvic circulation and restart menstrual periods was dancing with men. It had the additional advantage of leading to possible marriage and sexual intercourse 'with propriety'.[130]

Compared with other ailments seen at the Edinburgh Infirmary, the so-called 'cure' rate for amenorrhoea was around twenty percent, appallingly lower than the average sixty percent for other conditions managed in the teaching ward. Another forty-one percent of the patients were discharged 'relieved' while a fifth left on their own accord, presumably with their ailments unchanged or worsened by the treatments. Such unfavourable statistics reflect the difficulties Infirmary practitioners encountered in the treatment of amenorrhoea. In their opinion, the institutional environment failed to provide two effective and natural forms of treatment: fresh air and gentle exercise.[131] Cullen frankly admitted to his students: 'I have no command by my remedies over the menstrual flux to which time and a proper season are necessary'.[132] In some women, a better hospital diet may have assisted in temporarily restarting the menses well after their discharge from the institution, creating the perception that hospitalisation could be useful for menstrual irregularities.

Although practitioners believed that 'few women are so inexperienced as not to know when their evacuations exceed the natural limits',[133] nurses were dispatched to verify excessive vaginal bleeding and report their findings to the attending professor before daily rounds. Additional complaints were usually manifestations of chronic blood loss such as debility and pale skin, weak pulse and faintness, difficult breathing, cold and swollen limbs.[134] Physicians noted that the few poor women who sought admission primarily for 'flooding' or menorrhagia blamed exposure to cold for their symptoms. But this causality failed to stop practitioners from finding other causes. Miscarriages were always a real possibility. In a curious twist of the often-expressed notion that the warmth of the kitchen was an ideal location for women because of their cold nature, Cullen presented the case of a cook maid. He explained to students that her excessive menstrual bleeding had been caused by pelvic congestion because she had been forced to stand over an open fire for long hours preparing meals.[135] Once in the hospital, women suffering from menorrhagia remained there on average for four weeks, subjected to a medical regimen that sought to correct the presumed systemic debility. This included complete bed rest, cold drinks, a full diet with meat and diluted wine, supplemented with tonic remedies such as Peruvian bark and iron preparations. At the same time, the women faced the traditional triad of bloodletting, purgatives and emetics. The swollen legs and ankles were repeatedly massaged with warm water and hot towels.[136] While the patients' general health seemed to improve, the menstrual complaints persisted, leading to low rates of cure (25%).

Leucorrhoea, a vaginal discharge popularly known in Britain as the 'whites' or 'female weakness', was considered an embarrassing and 'universal complaint' afflicting women of all ages. Leading practitioners conceived the idea that both menstruation and leucorrhoea had similar origins in the uterus and possibly supplemented each other. They labelled the condition *menorrrhagia alba* (white menorrhagia). In fact, in several instances, the 'whites' would alternate with bouts of menorrhagia. For others, the troublesome condition was interpreted as another alternative natural drainage for females prone to fluid imbalances. This discharge sometimes preceded normal or excessively heavy and prolonged menstrual periods, or followed abortions or pregnancies. Those concerned about their fertility seemed particularly troubled by its periodic appearance since medical opinion associated this flux with systemic debility and barrenness. The usual suspects – excessive sexual activity, masturbation, a sedentary lifestyle, lack of sleep and too much coffee and tea drinking – were similarly blamed for the appearance of the 'whites'. Under ordinary circumstances, this flow was rarely brought to the attention of physicians and would seldom have required hospitalisation unless more serious symptoms were associated with it. Similar 'unclean' discharges were noted from vaginal and cervical ulcerations, venereal disease, the cervix of a prolapsed uterus, as well as following the vaginal insertion of pessaries. Given the diversity of causes, physicians complained that *fluor albus* – the traditional Latin term – was difficult to classify.

According to Cullen, 'weakly women of lax solids who have had many children and long laboured under ill health' were believed to be prime candidates for this disease.[137] This notion of systemic debility from frequent sexual relations and childbearing was similar to the ideas held by leading man-midwives of the period. Based on Cullen's pathogenesis of lax and spastic fibres, medical and surgical authors insisted the condition reflected an excessive discharge of lymphatic fluid from feeble uterine blood vessels incapable of sustaining their normal tone.[138] The number of recorded leucorrhoea cases admitted to the Edinburgh Infirmary remained extremely small. Their median age was thirty-one. In addition to their vaginal discharge, all hospital patients complained of fatigue – one woman blamed her condition on constantly carrying a heavy child in her arms. Another was exhausted from spending sleepless nights nursing another sick person. Others complained of digestive distress and pelvic pain.

Hospital physicians were always suspicious when confronted with reports of vaginal discharge because their decision to forgo internal pelvic examinations exposed them to deceit.[139] Instead, they looked for external signs of weakness such as a wasting body, a pale countenance, 'languid eyes' and 'body lassitude'. Given Scotland's harsh winters, coldness remained a key explanation. 'In this climate we have ample proof how effectual this cause is in weakening the body', declared one author.[140] Other women were suspected of harbouring a venereal disease, especially if the symptoms had appeared soon after sexual contact and the discharge appeared to be yellowish in colour. 'I am not without doubt as to the accuracy of the account given', declared Duncan in one 1795 case, adding that 'we have more apprehensions of gonorrhoea.'[141] Physicians had trouble making a differential diagnosis, since both the colour and quantity of the discharge were nearly similar. Once again, ward nurses were enlisted to ascertain the veracity of the patients' accounts. To confirm the presence of gonorrhoea, some practitioners looked for symptoms of painful urinary voiding.[142]

Women suffering from leucorrhoea were also subjected to a stimulant regimen 'to restore the system to its usual vigour'. The treatment consisted of nourishing meals, tonics, massage and exercise. The usual combination of emetics and cathartics were used to remove harmful matter from the digestive system. 'Lime water' – a calcium oxide solution – was frequently administered because of its astringent and diuretic properties. Some women were subjected to four to five vaginal irrigations per day with a solution of potassium aluminium sulphate and zinc sulphate – the latter was considered a potent astringent and cleansing agent.[143] Others employed decoctions of tormentil root and English oak bark, a less expensive substitute for the Peruvian variety. In one instance, Home decided to recommend electric sparks since the patient complained of pelvic pain radiating into the thighs.[144] In cases of suspected gonorrhoea that exhibited perineal ulcerations, Gregory offered a course of mercury pills and ointment. The average hospital stay for leucorrhoea lasted twenty-one days. At discharge most of the patients were considered 'cured' by their physicians.

Finally, the Infirmary also admitted a small contingent of women burdened with other gynaecological conditions, including an impending miscarriage, inflammation of the uterus, and suspected ovarian tumours. Two examples for each of these ailments appeared in students' casebooks. The miscarriages occurred in two married women, one of them in her fourth month, the other in her seventh month of pregnancy. The latter had sustained a fall, injuring her abdomen and she delivered a dead pair of twins within a week, only to die of postpartum infection six days later. The notebooks remain silent about any consultation or assistance from man-midwives or their female counterparts in the hospital. An autopsy disclosed a large amount of fluid in the abdomen, thorax and pericardium.[145] Two cases, labelled *hysteritis* or inflammation of the uterus occurred in 20-year-olds and appeared to be mild. The patients were admitted complaining of lower abdominal and back pains. This vague disease was given a separate genus among Cullen's inflammatory conditions but still considered distinct from puerperal fever. However, most explanations concerning its causes posited an increased arterial congestion in the uterus following delivery.[146] One of the women was examined and found to have a swollen and painful cervix. They were treated with purgatives, warm water massage and cupping. Both seemed to have recovered within a week.[147] By contrast, the women discovered with ovarian tumours (*hydrops ovarii*) never improved. All medical measures employed to reduce their abdominal swelling proved futile. Even contemporary surgeons such as John Hunter who performed abdominal tapping to remove fluid considered them incurable. One of the patients was a 12-year-old girl who remained at the Infirmary for nearly six weeks. She died a day after being discharged and her body was brought back for dissection. The autopsy disclosed the presence of a dark bloody fluid in the abdomen together with an enormously enlarged right ovary weighing about twenty pounds that had pushed up the bowels towards the diaphragm and created strong adhesions to the liver.[148] Like all conditions afflicting women, clinical experience with this assortment of distinctively 'female troubles' at the Edinburgh Infirmary seemed to confirm the presumptive systemic fragility and vascular imbalance characteristic of female bodies.

Conclusion

After arriving in the Infirmary's teaching ward, Euphemia McKay repeated her story to the attending staff. She was thirsty. Her pulse rate was fifty-four and said to be of 'ordinary strength'. Her skin felt cool, the tongue appeared clean on inspection. Like many poor patients, she was probably vague about her 'reckoning' because regularity was seldom part of their experience. Placed in a difficult position, Infirmary physicians nevertheless bowed to popular demands for treatment. From the start, Gregory was quite aware of the difficulties in achieving a cure. 'Prognosis here is unfavourable', he admitted to his students, 'and in all cases of this disease we must trust more to time and nature than art.' His cautious activism consisted in successive rounds of diet, drugs and physical methods that seldom seemed to find their intended target. He first proceeded to order gum pills, considered an effective emmenagogue and antispasmodic compound designed to relieve the suspected spasms afflicting the uterine arteries. Warm fomentation of the lower extremities was meant to shift blood into the pelvis and legs in addition to stimulating Euphemia's entire body.

Two days later, the professor ordered a more potent stimulus to increase the tone of the arterial system: the application of electricity to the patient's lower abdomen. Gregory cautioned that the electricity 'be applied in such a manner as not to shock the delicacy of the tender females'. For him, electricity was 'the most valuable remedy [to] boast of in restoring the menses.' The sparks were not directly administered to the skin but through her flannel nightgown. Also soon after admission, Euphemia received some of the traditional remedies, including a tincture containing the roots of black hellebore – *helleborus niger* – a drastic and toxic cathartic. The idea was to stimulate the intestines, especially the rectum, in the hope of achieving a similar effect on the nearby uterus. Unfortunately, the compound had significant side effects that caused the patient to experience nausea, abdominal cramps and diarrhoea. The other customary compound was *rubia tinctorum*. For generations, women had been familiar with this remedy, employing it as part of their domestic healing practices. Gregory, however, unlike Home, admitted to his students that he 'never observed any good effects from it', suggesting that his decision to prescribe this draught was solely made to please the patient for lack of more effective alternatives.

Towards the end of the first week in the hospital, this 'drenching' with medicines continued unabated. Euphemia received another potent emmenagogue to improve the vigour of her body systems: sabine. The subsequent addition of ipecac powders and aloes in wine to relieve internal bodily obstructions exacerbated her nausea and prolonged the diarrhoea, prompting the administration of opium pills to control them. A new round of mercury pills with opium came next, expected to stimulate the uterus directly responsible for the menstrual obstruction. Warm enemas containing laudanum were intended to achieve this objective through the rectum's proximity to the uterus and its vascular connections. For Gregory, exercise was one of the best remedies when the stubborn menses remained absent. In lieu of horseback riding, hospital patients were asked to perform housekeeping chores and feed bedridden patients. At the Infirmary, Euphemia may also have used a pair of dumbbells or been placed in a 'swing chair' or on a wooden rocking horse. Still, nothing seemed to help.

By early December, such therapeutic failures undoubtedly encouraged Gregory to try a more aggressive and extreme measure: arterial compression. He admitted that this method – known as 'a remedy which few will submit to' – was fraught with dangers such as impaired leg circulation and abdominal pain.[149] Nevertheless, with Euphemia's apparent consent, the procedure was carried out for three consecutive evenings without any benefit. In the end, Gregory lost all hope for achieving a cure. 'Our time has been this winter so much engaged in a variety of business', explained a medical student, 'that we have not been able to treat our case with all that scrupulous exactness and attention that we could have wished or which it deserves'.[150] After remaining for thirty-one days at the Edinburgh Infirmary, Euphemia McKay was allowed to leave. The holidays were approaching. Before departing from the teaching ward on 11 December 1785, she was provided with twelve additional doses of the magical madder root extract. Her discharge from the hospital was officially proclaimed 'improper'. This label, applied to many teaching cases, sought to indicate that the case had been found unsuitable for further hospital treatment. The Infirmary's General Register of Patients, however, recorded the patient as leaving 'relieved', a more favourable category designed to improve the hospital official statistics. Perhaps Euphemia shared with other contemporary hospital patients the notion that 'had cure been possible, [the physician] must have performed it'.[151]

In spite of obvious therapeutic failures, the formulations and actions of contemporary elite physicians and their students in support of the ongoing medicalisation of gynaecology cannot be ignored. As males, they had no personal experience on which to rely when judging the behaviours of female bodies in health and disease. Clearly impotent in most cases to reverse disorders they could neither accurately diagnose nor understand, these physicians nevertheless attempted to fulfil their roles as healers.[152] As such they provided legitimacy and reassurance to women and their complaints. Moreover, continuous clinical exposure forced practitioners to seek a further understanding of differences between the sexes. During the eighteenth century, menstruation and its physiopathology acquired new importance in the explanation and management of all diseases afflicting women. Ascertaining a female's menstrual status was now perceived to be the key to a better understanding of other gendered complaints. In fact, most disorders were defined in relation to this periodic phenomenon. By aligning menstrual regularity with new theories of nervous excitability and disease classification, physicians created a basic body of explanatory schemes that not only lent greater credibility to women's suffering but also enhanced professional medical authority. More importantly, such constructions accentuated the deleterious nature of menses as phenomena that often made women sick and more vulnerable to disease. This prejudicial coding of menstruation caused widespread apprehension among women and eventually led to formulations such as 'the curse'.[153] Poor women, in turn, further contributed to these negative judgements because of their genuinely compromised physical status as well as the fragmentary and distorted presentation of their complaints designed to impress and manipulate hospital managers and physicians.

Edinburgh's clinical experiences failed to produce substantial revisions in medical theory. A façade of lax fibres and nerves could not hide the fact that gynaecology dealt mostly with disturbed bodily fluids. Females were still soft and spongy creatures, slaves to the ebbs and flows of menstrual blood that was endowed with mysterious powers. Hospital cases tended to confirm and solidify such ancient preconceptions. Exposure to the ills of lower-class women only reinforced traditional stereotypes of female feebleness, irritability and emotionality. Based on social status, both the excesses of high and low living were said to affect women's sexual functioning. In the process, affluent females were denounced for their high living while their less fortunate sisters were blamed for being malnourished and working too hard. On balance, these medical formulations – widely published in texts and popular manuals – seemed arbitrary and contradictory. Yet, male physicians who sought to support morality and social values consonant with contemporary perceptions of a healthy life-style articulated them (Chapter 4).

In a telling comment that illustrates the Enlightenment's idea of sex as a natural and healthy activity, Gregory expressed his disappointment about the outcome of Euphemia's case. Summarising her case before the students, he explained that 'after exhausting my artillery, I sent her out to her husband who I thought might do more for her than I could.'[154] This traditional therapeutic indication exemplified the ambiguities and contradictions that still surrounded the explanation and institutional management of female disorders in Edinburgh. It also reflected the deep sense of frustration of professionals who realised that while contemporary medical dogma continued to demand menstrual regularity as an essential factor in women's health, their deserving poor patients' irregularities and complaints appeared intractable. In the end, eighteenth-century 'medical' gynaecology as practised in Edinburgh remained a poorly defined and understood field of medicine, a mirror of equivocal scientific knowledge, social barriers and traditional cultural biases.

Notes

1. J. Friend, *Emmenologia*, trans. from Latin by T. Dale (London: T. Cox, 1729), 1.
2. The initial clinical details were presented by a medical student, John Craven, to the Royal Medical Society of Edinburgh. See *Dissertations Read to the Royal Medical Society, Edinburgh (Diss. RMS)*, 95 vols (Edinburgh: 1751–1833), MSS Collection, Edinburgh University Library, Vol. 20 (1786–7), 263–77. For the voice of contemporary female patients, see B. Duden, *The Woman Beneath the Skin: A Doctor's Patients in Eighteenth–Century Germany*, trans. T. Dunlop (Cambridge: Harvard University Press, 1991).
3. Case of Euphemia McKay, in James Gregory, Clinical Cases of Dr Gregory in the Royal Infirmary of Edinburgh taken by Nathan Thomas (Edinburgh: 1785–6), MSS Collection, Edinburgh University Library.

4. For details, R. Porter, 'History of the Body', in P. Burke (ed.), *New Perspectives on Historical Writing* (Cambridge: Polity Press, 1991), 206–32.
5. H. Smith, 'Gynecology and Ideology in Seventeenth-Century England', in B.A. Carroll (ed.), *Liberating Women's History* (Urbana: University of Illinois Press, 1976), 97–114; A. Eccles, *Obstetrics and Gynecology in Tudor and Stuart England* (Kent: Kent State University Press, 1982).
6. The best account is A.M. Lord, '"To Relieve Distressed Women:" Teaching and Establishing the Scientific Art of Man-Midwifery or Gynecology in Edinburgh and London, 1720-1805', PhD dissertation, University of Wisconsin–Madison, 1995; see also M.E. Fissell, 'Gender and Generation: Representing Reproduction in Early Modern England', *Gender and History,* 7 (1995), 433–56. For a broad overview of contemporary medical publications, see J.V. Ricci, 'Gynaecology During the Eighteenth Century', in *The Genealogy of Gynaecology* (Philadelphia: Blakiston, 1950), 338–469.
7. See C. Smith-Rosenberg and C.E. Rosenberg, 'The Female Animal: Medical and Biological Views of Woman and Her Role in Nineteenth-Century America', *Journal of American History,* 60 (1973), 332–56; V. Bullough and M. Voght, 'Women, Menstruation and Nineteenth-Century Medicine', *Bulletin of the History of Medicine,* 47 (1973), 66–82.
8. A complete study of this invaluable source of clinical information can be found in G.B. Risse, *Hospital Life in Enlightenment Scotland: Care and Teaching at the Royal Infirmary of Edinburgh* (New York: Cambridge University Press, 1986).
9. For details, L. Jordanova, *Sexual Visions: Images of Gender in Science and Medicine Between the Eighteenth and Twentieth Centuries* (New York: Harvester Wheatsheaf, 1989); and E. Fox Keller, *Reflections on Gender and Science* (New Haven: Yale University Press, 1985).
10. I am grateful to Alexandra Lord for this insight. See Lord, *op. cit.* (note 6), 263.
11. A. Rousselle, 'Images Médicales du Corps: Observation Feminine et Ideologie Masculine: Le Corps de la Femme d'Après les Médecins Grecs', *Annales: Économies, Sociétés, Civilisations,* 35 (1980), 1098–115.
12. A.E. Hanson, 'Continuity and Change: Three Case Studies of Hippocratic Gynecological Therapy and Theory', in S.B. Pomeroy (ed.), *Women's History and Ancient History* (Chapel Hill: University of North Carolina Press, 1991), 73–110.
13. Details in H. King, *Hippocrates' Woman: Reading the Female Body in Ancient Greece* (London: Routledge, 1998); and L. Dean-Jones, *Women's Bodies in Classical Greek Science* (Oxford: Clarendon Press, 1994).
14. See R. Frisch, 'Demographic Implications of the Biological Determinants of Female Fecundity', *Social Biology,* 22 (1975), 17–22.

15. This information is based on a recent paper by Helen King, 'The Masculine Birth of Gynaecology' delivered at the 76th annual meeting of the American Association for the History of Medicine in Boston, 1–4 May 2003.
16. I. McLean, *The Renaissance Notion of Woman* (Cambridge: Cambridge University Press, 1980), 28–46.
17. R. Porter and L. Hall, *The Facts of Life: The Creation of Sexual Knowledge in Britain, 1650-1950* (New Haven: Yale University Press, 1995), 33–64. See also P.G. Bounce (ed.), *Sexuality in Eighteenth-Century Britain* (Manchester: Manchester University Press, 1982).
18. For details, N. Tuana, 'In Man's Control', in *The Less Noble Sex: Scientific, Religious, and Philosophical Conceptions of Woman's Nature* (Bloomington: Indiana University Press, 1993), 155–67.
19. For a discussion of gender differences, T. Laqueur, *Making Sex: Body and Gender From the Greeks to Freud* (Cambridge: Harvard University Press, 1990).
20. P.H. Nidditch (ed.), J. Locke, *An Essay Concerning Human Understanding*, (1690) (Oxford: Clarendon Press, 1975). For details, P. Foot, 'Locke, Hume and Modern Moral Theory: A Legacy of Seventeenth- and Eighteenth-Century Philosophies of Mind', in G.S. Rousseau (ed.), *The Languages of Psyche: Mind and Body in Enlightenment Thought* (Berkeley: University of California Press, 1990), 81–104.
21. An English translation of Newton's *Opticks* appeared in 1717.
22. W. Bynum, 'Cullen and the Nervous System', in A. Doig *et al.* (eds), *William Cullen and the Eighteenth-Century Medical World* (Edinburgh: Edinburgh University Press, 1993), 152–62.
23. A useful synthesis is presented in G.J. Barker-Benfield, *The Culture of Sensibility: Sex and Society in Eighteenth-Century Britain* (Chicago: University of Chicago Press, 1992), 1–36.
24. G.B. Risse, 'Medicine in the Age of Enlightenment', in A. Wear (ed.), *Medicine in Society: Historical Essays* (Cambridge: Cambridge University Press, 1992), 155–67.
25. Friend, *op. cit.* (note 1), 3.
26. John Gregory, *A Father's Legacy to His Daughters* (Boston: J. B. Dow, 1834), 32. This work was first published in 1774 by Gregory's son James shortly after the author's death.
27. J. Leake, *Medical Instructions Towards the Prevention and Cure of Chronic Diseases Peculiar to Women,* 5th edn (London: R. Baldwin, 1785), 246–7.
28. Consult O. Moscucci, 'Introduction', in *The Science of Woman: Gynaecology and Gender in England, 1800–1929* (Cambridge: Cambridge University Press, 1990), 5. For medical models of womanhood see also P. Hoffman, *La Femme dans la Pensée des Lumières* (Paris: Ophrys, 1977), 42–81.

29. Such professional concerns were evident in the contemporary literature on the subject, including a six-volume treatise written by the French physician Jean Astruc (1684–1766) published between 1761 and 1765 and translated into English by 1767. Astruc's largely speculative work was representative of what could be characterised as a text of 'medical gynaecology' containing a series of explanations of female physiology that upheld traditional biases.
30. W. Buchan, *Domestic Medicine*, rev. (New York: R. Scott, 1812), 77.
31. W. Cullen, Correspondence, XXI vols (Edinburgh, 1755–90). MSS Collection, Royal College of Physicians, Edinburgh, Vol. XV.
32. Buchan, *op. cit.* (note 30), 78–7.
33 . Anonymous, *The Ladies Dispensatory: Every Woman Her Own Physician*, 2nd (London: J. Hodges, 1740), preface, III.
34. The almost complete reliance on clinical histories for arriving at a diagnosis was pointed out by S.J. Reiser, *Medicine and the Reign of Technology* (New York: Cambridge University Press, 1978); 1–22; see also G.B. Risse, 'A Shift in Medical Epistemology: Clinical Diagnosis, 1770–1828', in Y. Kawakita (ed.), *History of Diagnostics, Proceedings, 9th International Symposium on the Comparative History of Medicine – East and West* (Osaka: Tanaguchi Foundation, 1987), 115–47.
35. P. Mac Flogg'em (pseud.), *Aesculapian Secrets Revealed* (London: C. Chapple, 1813), 141.
36. W. Cullen, *Nosology, Or a Systematic Arrangement of Diseases* (Edinburgh: 1800), 16–17.
37. W. Hunter, *Two Introductory Lectures* (London, 1784), 35; see R. Porter,. 'William Hunter: A Surgeon and A Gentleman', in W.F. Bynum and R. Porter (eds), *William Hunter and the Eighteenth-Century World* (Cambridge: Cambridge University Press, 1985), 7–34.
38. R. Porter, 'A Touch of Danger: The Man-Midwife as Sexual Predator', in G.S. Rousseau and R. Porter (eds), *Sexual Underworlds of the Enlightenment* (Manchester: Manchester University Press, 1988), 206–32.
39 . For a recent overview of the anthropological literature on the subject see T. Buckley and A. Gottlieb, 'A Critical Appraisal of Theories of Menstrual Symbolism', in T. Buckley and A. Gottlieb (eds), *Blood Magic: The Anthropology of Menstruation* (Berkeley: University of California Press, 1988), 3–50.
40. Galen wrote that 'a woman who is well cleansed is not seized with gouty or arthritic or pleuritic or peripneumonic diseases and neither epilepsy nor apoplexy nor suspension of breathing nor loss of speech occur at any time if she is properly cleansed'. See Galen, 'On Venesection Against Erasistratus', in *Galen On Bloodletting*, trans. P. Brain (Cambridge: Cambridge University Press, 1986), 26.

41. D. Jacquart and C. Thomasset, 'Impure Matter', in *Sexuality and Medicine in the Middle Ages*, trans. M. Adamson (Princeton: Princeton University Press, 1988), 71–8; see also S.J. Cohen, 'Menstruants and the Sacred in Judaism and Christianity', in S.B. Pomeroy (ed.), *Women's History and Ancient History* (Chapel Hill: University of North Carolina Press, 1991), 273–99.
42. M. Stolberg, '"A Woman's Hell"? Medical Perceptions of Menopause in Pre-Industrial Europe', *Bulletin of the History of Medicine*, 73 (1999), 404–28.
43. G. Pomata, 'Menstruating Men: Similarity and Difference of the Sexes in Early Modern Medicine', in V. Finucci and K. Brownlee (eds), *Generation and Degeneration: Tropes of Reproduction in Literature and History from Antiquity to Early Modern Europe* (Durham: Duke University Press, 2001), 109–52.
44. P. Crawford, 'Attitudes to Menstruation in Seventeenth-Century England', *Past & Present*, 91 (1981), 47–73.
45. R. Martensen, 'The Transformation of Eve: Women's Bodies, Medicine and Culture in Early Modern England', in R. Porter and M.Teich (eds.), *Sexual Knowledge, Sexual Science: The History of Attitudes To Sexuality* (Cambridge: Cambridge University Press, 1994), 107–33; see also R.G. Frank, 'Viewing the Body: Reframing Man and Disease in Commonwealth and Restoration England', in W.G. Marshall (ed.), *The Restoration Mind* (Newark: University of Delaware Press, 1997), 65–110; and R. Martensen, *The Brain Takes Shape: An Early History* (New York: Oxford University Press, 2004).
46. H. Manning, *A Treatise on Female Diseases* (London: R. Baldwin, 1771), 45–60.
47. More details in E. van de Walle, 'Flowers and Fruits: Two Thousand Years of Menstrual Regulation', *Journal of Interdisciplinary History*, 28 (1997), 183–203.
48. J. Ball, *The Female Physician or Every Woman Her Own Doctress* (London: L. Davis, 1770), 17.
49. J. Carver, 'What are the Most Probable Causes of Menstruation in the Human Species?', *Diss. RMS*, Vol. 14 (1782–3), 299–317; see also the medical dissertation by D. Thomson, *De Menstruis* (Edinburgh: Donaldson & Reid, 1765).
50. W. Cullen, *First Lines of the Practice of Physic*, new, IV vols (Edinburgh: C. Elliot, 1786), Vol. III, 32; see also W. Cullen, 'Clinical Lectures' (Edinburgh: 1772–3), MSS Collection, Royal College of Physicians, Edinburgh, 514.
51. A. Hamilton, *A Treatise for the Management of Female Complaints and of Children in Early Infancy* (Edinburgh, 1792), 130–1.
52. Buchan, *op. cit.* (note 30), 308; Leake, *op. cit* (note 28), 50. This fact is confirmed in Edinburgh's student casebooks. Moreover, a check of hospital

cases places the average age for menarche at 15.5, the youngest patient being 14, the oldest 19 years old.

53. Cullen, *First Lines, op. cit.* (note 50), Vol. III, 37; W. Nisbet, *The Clinical Guide* (London: J. Johnson, 1800), 5–10.
54. J. Astruc, *A Treatise on all the Diseases Incident to Women* (London: M. Cooper, 1743), 17.
55. John Ball, author of a self-help manual, observed that 'dainty and luxurious women who feed high and live sedentary lives have the first appearance of these [menses] earlier than working people'. See Ball, *op. cit.* (note 48), 13. These judgements tend to be supported by new findings regarding the linkage between critical amounts of fat tissue and the onset of menstrual cycles. See R.E. Frisch, 'Population, Food Intake and Fertility', *Science,* 199 (1978), 22–30.
56. Cullen, *First Lines, op. cit.* (note 50), Vol. III, 34.
57. W. Cullen, Clinical Lectures Delivered for John Gregory, February–April 1772 (Edinburgh, 1772), MSS Collection, Royal College of Physicians, Edinburgh, 2.
58. Anonymous, *The Edinburgh Practice of Physic, Surgery, and Midwifery,* new, 5 vols (London: G. Kearsley, 1803), Vol. II, 576. If the young woman had additional symptoms of lassitude, back pains, palpitations, difficult breathing, dyspepsia, swelling of the feet and, above all, a characteristic pale, greenish complexion, a diagnosis of chlorosis or 'green sickness' was in order. For an overview and attempts to explain the disorder in modern times see R.P. Hudson, 'The Biography of Disease: Lessons from Chlorosis', *Bulletin of the History of Medicine,* 51 (1977), 448–63.
59. Friend, *op. cit.* (note 1), 108–9.
60. Cullen, *First Lines, op. cit.* (note 50), Vol. III, 42; see also the case of Mary Gunn, in James Gregory, Clinical Notes and Lectures, Edinburgh 1779–80, MSS Collection, Royal College of Physicians, Edinburgh.
61. *Ibid.*, Vol. III, 33–4.
62. *Ibid.*, Vol. III, 32; Cullen, Clinical Lectures, *op. cit.* (note 50), 514.
63. Cullen, *First Lines, op. cit.* (note 50), Vol. III, 32–3; Nisbet, *op. cit.* (note 53), 2–5.
64. Cullen, *First Lines, op. cit.* (note 50), Vol. III, 11–15. Among published doctoral dissertations on this condition are D. Daly, *De Menorrhagia in Non Gravidas* (Edinburgh: Balfour & Smellie, 1774); and A. Sayers, *De Menorrhagia* (Edinburgh: Balfour & Smellie, 1782).
65. J. Brown, *The Elements of Medicine,* new rev. edn by T. Beddoes, II vols (London: J. Johnson, 1795), Vol. II, 200.
66. Leake, *op. cit.* (note 27), 82–4; Manning, *op. cit.* (note 46), 130.

67. As James Gregory remarked, 'women of quality have more of the menstrual flux than country women, hence the bareness of such'. See the case of Mary Gunn, in Gregory, *op. cit.* (note 60).
68. A. Lord, 'The Great Arcana of the Deity': Menstruation and Menstrual Disorders in Eighteenth-Century British Medical Thought, *Bulletin of the History of Medicine*, 73 (1999), 38–63.
69. Buchan, *op. cit.* (note 30), 309.
70. The Edinburgh student notebooks contain twenty-two cases in which the diagnosis of amenorrhoea was linked with so-called pectoral complaints. Most of them suffered from phthisis. Many of the women admitted with a diagnosis of 'dropsy' and 'anasarca' were also said to suffer 'suppressed menses'.
71. The letter was dated 13 July 1779; see Cullen, *op. cit.* (note 31), Vol. XII.
72. Ball, *op. cit.* (note 48), 15.
73. Case of Christy McDonald, in A. Duncan Sr, Clinical Reports and Commentaries, February to April 1795, presented by A. Blackhall Morison (Edinburgh: 1795), MSS Collection, Royal College of Physicians, Edinburgh.
74. Buchan, *op. cit.* (note 30), 310, and Leake, *op. cit.* (note 27), 65.
75. J. Fothergill, 'On the Management Proper at the Cessation of the Menses', reprinted in F. Churchill (ed.), *Essays on the Puerperal Fever and Other Diseases Peculiar to Women* (Philadelphia: Lea and Branchard, 1850), 425. See G.S. Plaut, *Dr. John Fothergill and Eighteenth-Century Medicine* (London: Royal Society of Medicine, 1993).
76. Letter dated 22 January 1777 in Cullen, *op. cit.* (note 31), Vol. VIII.
77. *Ibid.*, Vol. XIII.
78. A. Hamilton, *The Family Female Physician* (Worcester, Mass., 1793), 99.
79. Leake, *op. cit.* (note 27), 94.
80. *Ibid.*, 89; see also Ball, *op. cit.* (note 48), 233. Cullen tried to be reassuring: 'this change in constitution is seldom made without some disorder but it is not always necessary to proceed to remedies for what nature and time will better set to rights', he wrote in the late 1770s. Cullen, *op. cit.* (note 31), Vol. XII.
81. Much of this information on sexual activity was obtained from offences reported to the Kirk sessions and available in church archives. See L. Leneman and R. Mitchison, *Sin in the City: Sexuality and Social Control in Urban Scotland, 1660–1780* (Edinburgh: Scottish Social Press, 1998), 50–68.
82. Details in R. Mitchison, *Life in Scotland* (London: Batsford, 1978).
83. C. Hoolihan, 'Thomas Young, M.D., 1726–83, and Obstetrical Education', *Journal of the History of Medicine*, 40 (1985), 327–45.

84. See A. Wilson, 'William Hunter and the Varieties of Man-Midwife', in Bynum and Porter, *op. cit.* (note 37), 343–69; see also by this author *The Making of Man-Midwifery: Childbirth in England, 1660–1770* (Cambridge: Harvard University Press, 1995).
85. John Gregory, *Lectures on the Duties and Qualifications of a Physician* (Edinburgh, 1772), 49–50.
86. James Gregory, *Memorial to the Managers of the Royal Infirmary* (Edinburgh: Murray and Cochrane, 1800), 185–6.
87. The controversy has been examined by Michael Barfoot in an unpublished paper 'Pedagogy, Practice and Politics: The Gregory–Bell Dispute and the Nature of Early Nineteenth-Century Edinburgh Medicine'.
88. A. Hamilton, *Outlines of the Theory and Practice of Midwifery* (Edinburgh:. 1784), IV.
89. James Gregory, *Answer to Dr. James Hamilton Jr* (Edinburgh, 1793).
90. A. Hamilton, *A Treatise for the Management of Female Complaints and of Children in Early Infancy* (Edinburgh: P. Hill, 1792), preface.
91. J. Aikin, *Thoughts on Hospitals* (London: J. Johnson, 1771), 57.
92. G.B. Risse, '"Doctor William Cullen, Physician, Edinburgh": A Consultation Practice in the Eighteenth Century', *Bulletin of the History of Medicine,* 48 (1974), 338–51.
93. I. Loudon, *Medical Care and the General Practitioner, 1750–1850* (Oxford: Clarendon Press, 1986).
94. Aikin, *op. cit.* (note 91), 57.
95. See, for example, the selected admissions list from the Newcastle and Manchester Infirmaries in 1750 published by J. Woodward in his book *To Do the Sick No Harm, A Study of the British Voluntary Hospital System to 1875* (London: Routledge and Kegan Paul, 1974), 160–2.
96. Mac Flogg'em, *op. cit.* (note 36), 76.
97. Cullen, Clinical Lectures, *op. cit.* (note 50), 160.
98. Leake, *op. cit.* (note 27), 141.
99. Buchan, *op. cit.* (note 30), 310; and Leake, *op. cit.* (note 27), 52–3.
100. Case of Margaret Emery, in James Gregory, Clinical Reports 1 November 1795 – 1 February 1796 (Edinburgh, 1795–6), MSS Collection, Edinburgh University.
101. Cullen, Clinical Lectures, *op. cit.* (note 50), 8.
102. Buchan, *op. cit.* (note 30), 311. See also the case of Euphemia Hutchinson, in T.C. Hope, Clinical Casebook (Edinburgh 1876–97). MSS Collection, Royal College of Physicians, Edinburgh.
103. Some of these circumstances are described in an anonymous publication: *Remarks on the Situation of the Poor in the Metropolis* (London: R. Noble, 1801).

104. For France, L. Wilson, *Women and Medicine in the French Enlightenment* (Baltimore: Johns Hopkins University Press, 1993), 166.
105. This becomes clear from a careful perusal of the casebooks. A further sign of this institutional policy was a 1758 ban on surgery in the Infirmary's 'public theatre' if the 'privy parts of women are exposed'. See Royal Infirmary of Edinburgh, Minutes of Managers, MSS Collection, Edinburgh University Library, Vol. III, 6 February 1749–29 December 1760, 315.
106. M. Pelling, 'Compromised by Gender: The Role of the Male Medical Practitioner in Early Modern England', in H. Marland and M. Pelling (eds), *The Task of Healing: Medicine, Religion and Gender in England and the Netherlands, 1450–1800* (Rotterdam: Erasmus Publications, 1996), 107–12. On bedside rituals, R.L. Engle and B.J. Davis, 'Medical Diagnosis: Present, Past and Future', *Annals of Internal Medicine,* 112 (1963), 512–43.
107. M.E. Fissell, 'Innocent and Honorable Bribes: Medical Manners in Eighteenth-Century Britain', in R. Baker, D. Porter and R. Porter (eds), *The Codification of Medical Morality* (Dordrecht: Kluwer, 1993), 19–45.
108. If new patients were currently menstruating – the expression was 'had the catamenia upon her' that fact was recorded in Latin as *catamenia adsunt* (menses present). See, for example, the case of Peggy McKenzie, in James Gregory, Clinical Cases (Edinburgh, 1787–8), MSS Collection, National Library of Medicine, Bethesda, Maryland, USA.
109. 'They are so strongly persuaded that physicians running counter to any strong prejudice do it at their peril', explained Cullen to the students. Cullen complained that 'they [women] are persuaded that blooding is practised with hazard during the flow of menses'. See Cullen, Clinical Lectures, *op. cit.* (note 50), 161–2.
110. *Ibid.*, 157.
111. Case of Peggy McKenzie, in Gregory, *op. cit.* (note 108).
112. There were no fatalities among the gynaecological cases included in this study. In one instance, a patient died at home one day after discharge from the hospital and her body was brought back for an autopsy, but the results were not recorded.
113. F. Home, *Clinical Experiments, Histories, and Dissections*, 3rd edn (London: J. Murray, 1783), 409–10. Several Edinburgh students wrote their dissertations on this condition. See, for example, R. Harding, *De Amenorrhoea* (Edinburgh: Balfour and Smellie, 1783); and B. Coyne, *De Amenorrhoea* (Edinburgh: Stewart, 1803).
114. Manning, *op. cit.* (note 46), 73.
115. A. Duncan, Sr, *Observations on Medical Jurisprudence*, Delivered in Lectures in the University of Edinburgh, taken in notes by David Pollock, II vols. (Edinburgh, 1797–8), Vol. I, 152–3.

116. James Gregory, 'Hysteria', a lecture delivered to medical students in the academic year 1788–9, MSS Collection, National Library of Medicine, Bethesda, Maryland, USA, 104.
117. J. Craven, 'Amenorrhoea', *Diss. RMS*, Vol. 20 (1786–7), 266.
118. Cullen, Clinical Lectures, *op. cit.* (note 50), 157–73.
119. Cullen, *op. cit.* (note 57), 5.
120. G.B. Risse, 'The Road to Twentieth-Century Therapeutics: Shifting Perspectives and Approaches', in G.J. Higby and E.C. Stroud (eds), *The Inside Story of Medicines: A Symposium* (Madison: American Institute for the History of Pharmacy, 1997), 51–73.
121. Cullen, *op. cit.* (note 57), 6.
122. Cullen, *First Lines, op. cit.* (note 50), vol III, 40–8; see also Brown, *op. cit.* (note 65), Vol. II, 210; and Leake, *op. cit.* (note 27), 58–9.
123. Home, *op. cit.* (note 113), 419–37.
124. Cullen, *op. cit.* (note 57), 12–13.
125. For similar treatments across the Atlantic see S.S. Klepp, 'Colds, Worms, and Hysteria: Menstrual Regulation in Eighteenth-Century America', in E. Van de Walle and E. P. Renne (eds), *Regulating Menstruation: Beliefs, Practices, Interpretations* (Chicago: University of Chicago Press, 2001), 22–38.
126. Home, *op. cit.* (note 113), 417–9.
127. Case of Elizabeth Innes, in F. Home, *Clinical Cases*, copied by J.T. Shaaf (Edinburgh, 1788–9), MSS Collection, National Library of Medicine, Bethesda, Maryland.
128. Home, *op. cit.* (note 113), 411–6.
129. Cullen, *First Lines, op. cit.* (note 50), Vol. III, 41; and Ball, *op. cit.* (note 48), 15.
130. Brown, *op. cit.* (note 65), Vol. II, 210.
131. See explanations given by Duncan Sr. in the case of his patient Betty Jameson, in Duncan Sr, *op. cit.* (note 73).
132. Cullen, Clinical Lectures, *op. cit.* (note 50), 614.
133. Manning, *op. cit.* (note 46), 116.
134. Anon., *op. cit.* (note 58), Vol. I, 338.
135. Cullen, Clinical Lectures, *op. cit.* (note 50), 625.
136. Cullen, *First Lines, op. cit.* (note 50), Vol. III, 17–19.
137. Anon., *op. cit.* (note 58), Vol. I, 344–5.
138. Cullen, *First Lines, op. cit.* (note 50), Vol. III, 24–30, and Leake, *op. cit.* (note 27), 98–107.
139. 'The reality of this [complaint] depended on the veracity of the patient and the nurse's account'. See case of Sarah Forbes, in Duncan Sr, *op, cit.* (note 73).
140. J. Lane, 'Leucorrhoea', *Diss. RMS*, Vol. 20 (1786–7), 229.

141. Case of Isabel Morrison, in Duncan Sr, *op. cit.* (note 73).
142. Late in the century, both gonorrhoea and syphilis were finally declared to be separate diseases. See B. Bell, *A Treatise on Gonorrhoea Virulenta and Lues Venerea,* 2 vols (Edinburgh, 1793).
143. Cullen, *First Lines, op. cit.* (note 50), Vol. III, 26; see also the cases of Sarah Forbes and Isabel Morrison in Duncan Sr, *op. cit.* (note 73).
144. Case of Christian Steel, in F. Home, Cases of Patients in the Royal Infirmary Under the Care of Francis Home, MD (Edinburgh, 1780–1), MSS Collection, Royal College of Physicians, Edinburgh.
145. Case of Betty Grant, in James Gregory, Clinical Cases (Edinburgh, 1787), MSS Collection, National Library of Medicine, Bethesda, Maryland, USA.
146. Anon., *op. cit.* (note 58), Vol. I, 446–9.
147. Case of Margaret McBean, in Home, *op. cit.* (note 127); and Marion Dickson, in F. Home, *Clinical Cases from the Royal Infirmary and Reports, by Robert Dunlop* (Edinburgh, 1786–7), MSS Collection, Edinburgh Room, Edinburgh City Library.
148. Case of Ann Dick, in James Gregory, Clinical Lectures and Cases, copied by John T. Shaaf (Edinburgh, 1789), MSS Collection, National Library of Medicine, Bethesda, Maryland, USA.
149. Case of Euphemia McKay, in Gregory, *op. cit.* (note 3).
150. Craven, *op. cit.* (note 2), 277.
151. J. Wilde, *The Hospital: A Poem in Three Books Written in the Devon and Exeter Hospital, 1809* (Norwich: Stevenson, Matchett and Stevenson, 1810), 56.
152. See quotations from John Gregory's ethical stance in G.B. Risse, 'Patients and their Healers: Historical Studies in Health Care', in N.K. Bell (ed.), *Who Decides? Conflicts of Rights in Health Care* (Clifton: Humana Press, 1982), 36–8.
153. For a useful overview, J. Delaney, M.J. Lupton and E. Toth, *The Curse: A Cultural History of Menstruation,* rev. edn (Chicago: University of Illinois Press, 1988); and articles in A.J. Dan and L.L. Lewis (eds), *Menstrual Health in Women's Lives* (Urbana: University of Illinois Press, 1992).
154. Case of Euphemia McKay, in Gregory, *op. cit.* (note 3).

9

Mind–Body Enigma:
Hysteria and Hypochondriasis at the Edinburgh Infirmary

During the eighteenth century, hysteria and hypochondriasis were considered fashionable 'neuroses' caused by an affluent, civilised life-style. In a most unique way, both disorders entwined biological and mental, environmental, social and cultural aspects, creating representations of considerable medical complexity and uncertainty. This essay examines a paradoxical transfer of these traditional nosological labels to a new environment: the voluntary hospital. As observed at the Edinburgh Infirmary, physicians attempted to contextualise both diseases 'from below', branding famished women as hysterics while lethargic men became hypochondriacs. Their institutional progress and management expose the equivocal effects of hospitalisation and contingent nature of medical classifications.

Introduction

> Of all diseases incident to mankind, those of the nervous system are the most complicated and difficult to cure. A volume would not be sufficient to point out their various symptoms. They imitate almost every disease and are seldom alike in two different persons, or even in the same person at different times.
>
> William Buchan (1769)[1]

In the summer of 1781, John Hope (1725–86), physician-in-ordinary at the Edinburgh Infirmary for the past three years, accepted two young adults to the hospital's medical wards. At the time, Hope also held the professorship of botany at the University. Thanks to the survival of his patient journal from August to October of that year, we can reconstruct some of the details of his hospital activities. On 23 August, Angus Robertson, aged 27, asked to be admitted complaining of 'lowness of spirits', flatulence and insipid eructation. In spite of his vigorous physical appearance, this man related a history of unusual heart palpitations and constant oppression of his chest. The symptoms had started three weeks earlier and were similar to a previous bout nearly four years earlier; Hope's diagnosis: 'hypochondriasis'. A day later, 24 August, 18-year-old Ann Webster arrived with somewhat similar troubles. She complained of having had constant stomach pains, as well as episodes of anxiety and 'oppression of spirits' for the past two weeks, occurring mostly around noon and in the evening. Gurgling sounds in the lower abdomen and a sensation of 'balls rolling about', ascended towards the stomach and chest, producing a choking sensation in the throat. At that point, this young woman frequently experienced fits and fainting episodes lasting nearly twenty minutes. The digestive problems and fainting spells seemed to be linked to an abrupt interruption of her menses on the first day of her period. Hope labelled her case 'hysteria'.[2]

This essay focuses on the contours and treatment of conditions such as 'hysteria' and 'hypochondriasis' in an eighteenth-century hospital, the Royal Infirmary of Edinburgh. These fashionable diagnoses were usually bestowed upon affluent men and women. But the use of the same labels on the poor inmates of the charitable institution begs discussion. Hence, the investigation into these diagnoses first began in an effort to document and clarify the meaning of 'hysteria' and 'hysteric complaint'.[3] Hypochondriasis was later included because of its traditional association and symptomatic similarities with hysteria. Both conditions were believed to have originated in the abdomen below the rib cage or *hypo chondros* populated by organs such as the liver and spleen, uterus, bladder and intestines, and traditionally considered the seat of human vitality and emotions. Accounts of these ailments were also often class- and gender-biased and placed within the context of women's and men's health, leading to a variety of meanings throughout the course of history. Like other chapters, this study is based on rich archival sources: hospital registers, patient case histories, and student lecture notes.[4] While the texts present ambiguous medical interpretations of the patients' suffering, the case histories and lecture notes reveal the outlines of a more interactive relationship between ward physicians and their charges.

Languages of suffering: a genealogy of the 'vapours'.

As Roy Porter suggests, 'cultures, groups and individuals respond in different ways to life's pains and pressures'.[5] In doing so, they employ several idioms of suffering and sickness, including words, physical symptoms and emotional expressions. Much, of course, depends on disease conditions currently prevailing in any given society. In the past, rapid social and economic change, political turmoil and wars, migrations and urbanisation, natural disasters, as well as new technologies, created unique ecologies of disease responsible for epidemics and endemic, chronic afflictions (Chapter 5). Frustration and anxiety, resentment and fear, anger and sadness, all modify behaviour and affect the body. The distressed mind responds with somatic manifestations, conscious or unconsciously created, involving any or all organ systems. The reaction unleashes a great variety of symptoms, including pain, digestive disturbances, shortness of breath and heart palpitations. Because they suggest or simulate serious disorders, these representations trigger further concern and worry. Today, such behaviour and body dysfunction continue to be experienced and communicated within particular social frameworks, cultural contexts and languages of suffering.[6]

The attention on particular clusters of mental and physical distress eventually led to the identification and construction of numerous disease entities, among them two loosely defined sets of problems: 'hysterical' and 'hypochondriac' complaints. When bestowed on individuals, all disease labels had an important classificatory potential but their flexible character and arbitrariness also had nefarious consequences, entangling both sufferers and their healers into arbitrary sets of representation and relevance. In medicine, the assignment of particular names to certain afflictions was important in furnishing identity and *gravitas*, certainty and universality. Artificial pedigrees proved useful to physicians in making their much-awaited diagnostic pronouncements but changes in nomenclature have misled historians attempting to understand the successive metamorphoses and shifting meanings of particular terms to portray illness.[7] More than simply reflecting scientific medical choices, these constellations of physical and mental dysfunction should be observed through the lenses of contemporary culture and society.[8]

Often linked together, the status of 'hysteria' and 'hypochondriasis' as distinct human diseases has fluctuated throughout history and still continues to be debated today.[9] The term 'hysterical' denotes unbridled emotionality, while the description 'hypochrondriac' is reserved for one's obsessive preoccupation with health. Their very existence as specific entities with extensive and variable symptom complexes was often questioned. This led repeatedly to their identification as the great impersonators of other more serious ailments. Throughout history, these afflictions have been judged to be symbols of fashion and ridicule, emblems of refinement and frailty, signs of enhanced sensibility and lack of self-control, tools for empowerment as well as tokens of pride or submission. Created by physicians on the basis of popular beliefs, then subjected to multiple revisions and finally deconstructed, hysteria and hypochondriasis represent in some sense archetypal forms of bodily function and behaviour. Historical societies demanded causal explanations and measures designed to ameliorate or even cure troublesome physical and mental symptoms. Thus, both the public and medical profession were forced to create a rather speculative rationale that could interpret as well as validate the dysfunction.

In Classical Greece, some surviving Hippocratic texts described 'hysteric' episodes. They were typified as sensations of coldness, laboured breathing, suffocation, fainting and epileptic-like fits. When occurring in females, these symptoms were variously explained by the abdominal displacements of a dry and restless womb. In its search for moisture, the womb ascended from the lower abdomen towards the chest cage, hindering breathing and swallowing. As for the fits, they were said to be the result of an excess of black bile – already implicated in epileptic seizures. Later, in Roman times, the explanations shifted with an improved understanding of human anatomy. Galen gave new meaning to 'hysteric' complaints by blaming them on a fixed but plethoric womb filled with thick, poisonous blood and seed.[10] He also described another digestive symptom observed in both sexes. It was often identified as *morbus hypochondriacus* since its manifestations also centred primarily in the abdomen, presumably involving organs such as the liver and spleen. This illness featured left-sided pain in the loins, intestinal cramps and swelling accompanied by gastric bloating and heartburn. Within the prevailing humoralism, all symptoms resulted from a surplus of black bile obstructing abdominal organs, notably the spleen.[11] Within the classical schema, the spleen acted as 'a scavenger of nature'; a veritable filter preventing poorly cooked digestive humours from reaching the blood. Around 50AD according to Aretaeus, individuals who suffered from this condition also experienced some degree of lethargy and melancholia or mental depression.[12]

Female behaviour classified as 'hysterical' became infused with supernatural meaning during the rise of Christianity. The somatic displays were supposedly evidence of demonic possession. Fits and fainting spells fostered widespread concealment and deceit, permanently linking female conduct with potential representations of evil. Often portrayed as witches disguised as normal persons, 'hysterics' were persecuted and often burned at the stake.[13] Instead of following theological interpretations, seventeenth-century authors sought 'natural' explanations for hysteria. Cartesian mind–body dualism tilted the focus toward the body's structures and functions. Medical authors now employed iatrochemical concepts to explain the symptoms of both diseases.[14] In an effort to demystify hysteria, many physicians proposed that harmful 'vapours', created from menstrual obstructions and gastrointestinal fermentation, drifted through the body creating havoc when they reached the brain.[15] In 1667, Thomas Willis (1621–75) partially desexualised hysteria by claiming that it was actually a disease of nerves.[16] Willis' contemporary, Thomas Sydenham (1624–89) recognised symptomatic similarities in the construction of a male equivalent. For Sydenham, both hysteria and hypochondriasis were elite somatic and mental derangement, a result of heightened states of nerve-mediated sensibility created by contemporary 'civilised' life.[17]

Sydenham, who had repeatedly called for the establishment of 'natural histories' of disease, carefully mapped out the somatic features of hysterical and hypochondriac complaints. He found that both conditions shared a number of physical symptoms such as digestive complaints and – a pathognomonic sign – the periodic voiding of large amounts of clear, diluted urine. Sydenham pronounced hysteria the most common disease of his day with the brain and nerves its principal seat instead of the womb.[18] Sydenham based this assessment on his considerable clinical experience, which he gained by caring for mostly affluent private patients. He also found that the frequency of hysteria was 'no less remarkable than the multiformity of the shapes which it puts on. Few of the maladies of miserable mortality are not imitated by it.'[19] Sydenham warned practitioners that without 'skill and sagacity' they would often be deceived. In spite of the increasing focus on physical manifestations, the emotional roots of these disorders were not ignored. Robert Burton's (1577–1640) famous *Anatomy of Melancholy* (1621) had reinforced notions about the importance of the mind in health and disease by sympathetically portraying an array of mental states, including hysterical and hypochondriac 'melancholia'. Sydenham acknowledged that for patients suffering from hysteria and hypochondriasis, 'the mind sickens more than the body'. For him, both ailments resembled each other 'as one egg to another'. Hysterics were afflicted by 'commotions of the mind' including pain, anger, and 'incurable despair'. Hypochondriasis seemed similarly rooted in a 'dejection of spirits'. Anxiety and 'melancholy foreboding' dominated the miserable lives of its sufferers. In Sydenham's words, 'they are racked both in mind and body even as if life were a purgatory wherein they expiated and paid the penalty of crimes committed in a previous state'.[20]

Fanciful 'nervous distempers': a new British epidemic

In Britain, the growing popularity of hysteria and hypochondriasis as 'convulsive and spasmodic distempers' occurred within the new and fashionable culture of nerves. Prominent authors such as Richard Blackmore (1650–1729), Nicholas Robinson (1697–1775)[21], and George Cheyne (1671–1743) accepted a nerve-mediated pathology. Cheyne actually estimated that in his time nearly a third of all Britons came to suffer from ailments caused by disturbances of the nervous system involving both the body and the mind. Blackmore's own position on the spleen and vapours was outlined in his work *A Treatise of the Spleen and Vapours: Or Hypochondriacal and Hysterical Affections.* Robert Whytt (1714–66), a professor at the

University of Edinburgh, was quick to assert a nerve-mediated 'consensus' linking the brain, stomach and intestines. Malfunctions could start or end in the brain-or anywhere in between. Like others before him, Whytt concluded that 'vapours' and 'fits' occurred more frequently in women who naturally had greater sensibility and 'sympathy' due to the 'unusual delicacy or unnatural state of their nerves' (Chapter 8).[22] The presence of a uterus was also reintroduced into the chain of causality.[23] In addition to having a constitutional weakness, 'sensible' women in affluent circumstances were usually brought up to live lives that increased the risks for nervous diseases such as hysteria.[24] Among the dangers were lack of exercise, and menstrual troubles. Indeed, hysteria was categorised as the quintessentially feminine disease of tender, delicate bodies with sentimental and capricious minds. Thus, woman's bountiful sensibility could be an asset or a curse, making her emotionally unstable, vulnerable to seek pleasure as well as experience greater pain. Such cultural and scientific framing prompted a new wave of 'hysterisation'. The new vogue of medical theories used nervous models of explanation with the uterus returning to its former status of potential culprit.[25]

Two Edinburgh professors, William Cullen (1710–90) and James Gregory (1753–1821) also associated hysteria with gynaecological problems (Chapter 8). For every man afflicted with hysterical fits, Gregory speculated that ten thousand women suffered from such attacks.[26] Most of them were between the ages of fifteen and thirty-five. The basic reason for this lop-sided ratio was a perceived constitutional debility common to all females. Such debility generated greater bodily irritability, and absent or irregular menses, during the childbearing years (Chapter 8). Instead of viewing menstrual irregularities as possible effects of disease, most eighteenth-century physicians inverted the causal relationship and predicted that such disorders foreshadowed other serious ailments, including hysteria. Like Whytt, Cullen felt that hysteric fits could be linked to problems in other bodily systems, notably the 'prima via' or alimentary canal, but he refused to speculate about the precise pathways of this 'sympathy'. He strongly hinted, however, that both the uterus and ovaries were involved in triggering hysteric motions well before the appearance of gastrointestinal symptoms. The ultimate cause was placed on traditional notions of vascular plethora; as an excess of blood was deemed capable of enhancing nervous irritability.[27] This humoral idea was further advanced through the description of hysteric women as possessing a sanguine and plethoric constitution and a robust and vigorous habit. Ironically, these profiles were in flagrant opposition to the new image of delicate and debilitated females with fragile nerves.

Still popularly referred to as 'black fits', hypochondriasis sustained a similar transformation. Blackmore's 'English spleen' was conceived as another condition of debilitated nerves. This substituted for a traditional explanation that hypochondriasis was caused by noxious 'vapours' steaming from a melancholic spleen.[28] Also referred to as the 'hyp', the label was predominantly applied to affluent men of refinement – many 'advanced in life' – who were endowed with a melancholic temperament and were subject to frequent mood swings. Many were learned individuals, virtuosi and authors who worked in solitude, stuffing their brains through excessive reading of books. Their 'spirits' – an older term for the invisible matter believed to be circulating through the nerves – were calculated to be 'low', diminishing or 'sinking'. This mental outlook was aggravated during long British winters of dreary, cold weather. Homebound hypochondriacs also complained of heavy weight on their chests, indigestion with burning stomach sensations and flatulence. Some experienced cold sweats and palpitations, others complained of headaches and fainting spells or weakness and numbness in their limbs. A few unfortunate sufferers seemed to be in constant fear of death.[29]

Blackmore reached back to ancient humoralism as he attempted to explain the digestive uproar. He speculated that the suffocating stomach reflux, 'tumultuous belching', and rumbling intestines were caused by 'imprisoned underground vapours' struggling to find an outlet. 'Hyp' victims possessed a very acid stomach fluid described as capable of 'eroding linen'. Both hysteria and hypochondriasis seemed to share a number of gastro-intestinal manifestations frequently grouped under a separate label: 'dyspepsia'. This definition included a series of complaints ranging from lack of appetite to nausea, heartburn, belching and stomach pain. For Cullen and his followers, dyspepsia was considered to be another 'neurosis' causing systemic debility with particular loss of muscular tone in the stomach. This condition was responsible for the excessive secretion of gastric acid.[30] The main culprit for the acidity in the stomach was the excessive consumption of alcohol. In his contemporary survey of Scotland's health problems, John Sinclair had judged the replacement of ale with distilled liquors as one of the most destructive developments of the eighteenth century.[31] 'Dram' (liquor) drinking was an essential requirement for socialisation but it had nefarious effects on both the stomach and the mind. 'Disorderly passions of any kind', as well as 'uneasiness or vexation of mind' led to dyspeptic symptoms and by 'sympathy' generated hysteria and hypochondriasis.[32]

The issue whether hysteria and hypochondriasis were 'distinct disorders' or the same disease 'modified by temperament, sex and other circumstances' had already been raised by Sydenham. It remained a 'favourite topic of dispute' among eighteenth-century physicians. Most agreed that the characteristic choking sensation in the throat, shallow breathing and bouts of theatrical movements in women clearly pointed to a diagnosis of hysteria. More prevalent among males, 'hyp' also featured less spectacular fits and outbursts stemming from 'low spirits'. When Cullen published his disease classification in 1769, both hysteria and hypochondriasis were arranged within a new class of ailments termed the 'neuroses'. Neuroses were defined as generalised diseases involving changes in sensibility and motion without fever caused by the malfunction of the nervous system. Within this class, hysteria – in deference to its convulsive muscular contractions, was placed among the so-called spasmodic conditions, which also included tetanus, epilepsy, asthma, intestinal colic, and hydrophobia or rabies.[33] In turn, Cullen's nosology defined hypochondriasis as 'dyspepsia with languor, sadness and fear without any adequate causes in a melancholic temperament'. Therefore, he paired 'hyp' with other 'adynamic' diseases, such as syncope, dyspepsia and chlorosis.[34] Cullen admitted that the tag hysteria was 'extremely difficult' to define because of its 'many' and 'various' symptoms.[35] 'My first and chief care was to examine and distinguish the species of diseases in the patients themselves',[36] Cullen noted, explaining elsewhere that 'nosology is imperfect and far short of what it ought to be. Though what I have done is imperfect, I have published it because I thought it might be useful.'[37] In fact, to the consternation of colleagues who sought greater medical certainty in his disease classification, Cullen suggested that it was merely a work in progress. As more clinical information appeared in medical journals, he continued to search for new categories.[38]

Attesting to the popular characterisation of both illnesses, several medical theses were written in Edinburgh dealing with the clinical characteristics of hysteria and hypochondriasis.[39] In spite of these classificatory efforts, the earlier ambiguities remained, especially in the absence of convulsive episodes, leading Cullen to speak of intermediate instances of 'hypochondriac hysteria' in women with fits. Sullen men who were prone to tantrums could suffer from 'hysteric hypochondriasis'. Although no longer strictly gendered, the new constructions of hysteria and hypochondriasis continued to uphold stigmatising stereotypes of emotional female instability – reflected in fits – and other unruly but more forceful male outbursts.

In advancing their ideas, medical authors did not neglect the role of the mind. With 'sympathy' connecting various organ systems, both diseases were said to be 'imaginary', prominently influenced by the 'passions of the mind'. Feelings of fear, grief, anger and a 'train of misfortunes' could easily trigger hysterical fits and hypochondriac sadness. These manifestations could be forged to attract attention, allow manipulation, and create deception.

Excessive or insufficient sex was both viewed as an indirect factor in the appearance of hysteria. This was based on the widely held belief that a proper 'stimulus of love' guaranteed normal menstrual functions.[40] Cullen even described a special condition, the *hysteria libidinosa*, which he found in 'females who are liable to the nymphomania'. He defined this state an 'unrestrained desire for venereal enjoyment' caused by uterine irritability.[41] Other medical men wrote eloquently about the 'great proclivity to venery' among hysteric women, describing their lustful proclivities. Seductive gestures and 'libidinous speeches', and especially 'lascivious casting about their eyes' were said to accompany some hysteric fits.[42] Hypochondriacs, by contrast, seemed lonely, listless and disappointed, as well as suspicious of others. They displayed a 'want of resolution and activity with respect to all undertakings' as well as 'an apprehension of great evil'.[43] Cullen also blamed such persons for 'intemperance of all kinds, especially too early and excessive venery' in their lives.[44] Hypochondriasis was a disease of individuals with a 'turn of mind that was grave, serious, forward, selfish, unfeeling, full of doubt, distrust and caution'.[45]

Both hysteria and hypochondriasis were creations of the new consumer society and its growing obsession with health. In fact, these conditions became emblematic of urban living, as Enlightenment elites sought to pursue civility, sociability and knowledge. Men and women aimed to educate themselves, reading books and magazines – including medical ones – cultivating introspection and sensitivity while dosing themselves liberally with medicines.[46] The new quest for health preservation was endorsed and encouraged by the medical profession. Indeed, they gave information on how to stay healthy by avoiding detrimental living conditions and experiences. Prominent practitioners, including Cullen, became advisors to the rich and famous. Their professional authority lent credence to a comprehensive 'middle way' regimen of environmental and lifestyle practices aimed at preventing mental and physical collapse (Chapter 4).

Like other ailments, hysteria and hypochondriais became linked to a refined, upper-class life-style and 'the subject of raillery'.[47] Some practitioners considered 'nervous distempers' a badge of fancy and national pride; while critics singled them out as expressions of profligacy and hedonism, symbols of Britain's booming economic prosperity and material consumption.[48] In searching for plausible somatic causes, most eighteenth-century physicians condemned the deleterious effects of an affluent life-style, strongly recommending the return to more frugal tastes. Among the practices hurtful to women were dietary transgressions, real or surmised. Too much meat and gravy, exorbitant consumption of coffee, tea and alcohol, combined with excessive sex but not enough physical exercise in the outdoors, were highly dangerous (Chapter 4).[49] Swoons or fully developed fits could be particularly triggered in young virgins and widows who failed to follow the prescribed life-styles and social roles.

Because of their sedentary life-style and 'indolence', hypochondriacs were often censured for the 'excessive application to any particular pursuit'.[50] They ranged from young, shy students and bookworms to elderly grumpy, egotistical men obsessively attuned to every twitch in their bodies. Hypochondriasis, also known as the *morbus eruditorum* (disease of erudition) became popularly known as a hazard of literacy and learning. Physicians believed that hypochondriacs became anxious and miserable because of their tendency to introspection, melancholia and fixation on certain topics. Pursuing these matters with dogged determination, hypochondriacs neglected sleep, ate poorly and avoided physical exercise. Some were solitary drinkers, undisciplined eaters, and opium addicts. To prevent nervous deterioration, Cullen suggested these individuals embrace a moderate life-style and steady climate, guarding against the damp and cold winter air by staying indoors in towns and retiring to the countryside during summers in an effort to rebalance their passions. As with hysteria, social critics parodied the apparent disconnection between alleged suffering and minimal somatic manifestations of disease. In the end, all efforts designed to raise health consciousness and preach temperance created ideal conditions for the emergence of both illnesses. According to conventional medical wisdom, both men and women afflicted with fainting spells and bouts of depression had only themselves to blame for eschewing professional advice. In time, the inevitable result was nerve damage affecting all bodily systems, indirectly harming the mind. If symptoms persisted, melancholia, madness, dropsy, palsy, phthisis or 'some other fatal distemper' could easily follow.[51] To communicate and negotiate with physicians, contemporary women and men learned to express their discomfort and frustration in particular culturally and medically accepted physical terms. Thus, budding hysterics and hypochondriacs came to seek further professional advice, initiating an endless cycle of medical dependence.[52] In Foucault's view, this was just another aspect of the medicalisation process imposed on eighteenth-century life with its inherent shifts in power.[53]

Eighteenth-century medical views of hysteria and hypochondriasis revealed a number of traditional biases about female and male susceptibility to disease. Couched in the language of 'nerves' and 'sympathies' instead of traditional 'humours' and 'vapours', these illnesses mirrored the physical and mental problems of affluent sectors of society. Both ailments became popular and were, in fact, considered cultural metaphors of civilised and refined Georgian Britain.[54] But could these 'fashionable distempers' also occur among the less affluent sectors of society? Let us turn to the archival evidence.

Hysteria and hypochondriasis at the infirmary: patients' representations and diagnostic challenges

Socially marginalised and economically disadvantaged groups, including women, the elderly, and destitute, have traditionally carried a greater burden of disease. Historically feeble through malnutrition and ravaged by a variety of infectious and chronic illnesses, the 'deserving' poor came to view all bodily manifestations of sickness with greater concern. Disability could signal the end of employment and a life of homelessness and despair, ultimately spiralling towards death. Inconsistencies in the assignment of these nosological labels were common due to the fluid boundaries between hysteria and hypochondriasis. There remained a lack of consensus among contemporary medical practitioners in spite of Cullen's widely promoted classification system.[55] Moreover, at the institutional level, clerical errors and omissions, as well as bureaucratic manipulations further compounded the confusion. Nevertheless, some simple statistical information obtained from the Edinburgh Infirmary records provides an approximate picture of events at the hospital. The first set of data was obtained from surviving folios of the Infirmary's General Register of Patients between the years 1770 and 1800.[56] As noted in Table 9.1 (overleaf), the diagnosis 'hysteria' or 'hysterical complaint' appeared rather infrequently in the registration charts except for the year 1785, averaging only slightly over 1% of all entries.[57] Significant fluctuations from year to year were due to the influx of other categories of patients including soldiers and seamen who were admitted by hospital managers for political and economic reasons.[58] Those diagnosed with hysteria were overwhelmingly female: of the 157 cases identified in the registers, 154 (98%) were women. More than half of inmates identified as hysteric was sent to the ordinary medical ward. About one in four were listed as being servants and placed in a ward specifically outfitted for them. The rest went to the teaching ward managed by local university professors. Most entered the institution during the winter months, December through to March.

In turn, Infirmary admissions in the General Register under the category 'hypochondriasis' are summarised in Table 9.2 (overleaf) between 1770 and 1800. Their number was quite small – about 0.5% – perhaps because Infirmary Practitioners often employed other diagnostic labels such as dyspepsia, and melancholia to characterise similar complaints. Although admissions doubled in certain years like 1778 and 1788, no discernible trends can be detected. Nearly 75% of the patients were males. Like their

Table 9.1

Royal Infirmary of Edinburgh
General Register of Patients, 1770–1800:
Cases labelled 'Hysteria' or 'Hysteric Complaint'

Year	Admissions	Cases	Percentage	Females	Males
1770	1,170	16	1.3%	16	-
1775	1,795	25	1.3%	24	1
1780	2,100	24	1.1%	22	2
1785	1,737	62	3.5%	62	-
1790	1,768	11	0.6%	11	-
1795	1.620	14	0.8%	14	-
1800	1,836	05	0.2%	05	-
Totals	12,026	157	1.3%	154	3

hysteric counterparts, individuals specifically identified as suffering from hypochondriac complaints arrived mostly during the winter months. Two-thirds of the patients went into the ordinary medical ward; the rest were evenly divided between the servant and teaching wards. A few males were directly shipped to the soldiers and seamen's wards.

The second, and by far more important information source regarding hysteria came from fourteen student casebooks containing complete clinical histories copied from the Infirmary's teaching ward (Chapter 7). Between the years 1771 and 1799, these notebooks reveal the presence of thirty patients – all women – officially classified as suffering from hysteria. The group barely constituted 6.7% of all female admissions to that ward, but it should be noted that several patients with similar symptoms were admitted under the labels amenorrhoea, dyspepsia, and melancholia. A composite patient profile reveals their mean age was about twenty-three, slightly below the norm calculated for all other hospitalised women.[59] The available historical evidence does not support Foucault's statement that lower-class women managed to escape 'hysterisation'.[60] On admission, some individuals seemed genuinely concerned or frightened by their sensations of suffocation, fits, and blackouts. Others simply worried about their digestion or suffered menstrual irregularities that could be associated with early pregnancy. In fact, most of the women who provided a menstrual history revealed that their menses had stopped (Chapter 8). When 20-year-old Peggy Bonella petitioned for admission, she told physicians a typical story: she had experienced bouts of headaches, palpitations, weakness and vertigo, together

Table 9.2

Royal Infirmary of Edinburgh
General Register of Patients, 1770–1800:
Cases labelled 'Hypochonriasis

Year	Admissions	Cases	Percentage	Females	Males
1770	**1,170**	**4**	**0.3%**	**-**	**4**
1775	**1,795**	**15**	**0.8%**	**9**	**6**
1780	**2,100**	**9**	**0.4%**	**8**	**1**
1785	**1,737**	**6**	**0.3%**	**1**	**5**
1790	**1,768**	**12**	**0.6%**	**11**	**9**
1795	**1.620**	**8**	**0.5%**	**14**	**5**
1800	**1,836**	**15**	**0.8%**	**05**	**10**
Totals	**12,026**	**69**	**0.57%**	**29**	**40**

with general quivering of her body. According to the clerk recording her story, she also seemed 'inclined to dwell on her complaints'.[61] Other patients spoke of contracted hands, 'heavy balls ascending from the pit of the stomach', followed by shallow breathing and choking sensations. Next came frenzied outbursts followed by 'gentle faints' or seizures, and temporary loss of consciousness. A 15-year-old spoke of a 'globus' rising from the stomach to the throat, with a sensation not unlike 'the creeping of an animal on its hind legs' moving from her ankle to the knee.[62] Women had no monopoly on hysteric complaints, of course, but it was easier for them to portray themselves as weak and helpless. A young male miner complained of similar sensations arising from his lower abdomen and surging to the pit of the stomach, causing him to briefly faint.[63]

Only a handful of patients with hypochondriasis were listed in student notebooks. Therefore, they defy generality. All of them were males, two already in their forties, the others in their late twenties and thirties. All had been frequently exposed to cold and moisture, which was a typically prevailing condition in Scotland. Most of the men's complaints were defined as dyspeptic, combined with 'lowness of spirits' or 'depressing passions'. The hypochondriasis label was applied to those who always considered themselves 'in the greatest danger from very slight causes'.[64] Since the disease was believed to simulate other conditions, two of the arrivals also displayed symptoms suggestive of venereal disease. One of the patients, John Lumsden blamed his multiple complaints on an episode of gonorrhoea six months earlier – 'the only one to which he could refer his complaints' when in reality the 'primary affection' seemed to reside in his mind.[65] The other patient, 44-year-old James Plank, was a notorious 'worrier' whose 'anxiety for his health' added 'not a little to his complaints'. This man grumbled about flatulence and insipid eructation, copious salivation and vomiting after meals. He had been previously hospitalised in several London hospitals apparently 'without finding relief'.[66] A depressed 38-year-old fisherman from the Shetland Islands reported aches and pains localised in the chest but also travelling from the abdomen to the throat. Frequent belching, an uneasy stomach, as well as disturbed sleep were also among his symptoms. His attending physician, James Home (1758–1842), considered the complaints 'altogether the creature of his own brain'.[67]

The frequency of servants among those identified as hysterics both in the General Register of Patients and student notebooks, requires further review. Friendly social relations with domestic workers were an important component of polite society.[68] Their arrivals at the hospital suggest that Edinburgh employers took advantage of their ability to issue admission letters and exploit the existence of a separate servant ward in the Infirmary to rid themselves of sick and troublesome employees (Chapter 1). Conversely, disgruntled or fearful employees may have feigned the fits to protect themselves from mistreatment by their superiors. Since the average duration of recurring symptoms was several months, 'hysteric complaints' seemed perhaps a convenient description for a broad spectrum of recurring, interpersonal conflicts with female workers who failed to please their masters.

While much of the medical attention centred on the somatic manifestations described by those wishing to be admitted, behavioural and environmental factors were also readily identified. A number of individuals admitted as suffering from hysteria mentioned the presence of anguish, 'depression of spirits', or more specifically, 'shock from sudden death of husband'.[69] An unmarried teenage servant, Janet Nisbet, had been 'seized with a sense of globus after suffering an affront'.[70] According to the records, another inmate 'possessing an exquisite susceptibility of mental impression' became hysterical 'after a violent fright'.[71] Peggy Thompson, a patient of John Gregory, claimed that her fits had started after an incident in which another young woman scolded her.[72] Cullen's John Craig, the hysteric miner, began his erratic conduct following a frightful accident in a coal pit when his candle went out and he had great difficulty finding his way out of the dark shaft.[73] According to Andrew Duncan Sr, one of the professors managing the teaching ward, James Smyth's hypochondriac illness was the product of excessive self-absorption.[74] Additionally, the 'lonely manner of life and indifferent living' caused the multiple complaints and depression of the sailor from the Shetlands.

At first glance, the assignment of diagnostic labels such as hysteria and hypochondriasis to Edinburgh's deserving poor is somewhat puzzling.[75] Burton and others had advanced the notion that the 'vulgar' were constitutionally robust or 'coarse' enough to avoid falling prey to 'weak' nerves. Sydenham had exempted 'those who lead a hard and hardy life' from becoming hysteric,[76] although a few cases had been reported.[77] In explaining the appearance of nervous diseases among the poor, Georgian practitioners came to believe that people, regardless of class and gender, were subjected to the risks of urban living. Deleterious habits and disturbances of sensibility were no longer limited to class and gender.[78] In violation of their social contract 'people of no rank and slender means presume to intrude on the province of their superiors by fashionably ruining themselves, their families and connections', observed one Edinburgh graduate.[79] In fact, a prominent English physician, John C. Lettsom (1744–1815), remarked that servants through 'continual intercourse with people of decent manners' had acquired a 'delicacy of body and sensibility of mind' similar to that displayed by their employers.[80] In Edinburgh, one 'young lady' who arrived at the Infirmary was described of possessing 'a remarkably delicate habit of body'.[81] On the other hand, to gain admission, some of the arriving Infirmary patients, especially domestic servants, deliberately or perhaps unconsciously imitated the symptoms and manners of their affluent mistresses.[82] Working males portrayed as hypochondriacs seemed obsessed or depressed – or so it appeared – from suffering with venereal diseases – as demonstrated by John Lumsden earlier.

Most patients admitted with hysteria or hypochondriasis appeared to suffer from milder digestive conditions along with the general malaise associated with their lower-class status. Although all power and authority remained with the medical staff, patients seemed to be ready to negotiate with and manipulate Infirmary physicians standing between them and what was perceived during the winter months as 'the warmth of the house'.

The arrival of poor people in dispensaries and hospital wards with certain patterns of physical and mental complaints, it appears, compelled admitting practitioners to assign diagnoses such as hysteria and hypochondriasis. In so doing, they were forced to expand the range of causes previously established for those diseases in private patients. One author, Andrew Wilson, explained that hysteria could indeed afflict 'persons who live low, are exposed to much cold, who are wanting to themselves either through negligence, parsimony or poverty'.[83] Dyspepsia, popularly known in Scotland as 'waterbrash', was considered a frequent companion of hysteria and hypochondriasis among 'people in lower life'. According to medical authors, part of the reason was their meagre diet of milk and starches – 'potatoes form a great part of their subsistence'[84] – while all 'animal food' was virtually unavailable during winters. Seasonal starvation and exhaustion were ubiquitous. Another characteristic was the frequent consumption of 'ardent spirits' especially among the poor.[85] In Edinburgh, alcohol consumption was rampant, especially during 'high jinks' or drinking bouts.[86] Tea drinking was equally nefarious, suspected of swelling the ranks of the dyspeptic poor who 'stint themselves in so many essential necessaries of life to procure this article of luxury'. Sinclair condemned the coarse black tea sold to the masses as 'miserable and unwholesome', bound to ruin any stomach particularly if taken very strong and hot without milk or sugar.[87]

Was the hospital an appropriate place for admitting people presumed to suffer from such fashionable neuroses? According to James Gregory, there was widespread recognition that the hospital environment usually conspired against a cure of hysteria. 'This disease is very disagreeable to the practitioner especially in a hospital where exercise, air and the employment of mind are precluded', he declared. Despite efforts to ventilate the crowded and noisy wards, the ambience remained vitiated. Deadly contagion lurked. For this reason, Gregory claimed to accept as few hysteric patients as possible, explaining that 'more have been seized with this disease in the hospital than have been cured in it'.[88] Another professor, Andrew Duncan Sr, expressed similar reservations. Speaking to medical students in 1795, Duncan Sr. explained that:

> [A hospital] is a bad place for hypochondriasis.... [Patients] have too much time to brood over their complaints... their companions are affected with real diseases so that they suppose themselves affected with all the complaints they hear of.[89]

Among other reasons given by physicians who hesitated to admit hysterics was the threat of a disciplinary breakdown in the institution. By 'force of imitation' and 'association of ideas' patients with frequent fits had the potential of triggering similar attacks of disruptive behaviour among other inmates being treated for different ailments. In his treatise, Robert Whytt had already warned about this excess in sensibility and sympathy: 'it has frequently happened in the Royal Infirmary here that women have been seized with hysteric fits from seeing others attacked with them'.[90] In late-December 1771, Peggy McKay, a 14-year-old girl originally admitted with a fever, experienced three separate fits during the night after witnessing the hysterical attack of a roommate.[91] On another occasion Gregory had to contend with six women – half of the female teaching ward – who were all having fits during the same night, undoubtedly creating quite an uproar, especially since no nurses were routinely available during the nightshift.[92]

Such 'hysterical contagion – explained as a sympathetic effect akin to yawning or vomiting – was not infrequent at the time. 'Swoons and hysterics' were widely reported during emotional church assemblies and theatrical performances.[93] If anything, hospitals seemed to actually breed hysteria and the hyp instead of curing them.

To obtain temporary shelter and better nourishment, many candidates for admission to the Infirmary resorted to a shopping list of disparate complaints that would persuade physicians screening arrivals to authorise admission. Exaggerations, 'misrepresentations' and outright deceptions were not uncommon (Chapter 1).[94] Given the frequency of patients trying to gain access to the Edinburgh Infirmary, it was never easy to assess the veracity of their stories. This was especially true during the cold winter months, a period that coincided with the academic year and operation of the teaching ward.[95] The Infirmary profited from the sale of tickets to medical students wishing to attend medical rounds and clinical lectures; therefore professors were keen to admit interesting patients (Chapter 7). Since both hysteria and hypochondriasis presented themselves through a variety of symptoms, the deserving poor vying for a bed took full advantage of this situation expecting that their complaints would make for excellent teaching cases. 'I take a great number of these patients so that we may see it [hysteria] in its different shapes', explained Gregory. He believed that hysteria presented itself each year in new guises that were 'apt to deceive the young practitioner'. To avoid deceit and diagnostic confusion, students were encouraged to follow the course of such patients and learn the distinctions between hysteric and epileptic fits.[96]

Although the protean complaints suggestive of hysteria and hypochondriasis were often viewed with suspicion, most candidates 'deserving' admission claimed to be in genuine physical distress. Once the decision to accept the patient had been made, only time could tell whether the initial diagnosis proved correct. A 14-year-old boy admitted twice in 1780 claimed to suffer from daily fits and fainting. Each time the attending physicians became convinced that he was an impostor and threatened to apply a hot iron to his body. Miraculously cured, he was promptly expelled.[97] Cullen had a similar experience a few years earlier.[98] 'Whenever I find a patient falsifying his ailments as they may make me appear ridiculous in practice, I always think it proper to dismiss them', explained Cullen.[99] Tagged as suffering from hypochondriasis, another 17-year-old male was discovered to have 'exaggerated and to some degree misrepresented' symptoms. Duncan Sr, the attending physician, gave him the benefit of the doubt, explaining that the details of the patient's story were provided 'not indeed with a desire to deceive but from a propensity to imagine the worst'.[100] Admitted with numerous – and quite distressing – symptoms, John Menter was eventually suspected of 'conjuring up' some of his symptoms. After several days in the Infirmary, Duncan Sr concluded that 'more depends on his imagination than on any particular disease'. The condition, he explained, 'cannot be strictly called hypochondriasis because he did not labour under those particular symptoms, which characterise this disease as defined by nosologists'.[101] In another instance, the same professor commented on the clinical course of a 44-year-old labourer, telling students that 'it would have been better had he not been admitted for his complaints were mostly imaginary'.[102]

A majority of the Infirmary patients who were labelled hysterics and hypochondriacs simply complained of debility, lack of food or sleep, and anxiety. Another Edinburgh professor, Daniel Rutherford, defined two women hysteric for simply complaining of breathing difficulties, sometimes asthmatic in nature. These symptoms were usually ascribed to a variety of chest ailments, notably the feared pulmonary consumption or phthisis (Chapter 7).[103] Hypochondriac men, in turn, were 'indulging in gloomy thoughts', seeking solitude during dark and cold winters. Most had lost their appetites, experienced constipation, and became increasingly anxious about their health.[104] Edinburgh professors made much of their physical appearance, describing their dark complexion – private patients were usually pale – and 'spare countenance'. Some individuals reported experiencing chills, alternating with sudden flushing of the faces and chest palpitations. In this 'train of symptoms' there were also 'flying pains' in the limbs, as well as paroxysms of dry cough.[105]

Women seemed to be especially vulnerable to fits near the time of menstruation,[106] their imagination said to be 'wild and inconstant'.[107] A characteristic symptom was the so-called *clavus hystericus*, a sharp pain sensation described as if a nail had been driven through the head.[108] At other times, the afflicted women reported pain, swelling, and grumbling noises in the loins, especially on the left side, followed by a sensation of spasm routinely explained as if a ball was moving across the lower abdomen and heading upwards towards the stomach.[109] After much twisting, cramping, and belching, the imaginary ball continued its ascent into the chest. This movement would be accompanied by a rapid pulse, oppression, difficult breathing – *asphyxia hysterica* – until the sensation reached the throat where it impaired swallowing – *dysfagia hysterica* – and caused a sense of suffocation or 'globus'. A 35-year-old male admitted by James Gregory in 1783 described similar episodes.[110]

In many instances, hysteric patients 'took to the fits'. This pathognomonic sign was often a set of riotous motions. The individual experienced bouts of crying and convulsive laughing. Sufferers would flail their arms while others uttered 'alarming cries' that 'terrified the attendants'. One Infirmary patient was described as striking and kicking herself, as well as those around her, before falling to the ground and remaining there, apparently exhausted and unconscious.[111] Paroxysms usually fluctuated from fifteen to twenty-five minute episodes – repeated three or four times a day – to full hour spells with the stupefied patient foaming from the mouth just like during an epileptic seizure. The violent motions could lead to generalised muscular contractions accompanied by rigid bodily postures and, in the case of 14-year-old Cecilia McLean, the creation of bizarre arched postures.[112] Faced with such episodes, practitioners unsuccessfully struggled to establish a differential diagnosis between hysteria, epilepsy, as well as other forms of paralysis.[113]

Giddiness, swooning or fainting spells were considered valid substitutes for fits. Other patients simply complained of seeing 'floaters' before their eyes or experiencing 'dimmed' eyesight. Following the convulsions, patients quickly recovered their senses, voided large amounts of clear urine, or experienced residual muscular twitches as well as speech difficulties. Most seemed not to have had any recollection of their fits. Gregory, ever suspicious of the theatrical nature of these events, suggested the patients themselves deliberately induced them. Lecturing to students, he declared that for these patients 'there is a peculiar pleasure that attends the coming of the fit; analogous, I suppose, to that we experience in yawning, and that they really encourage them and bring them on'.[114] From the Edinburgh Infirmary casebooks, however, it seems obvious that only a minority of inmates described as hysteric actually displayed the characteristic fits.

Managing fits and rumblings: the gulf between medical theory and practice

Infirmary physicians considered both hysteria and hypochondriasis 'proper' diseases for hospital management despite the risks of admitting malingering individuals and its potential threat to institutional discipline. After all, the patients appeared to be in genuine distress and their complaints prevented them from carrying on their occupational responsibilities. Contemporary ethics formulated by John Gregory (1724–73) suggested that 'nervous complaints' should never be treated with ridicule or neglect because the suffering was real – although one can also detect physicians' veiled hostility towards such cases.[115] Most hospital practitioners agreed that these patients required 'a great deal of attention'. This was because of their alleged debilitated physical condition and mental distress. Edinburgh physicians managing cases at the Infirmary reached consensus on a three-pronged strategy for dealing with these ailments. The first was a strictly palliative program individually tailored to address the most bothersome symptoms, particularly the gastrointestinal complaints and hysteric fits so disruptive to hospital routine. To prevent repeated attacks, 'the most easy restraint is a waistcoat', declared Cullen.[116] With regard to hypochondriasis, 'medicines are of very little consequence in this disease and their frequent use does often great mischief', he warned. In his opinion, they were solely designed to 'remove a present fit or palliate a particular symptom but failed to strike at the root of this ailment'.[117]

Since gastrointestinal troubles were believed to be at the root of both hysteria and hypochondriasis, traditional stomach- and bowel-cleansing routines were initiated. The use of emetics such as ipecac and a great range of purgatives were administered with the goal of unburdening the digestive system of potentially harmful wastes. About half of the patients suffering from hysteria received cathartics, including rhubarb pills, Glauber salts (sodium sulphate), aloes, and even calomel, a mercurial. In hypochondriasis, the attending physicians administered a 'laxative course' with brisk cathartics including salt of tartar, jalap powder and an infusion of tamarinds with senna. They were usually prescribed – not always successfully – to specifically deal with constipation, abdominal cramps and gastric gas.[118] Following his admission in August 1781, Hope's hypochondriac, Angus Robertson, received such a course of 'cream of tartar' (sodium potassium tartrate) for his flatulence.[119] Since its first introduction in cases of mania at the Berlin Hospital, Duncan Sr claimed to have found tartar especially useful with beneficial effects across the mind–body divide. 'It is now a favourite remedy in mental affections with some London practitioners', he told students. When Duncan Sr persisted in administering this tartar solution to his patient John Smyth, the man soon refused to take the medicine from the nurse, thus breaching hospital rules and allowing the professor to dismiss him. 'I was not displeased to have this opportunity', admitted Duncan Sr, who may have deliberately sought such an outcome.[120] In fact, the aggressive employment of purgatives in hypochondriacs was often meant to 'tire' patients, testing their stamina and determination to remain in the Infirmary. In the case of John Menter, Duncan Sr commented that 'if he dislikes his medicines he will probably leave us', reiterating the widespread medical bias about the futility of treating this 'imaginary' disease in hospitals.

Because of the perceived nervous weakness in all bodily systems, physicians also used a group of so-called antispasmodic drugs. To prevent or reverse a blackout spell in hysteria, hospital physicians forced the inhalation of draughts containing ether or asafoetida, a resin endowed with an obnoxious odour designed to re-awaken patients from their slumber. The drug could also be administered in pills or in an emulsion. Tobacco fumes or burnt feathers similarly exposed to the nostrils helped bring hysterics back to consciousness. Painkillers (anodynes) and sedatives were also frequently prescribed in both diseases. The most favoured drug was opium, administered in various forms, including pills, tinctures and enema solutions. Hope's other patient, the hysteric Ann Webster, received an analgesic opiate draught in August 1781. Laudanum was the drug of choice in stopping hysteric fits, particularly if the condition of the patient's nervous system was considered quite delicate. However, physicians were aware that some of the patients seemed already addicted to this drug from its frequent domestic use. In fact, they blamed most symptoms of hysteria and hypochondriasis on this habit. Constipation and increased tolerance were frequent side-effects, and the attending physicians struggled to individually adjust dosages of the drug. Addiction to opiates and alcohol needed to be broken. Draughts made with powder from the root of valerian – a mild sedative – facilitated sleep in other anxious and depressed patients. Notes concerning the management of Ann Webster indicate that she also received this drug.

A second therapeutic effort aimed to prop up the patients' debilitated nervous system.[121] At the centre of this approach was the provision of a simple but nourishing full diet. Milk was recommended, however tea and coffee were discouraged because of their detrimental effects on the stomach. Eggs and meat were part of the strengthening plan. Alcohol was usually banned except for a few glasses of red wine diluted with water offered with dinner. Plentiful food was supplemented with tonic remedies such as bitters, Peruvian bark, musk and camphor preparations, as well as chalybeate (iron tartrate) and steel filings mixed in wine. All these were expected to further strengthen the bodily constitution, blood, stomach, and nerves.[122] Hope's patient, Ann Webster, received a course of 'stomach pills', containing a herbal mixture designed to warm and fortify that vital organ. Other measures, such as baths, could be equally stimulating. Webster took one and progress notes on her chart indicate that 'she found the bath agreeable and comfortable'.[123] A relaxing, warm-water bath was considered helpful in a variety of spasmodic conditions, but given the institutional limitations for the provision of hot water, hospital physicians compromised by merely ordering foot-baths. This *pediluvium* not only required minimal staff assistance, but its beneficial effects were expected to diffuse upward from the feet to the rest of the body, an important consideration particularly in hysteria if the patient's menses were also arrested.[124] As in several gynaecological conditions, practitioners tried very hard to restore the menstrual flow in women suffering from hysteria. They used warm water for the purpose of diminishing the presumptive uterine irritability (Chapter 8). If practitioners believed that patients displayed a marked constitutional debility, a complete immersion in cold water could be ordered to stimulate the entire body. In one 1797 report, hysteric fits were arrested by the shock of throwing a pitcher of cold water on Helen Christie, a 19-year-old servant under the care of Thomas C. Hope.[125] Not surprisingly, Infirmary inmates were seldom eager to take the recommended plunge, particularly during Edinburgh's winter months. They often negotiated compromises with caregivers by reducing such an immersion into a smaller tub – *semicupium* – for a partial bath or by simply placing their hands in cold water.

Two traditional measures, cupping and blistering, were popular stimulating physical methods employed in hysteria. The former consisted in the application of cups to the skin after heat or suction had removed air contained in them. Both Angus Robertson and Ann Webster had a number of such cups applied, Robertson to the chest, Webster to the region of her stomach. Blisters were small, deliberately produced skin sores through the application of caustics. Designed to extract potentially harmful humours from the sick body in classical humoralism, cupping and blistering had been reinterpreted according to the new tenets of nervous irritability. As a result, they were considered general stimulants.[126] In Edinburgh, the procedure consisted of the application of dressings on the skin, which were soaked in small quantities of mustard flour, garlic, or even diluted sulphuric acid. With the dressing firmly in place by a bandage, the irritated sites usually 'answered' within twelve to twenty-four hours by 'rising' and forming vesicles that physicians would periodically lance with a needle in order to drain the accumulating fluid. This painful practice had numerous drawbacks, including secondary infections. In 1785, one 20-year-old female patient under James Gregory's management actually experienced a 'hysteric fit on taking off the blisters'.[127] Blisters were considered most beneficial when created on sensitive areas including the neck,[128] the shaved crown of the head,[129] and occasionally the upper back between the shoulder blades. In one case of hysteria, the blister was applied to the sternum.[130] In hypochondriasis, blisters or dry-cupping were seldom employed except on painful areas of the abdomen and chest. On 28 August 1781, Angus Robertson's cups were replaced with a 'seton' – a running sore deliberately created through the placement of silk strings or horse hair in the incision. Not unexpectedly, some patients refused such treatments and promptly decided to leave the hospital.

Another fairly frequent treatment for hysteria was electricity. Within the new medical theories based on frail nerves, electricity was also considered a powerful stimulant. As early as 1750 the Edinburgh Infirmary had acquired its first static electrical apparatus operated by a surgical clerk.[131] Yet, physicians remained sceptical and divided about the utility of electricity.[132] Most patients sat on a chair and were subjected to the method of 'drawing sparks', as contact was made between the skin and the machine's wooden or metal tips. Connected to chain conductors, these points could be directed toward specific regions of the body, especially the throat, considered the seat of a suffocating 'globus'. Others were directed to the abdomen.[133] Patients simultaneously complaining of stopped menses and hysteria, usually received moderate electrical sparks over the lower abdomen in an effort to jump-start their menstrual flux. Patients occasionally reported the treatment as being painful.

Finally, bloodletting was occasionally prescribed if the hospital physicians portrayed particular hysteric patients as possessing a 'florid complexion', a sign of excessive blood in the system common to persons of 'sanguine temperament and constitution'. In one patient, successive venesections ordered over the course of five weeks by John Gregory amounted to twenty-eight ounces,[134] while another woman, under the care of Francis Home, lost eight ounces at the onset of her treatment.[135] Two others had leeches applied to their temples in an effort to diminish persistent headaches.[136] Cupping over the pit of the stomach was meant to stop gastric distress.[137] Such restraint may seem surprising given the views about the role of vascular congestion in the genesis of nervous irritability. Indeed, in a case presented by William Cullen during his clinical lectures, the withdrawal of three or four ounces daily was advocated until the fits would cease. After more than twenty ounces of blood had been withdrawn without improvement, Cullen finally desisted, commenting 'I am doubtful how far we can go on in this practice; it is incredible what a quantity of blood the human constitution will bear with impunity.'[138] In general, bloodletting was perceived to be an ineffective remedy since it actually tended to further weaken patients whose entire symptomatology was blamed on debility.

Patients were told to increase their physical activities by taking walks in the hospital's yard or using a pair of institutional dumb-bells. One of James Gregory's patients was ordered to exercise daily on a wooden 'bank' equipped with a spring mechanism – also variously referred to as an 'exercise machine' or 'spring deal'.[139] For others, a wooden horse was available to mimic the salutary effects ascribed to horseback riding. Finally, patients were supposed 'to be engaged in some business'.[140] In certain cases, this would have meant becoming involved in some of the daily hospital chores, including cleaning of the wards and feeding non-ambulatory patients. Some withdrawn hypochondriacs were watched closely to prevent suicide attempts.[141]

The third component of Edinburgh's therapeutic plan was the least successful: endeavours to remove some of the 'remote' causes believed to be involved in the genesis of both diseases. Given the alleged chronic nature of hysteria and hypochondriasis, this task of preventing the return of symptoms involved issues of environment, life-style and emotional status difficult to modify. 'Management of the mind' required 'much discretion', and the provision of 'distractions'. To be sure, inmates with hypochondriasis were temporarily 'withdrawn from any occupation which is attended with much anxiety and fatigue or which is exposed to accidental disappointments or failures', proclaimed one Edinburgh medical student.[142] 'We must content ourselves with amusing the mind of the patient as much as possible', recommended another who discussed a case of hysteria at the Royal Medical Society (Chapter 2).[143] But how could this be accomplished? Inmates were encouraged to put their minds at ease and leave their worries behind, a somewhat dubious proposition for persons who may have been virtually homeless or had lost their menial jobs on account of their fits.[144] According to James Gregory, the power of suggestion needed to be part of any improvement. 'It is a maxim I inculcate very strongly to my patients', he observed, 'to use the utmost endeavours to prevent the coming of the fits. I have often known it to succeed though my advice is not well received by many.'[145] In 1784, Gregory prescribed for one of his hypochondriac patients 'some pills of bread alone for no other intention than to amuse him'.[146]

As expected, hospital physicians proclaimed some treatments effective. In their reports and lectures, Edinburgh professors claimed that certain hysterical and hypochondriacal manifestations subsided during the course of hospitalisation. For many patients, complaints of 'globus' in the throat ceased to be reported. Such success could perhaps be credited to the strict regimentation of eighteenth-century hospital life in Britain. Indeed, inmates at the Edinburgh Infirmary were subjected to strict rules of conduct, posted in the wards.[147] Refusal usually resulted in voluntary or forced discharge from the institution. Harkening back to earlier needs for social control and isolation, institutional discipline was paramount to restrict loitering, avoid brawls, and impose a measure of silence. Threat of expulsion for 'irregularities' – often understood as non-compliance with rules and treatments – hung over every patient (Chapter 1). Just as important were the warnings issued by the attending physicians. The comment 'fit stopped by threat of cold bath' appears in a progress report of a patient being treated by Gregory.[148] Cullen's famous schedule of repeated and painful blisters was not only designed to test the veracity of patients' complaints but also their stamina and commitment to institutional treatment. Some patients, however, remained undaunted by the threats and retaliated by having more fits. In such cases, the episodes would prominently occur during medical rounds and at bedtime, as well as in the course of medical procedures, representing possible instances of patient defiance. One 20-year-old female patient, experienced an attack after being placed in a small tub filled with cold water. A similar outburst occurred following venesection as blood continued to ooze from her arm.[149] Other inmates had their fits during the painful application of blisters[150] or the administration of evil-tasting draughts prescribed by the attending physicians.

Conclusion

Discharged by John Hope, Ann Webster left the Infirmary on 1 September 1781 after a nine-day stay in the Infirmary. According to the General Register of Patients, the average hospital residence for patients suffering from hysteria between 1770 and 1800 was 26.5 days with considerable yearly fluctuations. Angus Robertson was dismissed two days later, after twelve days in the medical ward. He was given a bottle of 'stomach pills' and an irritating ointment to keep his ulcer flowing. The mean stay for individuals with hypochondriasis for the same decades was 20.3 days. In the teaching ward, hysteria cases remained for 23.2 days, significantly below the 32-day average calculated for all women inmates regardless of diagnosis. Not a single fatality was reported for both conditions. When Gregory was in charge, he kept hysteric patients for less than two weeks (13 days), but this shorter hospitalisation period cannot be correlated with greater therapeutic success. In fact, Gregory's cure rate was only 33.3%. In the eyes of Infirmary practitioners, the long-term prognosis of hysteria remained guarded since it was generally considered a chronic problem due to an intractable constitutional weakness and fragile nervous system.[151]

Less than half of the patients suffering from hysteria were discharged as 'cured' (49.6%), a statistic in sharp contrast with the 70% rate recorded for all Infirmary admissions between 1770 and 1800. Ann Webster was among them. Hypochondriac patients fared much worse, with only 15% considered cured. An additional third of the hysteric patients (36.9%) and nearly half of the hypochondriacs (46%) – Angus Robertson included – left 'relieved' – an ambiguous term that generally meant temporary improvement, lack of effective treatments, or an intractable ailment. On average only 10% of patients suffering from other conditions were placed in this discharge category. Finally, the hospital honoured patient requests to leave the institution, placing them in the category of 'dismissed by desire'. These were inmates who had become disillusioned or displeased with the results of their treatment. Here again, those labelled as suffering from hysteria left in greater numbers (7.6%) than the average 5.0% for other classifications.[152] The numbers for patients with hypochondriasis were even less encouraging. Of those departing the Infirmary, close to one in five left of their own volition. As a further sign of difficulties surrounding the management of these patients, the medical authorities dismissed nearly a fifth more (18.5%) with hysteria and hypochondriasis, branding them 'improper' candidates for further treatment, a bureaucratic term that included those feigning their symptoms. 'Went out as being an improper patient for the house', explained Gregory in reference to a patient suffering from hysteria admitted in 1783. He added that 'she showed a force of imagination or whimsical disposition.... I did not expect to relieve her and only took her into the ward for [student] inspection'.[153]

Although well below the average rankings published monthly by the Edinburgh Infirmary, the cure rates for hysteria and hypochondriasis were somewhat deceptive. In spite of the official statistics, Gregory conceded that most of his patients were 'leaving the house very little better than when admitted'.[154] There was also evidence that some of the women suffering from hysteria were subsequently re-admitted to the Infirmary for similar complaints. The official outcomes of James Gregory's hysteric patients – 30% cured, 58% relieved and 8% dismissed by desire – suggests more honest reporting and perhaps greater scrutiny of applicants for hospital admission in order to ferret out potential impostors. The shorter hospital tenure suggests that Gregory's patients may have had a more realistic understanding of the limits imposed on medical management. His status as an attending physician and Infirmary manager also explains his desire to maintain proper discipline in the women's teaching ward and avoid publicity detrimental to the institution (Chapter 1). In any event, whether the treatments were successful or not, patients admitted to the hospital with hysteria and hypochondriasis received a temporary respite before returning to their daily struggles. As one report indicated, most Infirmary patients were usually reluctant to leave the premises, often facing a destitute and homeless existence.[155] In recognition of this fact, the attending physicians from time to time purposely delayed discharging some of these patients. In early 1772, Cullen inherited a female patient labelled as suffering from hysteria who had originally been admitted to the teaching ward by the late John Gregory. Instead of discharging her – the medical regimen had failed to improve her symptoms – Cullen decided to postpone her discharge. He explained to his students that 'in consideration of the season' his clinical experience suggested it would be 'extremely inconvenient to dismiss patients from the warmth and shelter of this house to their own cold and starving habitations'.[156]

The study of hysteria and hypochondriasis demonstrates that both conditions were closely related and displayed an extensive lineage stretching back to Antiquity. Forged within humoral views of the human body, the theoretical underpinnings of these diseases had undergone extensive changes, shifting from an iatrochemical causality of vapours to a system of debilitated nerves. At its core, hysteria and hypochondriasis exposed the complex relationships between the spheres of soma and mind. In spite of clinical confusion and flexible nosological labels, both hysteria and hypochondriasis consolidated their prominence among nervous disorders. They belonged to Cullen's family of 'neuroses' derived from the newly minted pathology of nerves. Placing the blame on fragile nerves and debilitated bodily constitutions, physicians re-affirmed causality previously linked to the traditional inferiority of women. Embossed with these fashionable labels, their sufferings were duly legitimised. Persons 'liable to 'globus' were told their bodies, life-style, or both were at fault. The presumed 'imaginary' nature of these conditions challenged both the social order and medical skills.

When Edinburgh's deserving poor came to the Infirmary seeking relief from their numerous complaints, a small number of them where portrayed as suffering from hysteria and hypochondriasis, fashionable diagnoses usually bestowed on 'better sort' people. Traditional boundaries between them were redefined and causality expanded. This action was not only needed to bureaucratically justify admissions but also to design a course of treatment. Personal reputation – the very status as medical professionals and educators – was at stake. The eighteenth-century reality, as reflected in Edinburgh's clinical documentation, was quite different from the published medical views on both diseases. Women admitted to the hospital failed to conform to the stereotype of overindulgent females. Poor, young, a majority of them still unmarried, these patients seemed to suffer from deprivations consonant with their social class rather than the excesses of an affluent life. Lack of menstrual periods, lethargy and depression were probably the effects of widespread malnutrition and hunger. Both flatulence and bowel cramps may have been the effects of meagre diets based on oatmeal, barley, cabbage, and potatoes.[157] It was largely their physical debility, gastrointestinal complaints, repeated fainting spells and frequent stoppage of menses, that prompted 'hysterisation'. Those designated hypochondriacs were believed to be in similar circumstances. One of Duncan Sr's patients, identified as a porter, was characterised as 'a poor indigent man without house or family'. The professor then went on to explain that 'it is not unlikely that the causes to which he attributes his disease as cold and proper nourishment are those which contribute the principal part of or the whole of his disease'. Duncan Sr concluded that the patient 'seemed most to want shelter and protection during the wintry months and wholesome diet which he had no opportunity of obtaining by his labour'.[158]

Despite all the ambiguities and challenges to conventional medical theories, the multiple complaints were heard and subjected to treatment in hospitals. Recovery from hysteria and hypochondriasis was attempted through a strict regimen rhetorically designed to strengthen lax body fibres and rest the mind. To deal with these ailments, however, eighteenth-century practitioners fell back on a series of traditional dietary and behavioural recommendations designed for rich and poor alike. With the help of textbooks and popular manuals, these prescriptions were widely disseminated and accepted by people regardless of social position and income. At best, the rules provided encouragement. A carefully crafted plan carried the possibility of recovery, or at least promised to put a stop to the fits and depression. Duncan Sr suggested that physical and mental exertion would be the best remedy for one of his patients, a labourer: 'I think he will be better to return to his former occupation than by any remedies we could have given him during his stay in the house'.[159] At worst, these precepts consolidated the issue of personal responsibility in the genesis of these diseases and frustrated those who found it materially impossible to comply. Practitioners tended to justify and support the prevailing social and biological notions of gender with their medical care. For example, for patients with hysteria, a blueprint for matrimonial living was encouraged. Similarly, hypochondriacs were told to shed their narcissism and resume an active and useful life of work.[160]

In their quest for attention and relief, the prospective Infirmary patients were willing to put up with a regimen of diet, drugs and physical measures traditionally judged to be useful in promoting relief if not recovery. Responding to the needs of their patients, Edinburgh physicians mostly concentrated on the physical aspects of these diseases. They paid lip-service to notions that suggested control over the body's nervous function. Instead, they actually instituted a series of traditional treatments that ranged from irritating salts and purgatives to blisters and electric sparks. Their aim was to simply ameliorate a series of functional disabilities fraught with social consequences. Little could be done in the hospital about the mental status of their charges. Physicians simply told both male and female patients to lift their spirits and quit worrying about their health. Paradoxically, life in the hospital actually provided opportunities to verbalise emotional suffering with caregivers and fellow inmates. Solidarity and empathy could be beneficial (Chapter 1).

Historians have recently called for a multidisciplinary history of disease that blends medical and scientific perspectives with cultural and social dimensions including class, race and gender (Chapter 5).[161] This effort to contextualise hysteria and hypochondriasis 'from below' at the Edinburgh Infirmary during the second half of the eighteenth century tried to expose some of the paradoxes surrounding the construction of two popular neuroses in a particular place and time. Physicians redefined and expanded both diagnostic labels based on a reinterpretation of the clinical evidence gathered from poor hospital inmates. Constitutional and acquired debility, later frequently defined as 'asthenia' (Chapter 3) became inextricably linked to both hysteria and hypochondriasis with considerable consequences for their subsequent representation.[162] Among the key factors in this theoretical remodelling were new scientific insights into the functioning of the nervous system and its pervasive influence over all bodily phenomena. Moreover, the flexible notion of a nerve-mediated 'sensibility' and 'sympathy' preserved the traditional holism of the human body and mind, thus precluding for a time the need for strict clinico–pathological correlations that became the hallmark of French medicine decades later. When needed, the traditional speculations of uterine involvement in hysteria handily filled the gaps in medical knowledge. Finally, by broadening their clinical boundaries and causality, hysteria and hypochondriasis became diseases of inclusion, the great imitators of many other illnesses. In a most unique way, both disorders entwined biological and mental, environmental, social, and cultural aspects, creating representations of considerable medical complexity and ambiguity. By 1800, this construction process was firmly on its way, transforming hysteria and hypochondriasis into fashionable Victorian afflictions of the nerves before their eventual fragmentation and disappearance a century later.[163]

Notes

1 W. Buchan, *Domestic Medicine* (Edinburgh: Balfour, Auld and Smellie, 1769), 508. For details on Buchan, see C. Lawrence, ''William Buchan: Medicine Laid Open', *Medical History*, 57, 1 (1983), 22–42.

2. Cases of Angus Robertson and Ann Webster, in J. Hope, Cases of Patients in the Royal Infirmary of Edinburgh under the Care of John Hope MD (Edinburgh, 1781), MSS Collection, University of Edinburgh

3. G.B. Risse, 'Hysteria at the Edinburgh Infirmary: The Construction of a Disease, 1770–1800', *Medical History*, 32, 1 (1988), 1–22.

4. The sources used for this study are a number of student casebooks and lecture notes. The casebooks contained information from the official ledgers. For details, see G.B. Risse, *Hospital Life in Enlightenment Scotland: Care and Teaching at the Royal Infirmary of Edinburgh* (New York: Cambridge University Press, 1986), 7–59, 296–302.

5. R. Porter, 'The body and the Mind, The Doctor and the Patient', in S.L. Gilman *et al.*, *Hysteria Beyond Freud* (Berkeley: University of California Press, 1993), 228.
6. For details, B. Goodman, *When the Body Speaks its Mind* (New York: G.P. Putnam, 1994).
7. A typical example is I. Veith, *Hysteria: The History of a Disease* (Chicago: University of Chicago Press, 1965).
8. For an informative discussion of the historiography of hysteria, consult M.S. Micale, *Approaching Hysteria: Disease and Its Interpretations* (Princeton: Princeton University Press, 1995), 33–107.
9. See, for example, E. Bronfen, *The Knotted Subject: Hysteria and its Discontents* (Princeton: Princeton University Press, 1998); S. Baur, *Hypochondria: Woeful Imaginings* (Berkeley: University of California Press, 1980; and V. Starcevic and D.R. Lipsitt (eds), *Hypochondriasis: Modern Perspectives on an Ancient Malady* (Oxford: Oxford University Press, 2001).
10. H. King, 'Once Upon a Text: Hysteria from Hippocrates', in *Hippocrates' Woman: Reading the Female Body in Ancient Greece* (London: Routledge, 1998), 205–46.
11. G.E.R. Lloyd (ed.), *Hippocratic Writings*, trans. J. Chadwick and W.N. Mann (New York: Penguin Books, 1978).
12. See Aretaeus the Cappadocian, 'Causes and Symptoms of Chronic Diseases', in F. Adams (ed.), Aretaeus, *The Extant Works* (London, 1856), as quoted in E. Fischer-Homberger, 'Hypochondriasis of the Eighteenth Century – Neurosis of the Present Century', *Bulletin of the History of Medicine*, 46 (1972), 391–401.
13. For a recent discussion of the relationships between religion and hysteria see C. Mazzoni, *Saint Hysteria: Neurosis, Mysticism, and Gender in European Culture* (Ithaca: Cornell University Press, 1996).
14. For previous associations of hysteria and witchcraft, see M. MacDonald, *Witchcraft and Hysteria in Elizabethan London* (London: Tavistock/Routledge, 1991).
15. R. Brain, 'The Concept of Hysteria in the Time of William Harvey', *Proceedings of the Royal Society of Medicine*, 56 (1963), 317–24; and J. Wright, 'Hysteria and Mechanical Man', *Journal of the History of Ideas*, 41 (1980), 233–47.
16. R. Martensen, 'The Transformation of Eve: Women's Bodies, Medicine and Culture in Early Modern England', in R. Porter and M. Teich (eds), *Sexual Knowledge, Sexual Science: The History of Attitudes to Sexuality* (Cambridge: Cambridge University Press, 1994), 107–33.
17. J.M.N. Boss, 'The Seventeenth-Century Transformation of the Hysteric Affliction and Sydenham's Baconian Medicine', *Psychological Medicine*, 9

(1979), 221–34.

18. For an explanation of contemporary views, see G.S. Rousseau, 'Nerves, Spirits, and Fibres: Towards Defining the Origins of Sensibility, with a Postscript 1976', in *The Blue Guitar,* 2 (1976), 125–53.
19. Sydenham's ideas were expressed in his 'Epistolary Dissertation', a lengthy discussion in the form of a letter dated 20 January 1682 and written to William Cole, a colleague in Worcester. See T. Sydenham, *The Works of Thomas Sydenham, MD,* trans. R.G. Latham, 2 vols (London: Sydenham Society, 1850), Vol. 2, 85.
20. *Ibid.*, Vol. 2, 89.
21. N. Robinson, *A New System of the Spleen, Vapours, and Hypochondriack Melancholy* (London: A. Bettesworth, 1729).
22. R. Whytt, *Observations On the Nature, Causes, and Cure of the Disorders Which Have Been Commonly Called Nervous, Hypochondriac, or Hysteric* (Edinburgh: T. Becket & J. Balfour, 1765), V and 28. For details, R.K. French, *Robert Whytt: The Soul and Medicine* (London: Wellcome Institute for the History of Medicine, 1969), 31–45. Such 'nervous' pathogenesis was not exclusively British; see S.A.A.D. Tissot, *Traité des Nerfs et de Leurs Maladies,* 2 vols (Paris, 1778–80).
23. *Ibid.*, IV.
24. For the argument that such physiology and pathology blended with Scottish ideas and cultural values, consult C. Lawrence, 'The Nervous System and Society in the Scottish Enlightenment', in B. Barnes and S. Shapiro (eds), *Natural Order: Historical Studies of Scientific Culture* (London: Sage Publications, 1979), 19–40; see also J. Mullan, 'Hypochondria and Hysteria: Sensibility and the Physician', *The Eighteenth Century: Theory and Interpretation,* 25 (1984), 141–74.
25. By the term 'hysterisation', Michel Foucault meant that medicine now explained women's behaviour within new theoretical frameworks based on sensibility and nerves. See his *The History of Sexuality: An Introduction,* trans. R. Hurley (New York: Vintage Books, 1980), 104, 116–23.
26. J. Gregory, 'Hysteria' – a lecture delivered to medical students in the academic year 1788–9, MSS Collection, National Library of Medicine, Bethesda, Maryland, USA.
27. W. Cullen, 'Of Hysteria or the Hysteric Disease', in *First Lines of the Practice of Physic,* new edn, IV vols (Edinburgh: C. Elliott, 1788), Vol. IV, 93–106.
28. For more details about earlier beliefs regarding this organ see W. Pagel, *The Smiling Spleen: Paracelsianism in Storm and Stress* (Basel: Karger, 1984).
29. R. Blackmore, *A Treatise of the Spleen and Vapours: Or Hypochondriacal and Hysterical Affections* (London: J. Pemberton, 1725), 12.

30. Cullen, *op. cit.* (note 27), Vol. III, 217–25; see also A.P. Wilson's medical dissertation, *De Dyspepsia* (Edinburgh: Balfour and Smellie, 1792).
31. J. Sinclair, *Analysis of the Statistical Account of Scotland*, II parts (Edinburgh: A. Constable, 1825), reprint (New York: Johnson Reprint Corporation, 1970), part I, 142.
32. Cullen, *op. cit.* (note 27), Vol. III, 225.
33. W. Cullen, *Synopsis Nosologiae Methodicae* (Edinburgh: A. Kincaid and W. Creech, 1772). An English translation of this work first appeared in 1792 under the title *Synopsis and Nosology* (Hartfort, Conn.: N. Palten, 1792). For a brief background, see W.F. Knoff, 'A History of the Concept of Neurosis, with a memoir of William Cullen', *American Journal of Psychiatry*, 127 (1970), 120–4; and J. Lopez Piñero, *Historical Origins of the Concept of Neurosis*, transl. D. Berrios (Cambridge: Cambridge University Press, 1982), 1–15.
34. *Ibid.*, 31–2.
35. Cullen, *op. cit.* (note 27), Vol. II, 153.
36. Cullen, *op. cit.* (note 33), X.
37. W. Cullen, Clinical Lectures (Edinburgh: 1772–3), MSS Collection, Royal College of Physicians, Edinburgh.
38. W. Cullen, Clinical Lectures Delivered for John Gregory, February–April 1772 (Edinburgh, 1772), MSS Collection, Royal College of Physicians, Edinburgh, 75–80.
39. See, for example, J. Caldwell, *De Hysteria* (Edinburgh: Balfour and Smellie, 1780); and J. Mitchell, *De Hysteria* (Edinburgh: Balfour and Smellie, 1789). For hypochondriasis see J. Stark, *De Malo Hypochondriaco* (Edinburgh: Balfour and Smellie, 1783). Stark was the Senior President of the Royal Medical Society during the 1782–3 academic year, and prominently involved in a lawsuit against a local publisher. Two theses published earlier were by T. Cupples, *De Hypochondriasis Causis* (Edinburgh: Balfour and Smellie, 1777); and S. Baynes, *De Hypochondriasis* (Edinburgh: Balfour and Smellie, 1777).
40. Cullen spoke about the favourable effects derived from the 'exercise of venery'. See Cullen, *op. cit.* (note 27), Vol. III, 41. Another author suggested: 'Follow Hippocrates; a woman's best remedy is to marry and bear children', in John Ball, *The Female Physician: Or Every Woman Her Own Doctress* (London: L. Davis, 1770), 15.
41. Cullen, *op. cit.* (note 27), Vol. IV, 98.
42. One such author was W. Saunders, *Elements of the Practice of Physic* (London, 1784), 122; another W. Nesbit, *The Clinical Guide*, 3rd edn (Edinburgh: J. Watson, 1799), 97–100.

43. Cullen, *op. cit.* (note 27), Vol. III, 249–50.
44. W. Cullen, 'An Essay on the Hypochondriac Disease' (in a letter), Thomson/Cullen Papers, MSS Collection, Glasgow University Library, 33.
45. *Ibid.*, 18.
46. R. Porter makes this point, see his *Bodies Politic: Disease, Death and Doctors in Britain, 1650–1900* (Ithaca: Cornell University Press, 2001), 158–62.
47. Blackmore, *op. cit.* (note 29), 97–8. One of the most famous contemporary hypochondriacs was James Boswell (1740–95, a diarist and one of the Scottish literati. For details regarding his fits of depression, see F. Brady, *James Boswell: The Later Years, 1769–1795* (New York: McGraw–Hill, 1984).
48. Details in G.S. Rousseau, '"A Strange Pathology": Hysteria in the Early Modern World, 1500-1800', in Gilman *et al.*, *op. cit* (note 5), 91–221.
49. G. Cheyne, *The Natural Method of Curing the Diseases of the Body and the Disorders of the Mind Depending on the Body* (London: Strahan & Leake, 1773).
50. J. Buchan, 'Hypochondriasis', *in Dissertations Read to the Royal Medical Society, Edinburgh (Diss. RMS)*, 95 vols (Edinburgh, 1751–1833), MSS Collection, Edinburgh University Library, Vol. 24 (1789–90), 437.
51. W. Belcher, 'Hysteria', *Diss. RMS*, Vol. 25 (1790–1), 226. Some medical dissertations written on this topic were J. Caldwell, *De Hysteria* (Edinburgh: Balfour & Smellie, 1780); R. Groat, *De Hysteria* (Edinburgh: Balfour & Smellie, 1783); and J.S. Kerr, *De Hysteria* (Edinburgh: Balfour & Smellie, 1794).
52. M. Barfoot, 'Dr William Cullen and Mr Adam Smith: A Case of Hypochondriasis', *Proceedings of the Royal College of Physicians, Edinburgh*, 21 (1991), 204–14.
53. See especially Michel Foucault's *The Birth of the Clinic: An Archeology of Medical Perception*, trans. A.M. Sheridan Smith (New York: Pantheon, 1973); and his *Madness and Civilization: A History of Insanity in the Age of Reason*, trans. R. Howard (New York: Random House, 1965). For an excellent introduction to Foucault's writings, C. Jones and R. Porter (eds), *Reassessing Foucault: Power, Medicine and the Body* (London: Routledge, 1994), 1–16.
54. R. Porter, 'Civilisation and Disease: Medical Ideology in the Enlightenment', in J. Black and J. Gregory (eds), *Culture, Politics, and Society in Britain, 1660–1800* (Manchester: Manchester University Press, 1991), 154–83.
55. The same applies to other contemporary mental conditions. See R.A. Houston, *Madness and Society in Eighteenth-Century Scotland* (Oxford: Clarendon Press, 2000), 25.
56. See the surviving folios of the General Register, available from 1770 with the exception of one volume listing patients admitted between 28 March 1797

and 27 July 1799. All volumes are preserved in the MSS Collection, Edinburgh University Library. The diagnostic labels of 'hysteria' and 'hysteric complaint' were sorted out from all admissions listed for the year 1770 and then repeated for every five years until 1800. Sex was determined from the patients' first names. Ward, length of hospitalisation, and category of discharge were also collected from the same register. For more details, Risse, *op. cit.* (note 4), 50–6.

57. A small number of patients with hysteric complaints were officially labelled as suffering from 'dyspepsia', a stomach disorder, but included in this study.
58. See, for example, G.B. Risse, 'Britannia Rules the Seas: The Health of Seamen, Edinburgh, 1791–1800', *Journal of the History of Medicine*, 43 (1988), 426–46.
59. However, this average is somewhat deceiving since most of the persons admitted were teenagers. Sixty-three percent of all women listing their marital status were unmarried. The rest were about equally divided between married and widowed females.
60. Foucault, *op. cit.* (note 25), 121.
61. Case of Peggy Bonella, in J. Gregory, Clinical Cases, Men's Book and Women's Book (Edinburgh, 1785), MSS Collection, Royal College of Physicians, Edinburgh.
62. This description was provided by a 15-year-old girl, Betty Drysdale, in J. Gregory, Clinical Cases of Patients in the Royal Infirmary of Edinburgh (Edinburgh, 1787), MSS Collection, National Library of Medicine, Bethesda, Maryland, USA.
63. Case of John Craig, in W. Cullen, Clinical Cases and Reports taken at the Royal Infirmary of Edinburgh from Dr Cullen by Richard W. Hall (Edinburgh, 1773–4), MSS Collection, National Library of Medicine, Bethesda, Maryland, USA.
64. Case of A.B., in J. Buchan, *op. cit.* (note 50), 426.
65. On 17 March 1784, James Gregory admitted 35-year-old John Lumsden to the teaching ward 'constantly complaining of imaginary complaints particularly pain and swelling in the perineum'. The information is contained in *Medical Tracts I*, recorded by John Unthank, a student notebook in my possession.
66. Case of James Plank, in Duncan, Sr, Clinical Reports and Commentaries, February–April 1795, presented by A.B. Morrison (Edinburgh, 1795), MSS Collection, Royal College of Physicians, Edinburgh.
67. Case of Nichol Johnstone, in J. Home and A. Duncan, Jr., Case Notes and Clinical Lecture Notes (Edinburgh, 1808–9), MSS Collection, Edinburgh University Library.

68. J. Dwer, *Virtuous Discourse: Sensibility and Community in Late Eighteenth-Century Scotland* (Edinburgh: J. Donald, 1987), 95.
69. See case of Elizabeth Miller, in John Gregory, Clinical Cases of the Royal Infirmary of Edinburgh (Edinburgh, 1771–2), MSS Collection, Edinburgh University Library.
70. Case of Janet Nisbet, in F. Home, Clinical Cases From the Royal Infirmary and Reports, by R. Dunlop (Edinburgh, 1786–7), MSS Collection, Edinburgh Room, Edinburgh City Library.
71. R. Gray, 'Hysteria', *Diss. RMS,* Vol. 24 (1789–90), 1.
72. Case of Peggy Thomson, in Gregory, *op. cit.* (note 69).
73. Case of John Craig, in Cullen, *op. cit.* (note 63)
74. Case of James Smyth, in Duncan, Sr, *op. cit.* (note 66).
75. Michel Foucault emphasised that poor women were not concerned with their bodily care at a time when sexuality became a medical concern and women were subjected to 'hysterisation'. For a general overview of eighteenth-century medicine, see G.B. Risse, 'Medicine in the Age of Enlightenment', in A. Wear (ed.), *Medicine in Society: Historical Essays* (Cambridge: Cambridge University Press, 1992), 149–95. The social construction of disease is presented in a series of case studies in P. Wright and A. Treacher (eds), *The Problem of Medical Knowledge* (Edinburgh: Edinburgh University Press, 1982).
76. Sydenham, *op. cit.* (note 19), Vol. II, 85.
77. K.E. Williams, 'Hysteria in Seventeenth-Century Case Records and Unpublished Manuscripts', *History of Psychiatry,* 1 (1990), 383–401.
78. W. Buchan, *Domestic Medicine,* enlarged edn (New York: R. Scott, 1812), 62; see also J. Mullan, *Sentiment and Sociability: The Language of Feeling in the Eighteenth Century* (Oxford: Clarendon Press, 1988), 201–40.
79. J.M. Adair, *Essays on Fashionable Diseases* (London: T. P. Bateman, 1790), 3. Adair (1728–1802) was a prominent member and president of the Royal Medical Society during the 1788–9 session.
80. J.C. Lettsom, *On the Improvement of Medicine in London on the Basis of Public Good,* 2nd edn (London: J. Phillips, 1775), 28.
81. Gray, *op. cit.* (note 71), 1.
82. Micale called this 'psychological gentrification', *op. cit.* (note 8), 160. For more details about the status of female servants in Edinburgh, R.A. Houston, *Social Change in the Age of Enlightenment: Edinburgh, 1660–1760* (Oxford: Clarendon Press, 1994), 87–101.
83. A. Wilson, *Medical Researches: Being an Enquiry into the Nature and Origin of Hysterics in the Female Constitution* (London: Hooper & Robinson, 1777), 102.

84. Royal Infirmary of Edinburgh, *Report of a Committee on the State of the Hospital* (Edinburgh, 1818), 89.
85. Cullen, *op. cit.* (note 27), Vol. IV, 9–16.
86. F.W. Watkeys, *Old Edinburgh,* 2 vols (Boston: L. Page, 1908), Vol. 2, 192–3.
87 . Sinclair, *op. cit.* (note 31), part I, 142.
88. James Gregory, *op. cit.* (note 26).
89. Case of James Smyth, in Duncan, Sr, *op. cit.* (note 66).
90. Whytt, *op. cit.* (note 22), 86. In discussing one of his patients, Gregory made similar comments. See the case of Isabel Gray, in James Gregory, Clinical Cases in the Royal Infirmary of Edinburgh, taken by N. Thomas (Edinburgh, 1785–6) MSS Collection, Edinburgh University Library.
91. Case of Peggy McKay, in Gregory, *op. cit.* (note 65).
92. *Ibid.*; see also Whytt, *op. cit.* (note 22), 215. Similar instances of this imitative behavior – still today referred to as 'hysterical contagion' – were reported in nineteenth-century church assemblies and theatrical performances. A recent outbreak of what is now termed 'mass psychogenic illness' with very similar manifestations was blamed on the anxiety and stress of hospitalised patients who share common institutional space.
93. M. Lochhead, *The Scots Household in the Eighteenth Century* (Edinburgh: Moray Press, 1948), 281.
94. Case of Janet Nisbet, in Home, *op. cit.* (note 70).
95. For more information about hospitalisation at the Edinburgh Infirmary, consult Risse, *op. cit.* (note 4), 60–118.
96. Case of Isabel Gray, in James Gregory, *op. cit.* (note 90).
97. Case of C.M., in Cases of Francis Home (1780), MSS 2933, Wellcome Library, London.
98. Cullen, *op. cit.* (note 38).
99. Cullen, *op. cit.* (note 37), 64.
100. Case of Bell Robinson, in Duncan, Sr, *op. cit.* (note 66).
101. Case of John Menter, in *ibid.*
102 . Case of James Smyth, in *ibid.*
103. Cases of Margaret Paterson and Mary Taylor, in Daniel Rutherford, Clinical Cases (Edinburgh, 1799), MSS Collection, Royal College of Physicians, Edinburgh.
104. Buchan, *op. cit.* (note 50), 428. Other published dissertations on this topic were R. Wightman, *De Hypochondria* (Edinburgh: Balfour and Smellie, 1789); and J. Stark, *De Malo Hypochondriaco* (Edinburgh: Balfour and Smellie, 1783).
105. W. Belcher, 'Hysteria', *Diss. RMS,* Vol. 25 (1790–1), 224.
106. Cullen, *op. cit.* (note 27), Vol. IV, 97–8.
107. Gray, *op. cit.* (note 71), 4.

108. Whytt, *op. cit.* (note 22), 230.
109. See 'Hysteria', in Anonymous, *The Edinburgh Practice of Physic, Surgery, and Midwifery*, new edn, V vols (London: G. Kearsley, 1803), Vol. II, 439–40.
110. Case of John Lumsden, in Gregory, *op. cit.* (note 65).
111. Case of Elizabeth Miller, in Gregory, *op. cit.* (note 69).
112. Case of Cecilia McLean, in Gregory, *op. cit.* (note 90).
113. Risse, *op. cit.* (note 4), 153–7.
114. Gregory, *op. cit.* (note 26), 98.
115. Case of Isabel Gray, in Gregory, *op. cit.* (note 90); see also John Gregory, *Observations on the Duties and Offices of a Physician* (London: W. Strahan and T. Cadell, 1770), 23.
116. W. Cullen, Letter dated 5 May 1779 to a private patient, See his *Correspondence*, XXI vols (Edinburgh, 1755–90), MSS Collection, Royal College of Physicians, Edinburgh, Vol. XI.
117. Cullen, *op. cit.* (note 44), 38–9.
118. See case of James Smyth, in Duncan, Sr, *op. cit.* (note 66).
119. Hope, *op. cit.* (note 2).
120. Case of James Smyth, in Duncan Sr, *op. cit.* (note 66).
121. A., *op. cit.* (note 109), 441–2; see also B. Parr, 'Hysteria', in *The London Medical Dictionary*, rev. edn, II vols (Philadelphia: Mitchell, Ames & White, 1819), Vol. I, 784–5.
122. See Gregory, *op. cit.* (note 26), 103–5.
123. Case of Ann Webster, in Hope, *op. cit.* (note 2).
124. Gregory, *op. cit.* (note 26), 98–100.
125. The patient, Helen Christie, was a 19-year-old servant suffering from almost daily fits. See T.C. Hope, Clinical Casebook (Edinburgh, 1796–7), MSS Collection, Royal College of Physicians, Edinburgh.
126. For an overview, Risse, *op. cit.* (note 4), 210–1; see also Parr, 'Blisters', *op. cit.* (note 121), Vol. I, 254–6.
127. Case of Mary Morrison, in Gregory, *op. cit.* (note 90).
128. Case of Peggy Thykston, in Gregory, *op. cit.* (note 69).
129. *Ibid.*, case of Elizabeth Miller; see also the case of Renny Mathew, in James Gregory, Cases of Patients Under the Care of James Gregory, MD (Edinburgh: 1781–82), MSS Collection, Royal College of Physicians, Edinburgh. Her entire case is reproduced in Risse, *op. cit.* (note 4), 336–9.
130. Cases of Bell Robinson, in Duncan, Sr, *op. cit.* (note 66); Ann Webster, in Gregory, *op. cit.* (note 90); and Margaret Paterson, in Rutherford, *op. cit.* (note 103).
131. Royal Infirmary of Edinburgh, Minutes of Managers, MSS Collection, Edinburgh University Library, Vol. III, meeting 20 Apr 1750, 53.
132. Risse, *op. cit.* (note 4), 213–17; see also W. Cullen, 'On Electricity as

Applied to Medicine', in *Clinical Lectures Delivered on the Years 1765 and 1766* (London: Lea & Hurst, 1797), 243.
133. Case of Mary Morrison, in Gregory, *op. cit.* (note 90).
134. Case of Helen Thykston, in Gregory, *op. cit.* (note 69).
135. Case of Lilly Thompson, in F. Home, Cases of Patients under the Care of Francis Home (Edinburgh, 1780–1), MSS Collection, Royal College of Physicians, Edinburgh.
136. Case of Peggy Bonella, in Gregory, *op. cit.* (note 69).
137. Case of Ann Webster, in Hope, *op. cit.* (note 2).
138. Cullen, *op. cit.* (note 38), 191–2.
139. Case of Renny Mathew, in Gregory, *op. cit.* (note 129).
140. Case of Isabel Gray, in Gregory, *op. cit.* (note 90).
141. Case of Nichol Johnstone, in J. Home and A. Duncan Jr., *op. cit.* (note 67).
142. R.E. Taylor, 'Hypochondriasis', *Diss. RMS*, Vol. 34 (1793–4), 159.
143. Gray, *op. cit.* (note 71), 21.
144. Writing for a different audience, Whytt had recommended that 'the mind ought to be diverted and kept easy and cheerful as possible', adding that 'nothing hurts more the nervous system and particularly the concoctive powers than fear, grief, and anxiety'. See Whytt, *op. cit.* (note 22), 358.
145. Gregory, *op. cit.* (note 26), 97.
146. Case of John Lumsden, in Gregory, *op. cit.* (note 65).
147. Royal Infirmary of Edinburgh, *Rules* (Edinburgh: 1775).
148. Case of Isabel Gray, in Gregory, *op. cit.* (note 90).
149. Case of Helen Thykston, in John Gregory, *op. cit.* (note 69).
150. Case of Mary Morrison, in Gregory, *op. cit.* (note 90).
151. Whytt, *op. cit.* (note 22), 332.
152. The published statistics of admissions and discharges indicate that the Infirmary reported fairly steady discharge rates, published yearly in the January issue of *Scots Magazine*, a popular monthly covering political, social and literary events in Scotland.
153. Case of Rebecca Miller, in James Gregory, Clinical Lectures (Edinburgh, 1783), recorded by John Unthank, in Medical Tracts III, another student notebook in my possession.
154. Case of Mary Morrison, in Gregory, *op. cit.* (note 90).
155. R.I.E,, *op. cit.* (note 84), 9.
156. Case of Elizabeth Miller, in Gregory, *op. cit.* (note 69); and Cullen, Clinical Lectures (1772–3), recorded in Medical Tracts III, *op. cit.* (note 153).
157. Whytt, *op. cit.* (note 22), 414.
158. Case of John Menter, in Duncan, Sr, *op. cit.* (note 66).
159. *Ibid.*, case of James Smyth.
160. Referring to Nichol Johnstone, the melancholic fisherman from the Shetland

Islands who requested his discharge, James Home commented: 'the best thing would be his entering into our navy where he would have no idle time and plenty of regular exercise and company'. See his case in J. Home and A. Duncan Jr, *op. cit.* (note 67).

161. Micale, *op. cit.* (note 8), 286–94.
162. For John Brown's views on hysteria as an asthenic disease, see his *The Elements of Medicine*, trans. from Latin by the author, 2 vols (London: J. Johnson, 1795), Vol. 2, 230–1. For a summary of Brunonian or Brownian views, consult G.B. Risse, 'The Brownian System of Medicine: Its Theoretical and Practical Implications', *Clio Medica*, 5 (1970), 45–51.
163. See M.S. Micale, 'On the 'Disappearance' of Hysteria: A Study in the Clinical Deconstruction of a Diagnosis', *Isis*, 84 (1993), 496–526. I am indebted to Micale's early-twentieth-century analysis because it depicts the process outlined in this essay in reverse.

Eighteenth-Century Medical Scotland: A Select Bibliography

Manuscripts and dissertations

A Narrative of Some Late Injurious Proceedings of the Managers of the Royal Infirmary Against the Students of Medicine in the University of Edinburgh (pamphlet) (Edinburgh, 1785), MSS Collection, Edinburgh University Library.

Appeal for Funds Made in Behalf of Lord Provost, Magistrates and Council, for Funding of the Special Servants Ward at the Infirmary, Edinburgh, 31 January 1771 (pamphlet) National Library of Scotland.

W. Cullen, Consultation Correspondence, XXI vols (Edinburgh, 1755–90), MSS Collection, Royal College of Physicians, Edinburgh.

W. Cullen, Essay on the Preservation of Health, parts I-II, MSS, Thomson/Cullen Papers, Glasgow University Library.

W. Cullen, An Essay on the Hypochondriac Disease in a Letter, MSS, Thomson/Cullen Papers, Glasgow University Library.

W. Cullen, Clinical Lectures delivered for John Gregory, February–April 1772 (Edinburgh, 1772), MSS Collection, Royal College of Physicians, Edinburgh.

W. Cullen, Clinical Lectures (Edinburgh, 1772–3), MSS Collection, Royal College of Physicians, Edinburgh.

W. Cullen, Clinical Cases and Reports taken at the Royal Infirmary of Edinburgh from Dr Cullen by R.W. Hall (Edinburgh, 1773–4), MSS Collection, National Library of Medicine, Bethesda, Maryland, USA.

A. Duncan, Sr, Clinical Reports and Commentaries, February–April 1795, presented by A.B. Morison (Edinburgh, 1795), MSS Collection, Royal College of Physicians, Edinburgh.

Edinburgh Infirmary, General Register of Patients, MSS Collection, Edinburgh University Library.

Edinburgh Infirmary, Treasurer's Account Book, MSS Collection, Edinburgh University Library.

Edinburgh, Infirmary, Minute Books, MSS Collection, Edinburgh University Library.

M.D.L. Finlay, An Enquiry into the 'Ague' in Scotland, MD thesis, Edinburgh University, 1978.

James Gregory, Clinical Notes and Lectures (Edinburgh, 1779–80), MSS Collection, Royal College of Physicians, Edinburgh.

James Gregory, Cases of Patients Under the Care of James Gregory, MD (Edinburgh, 1781-82), MSS Collection, Royal College of Physicians, Edinburgh.

James Gregory, Clinical Cases of Dr Gregory in the Royal Infirmary of Edinburgh, taken by N. Thomas (Edinburgh, 1785–6), MSS Collection, Edinburgh University Library.

James Gregory, Clinical Lectures and Cases (Edinburgh, 1787), MSS Collection, National Library of Medicine, Bethesda, Maryland, USA.

James Gregory, 'Hysteria', a Lecture Delivered to Medical Students in the Academic Year 1788–9, MSS Collection, National Library of Medicine, Bethesda, Maryland, USA.

James Gregory, Clinical Reports, 1 November 1795–1 February 1796 (Edinburgh, 1795–6), MSS Collection, Edinburgh University Library.

John Gregory, Clinical Cases of the Royal Infirmary of Edinburgh (Edinburgh, 1771–2), MSS Collection, Edinburgh University Library.

J. Home, and A. Duncan Jr., Case Notes and Clinical Lecture Notes (Edinburgh, 1808–9), MSS Collection, Edinburgh University Library.

F. Home, Cases of Patients Under the Care of Francis Home (Edinburgh, 1780–1), MSS Collection, Royal College of Physicians, Edinburgh.

F. Home, Clinical Lectures Delivered in the Year 1769, taken by J. Goodsir (Edinburgh, 1769), MSS Collection, Royal College of Physicians, Edinburgh.

J. Hope, Cases of Patients in the Royal Infirmary Under the Care of John Hope, MD (Edinburgh, 1781), MSS Collection, Edinburgh University Library.

T.C. Hope, Clinical Casebook (Edinburgh, 1796–7), MSS Collection, Royal College of Physicians, Edinburgh.

D.D. McElroy, The Literary Clubs and Societies of Eighteenth-Century Scotland, PhD thesis, Edinburgh University Library, 1952.

Royal Medical Society, Edinburgh, Dissertations Read at the Royal Medical Society, MSS Collection, Edinburgh University Library (also available in microfilm form from Microfilm Ltd, Wakefield, West Yorkshire).

D. Rutherford, Clinical Cases (Edinburgh, 1799), MSS Collection, Royal College of Physicians, Edinburgh.

The State of Kelso Dispensary (Kelso: J. Palmer, 1778–1800), and other documents, Scottish Record Office, Edinburgh.

Primary sources

J. Aikin, *Thoughts on Hospitals* (London: J. Johnson, 1771).

Anonymous, *The History and Statutes of the Royal Infirmary of Edinburgh* (Edinburgh: Balfour & Smellie, 1749).

Anonymous, *Letters to the Patients in the Royal Infirmary of Edinburgh* (Edinburgh: J. Reid, 1772).

Anonymous, *The Ladies Dispensatory: Every Woman Her Own Physician*, 2nd edn (London: J. Hodges, 1740).

Anonymous, *The Edinburgh Practice of Physic, Surgery, and Midwifery*, 5 vols (London: G. Kearsley, 1803).

H. Arnot, *The History of Edinburgh* (Edinburgh: W. Creech, 1779).

G. Baker, *An Essay Concerning the Cause of the Endemial Colic of Devonshire* (London: J. Hughs, 1767).

T. Beddoes, *Essay on the Causes, Early Signs, and Prevention of Pulmonary Consumption for the Use of Parents and Preceptors* (Bristol: Biggs & Cottle, 1799).

T. Beddoes, 'Observations on the Character and Writings of John Brown, M.D.', in *The Elements of Medicine of John Brown, M.D.*, new edn, 2 vols (London: J. Johnson, 1795).

J. Bellers, *Essay Towards the Improvement of Physick* (London: J. Sowle, 1714).

J. Black, *Lectures on the Elements of Chemistry*, ed. J. Robison (Edinburgh: 1803).

W. Blizard, *Suggestions for the Improvement of Hospitals and Other Charitable Institutions* (London: H. L. Galabin, 1796).

J. Brown, *The Elements of Medicine of John Brown M.D.*, trans. from Latin by the author, 2 vols (London: J. Johnson, 1795).

W. Buchan, *Domestic Medicine*, 9th edn (London: A. Strahan, 1786).

J. Bull, *The Female Physician; or Every Woman Her Own Doctress* (London: L. Davis, 1770).

R. Chambers (ed.), *A Biographical Dictionary of Eminent Scotsmen*, 5 vols (Edinburgh: Blackie and Son, 1859).

G. Cheyne, *An Essay on Health and Long Life*, 2nd edn (London: G. Strahan, 1725).

G. Cheyne, *The English Malady, or A Treatise of Nervous Diseases* (London, 1733).

G. Cheyne, *The Natural Method of Curing the Diseases of the Body and the Disorders of the Mind Depending on the Body* (London: Strahan & Leake, 1773).

F. Clifton, *Tabular Observations, Recommended as the Plainest and Surest Way of Practicing and Improving Physick* (London: J. Brindley, 1731).

H. Clutterbuck, *An Account of a New and Successful Method of Treating those Affections which Arise from the Poison of Lead* (London: T. Boosey, 1794).

L. Cornaro, *Discourses on a Sober and Temperate Life*, trans. from Italian (Philadelphia: T. Dobson, 1791).

W. Creech, *Edinburgh Fugitive Pieces* (Edinburgh: G. Ramsay, 1815).

W. Cullen, *Clinical Lectures Delivered on the Years 1765 and 1766* (London: Lea & Hurst, 1797).

W. Cullen, *First Lines of the Practice of Physic*, new edn, 4 vols (Edinburgh: C. Elliot, 1785).

W. Cullen, *A Treatise of the Materia Medica*, 2 vols (Edinburgh: Elliot and Kay, 1789).

W. Cullen, *Nosology or a Systematic Arrangement of Diseases by Classes, Orders, Genera and Species*, trans. from Latin (Edinburgh: W. Creech, 1800).

A. Duncan Sr, *Elements of Therapeutics*, 2nd edn, 2 vols (Edinburgh: Drummond, 1773).

A. Duncan Sr. (ed.), *The Edinburgh New Dispensatory*, 2nd edn (Edinburgh: C. Elliot, 1789).

Edinburgh, *List of Members, Laws, and Library Catalogue of the Medical Society of Edinburgh* (Edinburgh: W. Aiken, 1820).

Edinburgh Infirmary, *An Account of the Rise and Establishment of the Infirmary for Sick Poor Erected at Edinburgh* (Edinburgh, 1730).

Edinburgh Infirmary, *Annual Report for the Year 1801* (Edinburgh: J. Hay, 1802).

Edinburgh Infirmary, *Report of a Committee on the State of the Hospital* (Edinburgh, 1818).

Edinburgh University, *List of Graduates in Medicine at the University of Edinburgh from MDCCV (1705) to MDCCCLXVI (1866)* (Edinburgh: Neill, 1867).

G. Fordyce, *A Second Dissertation on Fever* (London: J. Johnson, 1795).

E. Foster, *An Essay on Hospitals* (Dublin: W. G. Jones, 1768).

E. Gilchrist, *The Use of Sea Voyages in Medicine*, 2nd edn (London: A. Millar and D. Wilson, 1756).

W. Grant, *An Enquiry into the Nature, Rise and Progress of the Fevers Most Common in London* (London: T. Cadell, 1771).

James Gregory, *Memorial to the Managers of the Royal Infirmary* (Edinburgh: Murray & Cochrane, 1800).

James Gregory, *Additional Memorial to the Managers of the Royal Infirmary* (Edinburgh: Murray & Cochrane, 1803).

John Gregory, *Lectures on the Duties and Qualifications of a Physician* (London: W. Strahan and T. Cadell, 1772).

A. Hamilton, *The Family Female Physician* (Worcester, Mass: I. Thomas, 1793).

W. Hardy, *The Miner's Guide: Or Compleat Miner* (Sheffield: F. Lister, 1748).

C. Hatchett, *The Hatchett Diary: A Tour through the Counties of England and Scotland in 1796 Visiting their Mines and Manufactories*, ed. A. Raistrick (Truro: Barton, 1967).

J. Hill, *Hypochondriasis: A Practical Treatise* (1766), reprint (Los Angeles: Clark Memorial Library, 1969).

F. Home, *Clinical Experiments, Histories, and Dissections*, 3rd edn (London: J. Murray, 1783).

J. Johnson, *A Guide for Gentlemen Studying Medicine at the University of Edinburgh* (London: Robinson, 1792).

Kelso, *The State of Kelso Dispensary* (Kelso, J. Palmer/Union Press, 1780–1800).

J. Leake, *Medical Instructions Towards the Prevention and Cure of Chronic Diseases Peculiar to Women*, 5th edn (London: R. Baldwin, 1785).

J.C. Lettsom, *General Reflections on the Treatment and Cure of Fevers* (London, 1772).

J.C. Lettsom, *On the Improvement of Medicine in London on the Basis of Public Good*, 2nd edn (London: J. Phillips, 1775).

W. Lewis (ed.), *The Pharmacopoeia of the Royal College of Physicians at Edinburgh* (London: J. Nourse, 1748).

J. Lind, *Essay on the Diseases Incidental to Europeans in Hot Climates* (London: T. Becket, 1768).

R.J. Mackintosh, *Memoirs of the Life of the Right Honorable Sir James Macintosh*, 2 vols (London: E. Moxon, 1835).

W. Maitland, *The History of Edinburgh* (Edinburgh: Longman & Cadell, 1779).

S. Mason, *The Nature of an Intermittent Fever and Ague Consider'd* (London: J. Hodges, 1745).

J. Maubray, *Female Physician, Containing All the Diseases Incident to That Sex* (London: J. Holland, 1724).

R. Morton, *Phthisiologia or A Treatise of Consumption* (London: W. and J. Innis, 1720).

G. Motherby, *A New Medical Dictionary or General Repository of Physick*, 3rd edn (London: J. Johnson, 1791).

W. Nesbit, *The Clinical Guide*, 3rd edn (Edinburgh: J. Watson, 1799).

T. Newte, *A Tour in England and Scotland in 1785* (by an English Gentleman) (London: Robinson, 1788).

W. Nisbet, *The Clinical Guide* (Edinburgh: J. Watson, 1793).

N. Niving, *Jesus Christ in the Poor: Or the Royal Infirmary of Edinburgh Recommended to the Charity of Well-Disposed Christians* (Edinburgh: Sands, Brymer, Murray & Cochran, 1739).

W. Nolan, *An Essay on Humanity, or A View of Abuses in Hospitals* (London: J. Murray, 1786).

B. Parr, *London Medical Dictionary*, 2 vols (Philadelphia: Mitchell, Ames and White, 1819).

T. Pennant, *A Tour of Scotland, MDCCLXIX*, 4th edn, 2 vols (Dublin: A. Leathley, 1775).

T. Percival, *Observations and Experiments on the Poison of Lead* (London: J. Johnson, 1774).

S. Pett, *De Colica Pictonum* (Edinburgh: W. Creech, 1793).

Philanthropus, *A Letter from a Gentleman in Town to His Friend in the Country, Relating to the Royal Infirmary of Edinburgh* (Edinburgh, 1738).

Philasthenes, *A Letter from a Gentleman in Town to His friend in the Country, Relating to the Royal Infirmary of Edinburgh* (Edinburgh, 1739).

B. Ramazzini, *Diseases of Tradesmen* (New York: Medical Lay Press, 1933).

W. Saunders, *Elements of the Practice of Physic* (London, 1780).

J. Sinclair, *Analysis of the Statistical Account of Scotland*, 2 parts (Edinburgh: A. Constable, 1825).

J. Sinclair, *The Statistical Account of Scotland, Drawn up from Communications of the Ministers of the Different Parishes*, XXI vols (Edinburgh: W. Creech, 1791–9).

T. Somerville, *My Own Life and Times, 1741–1814* (Edinburgh: Edmonston and Douglas, 1861).

J. Stedman, *The History and Statutes of the Royal Infirmary of Edinburgh* (Edinburgh: Balfour and Smellie, 1778).

[W. Stroude],'History of the Royal Medical Society', in *List of Members, Laws and Library Catalogue of the Medical Society of Edinburgh* (Edinburgh: Aitken, 1820), XIII-LXVII.

J. Thomson (ed.), *The Works of William Cullen, MD*, 2 vols (Edinburgh: Blackwood, 1827).

R.J. Thornton, *The Philosophy of Medicine: Or Medical Extracts on the Nature of Health and Disease*, 4th edn, 5 vols (London: C. Whittingham, 1799).

T. Tronchin, *A Treatise on the Colica Pictonum or the Dry Belly Ache*, trans. from Latin and ed. R. Schomberg (London: W. Johnston, 1764).

R. Whytt, *Observations On the Nature, Causes, and Cure of the Disorders Which Have Been Commonly Called Nervous, Hypochondriac, or Hysteric* (Edinburgh: T. Becket & J. Balfour, 1765).

J. Wilde, *The Hospital: A Poem in Three Books* (Norwich: Stevenson, Matchett & Stevenson, 1810).

C. Wilson, 'Statistical Observations on the Health of the Labouring Population of the District of Kelso in Two Decennial Periods, From 1777 to 1787 and from 1829 to 1839', *Proceedings of the Border Medical Society*, (1841), 47–85.

J. Wilson (surgeon at Durrisdeer), 'An Account of the Disease called Mill Reek by the Miners at Leadhills', in a letter to A. Monro, *Essays and Observations, Physical and Literary*, I (1754), 459–66.

Secondary sources

R.G.W Anderson and A.D.C Simpson (eds), *The Early Years of the Edinburgh Medical School* (Edinburgh: Royal Scottish Museum, 1976).

D.T. Andrew, *Philanthropy and Police: London Charity in the Eighteenth Century* (Princeton, NJ: Princeton University Press, 1989).

R. Baker *et al.* (eds), *The Codification of Medical Morality: Historical and Philosophical Studies, Medical Ethics and Etiquette in the Eighteenth Century* (Dordrecht: Kluwer, 1993).

M. Barfoot, 'Brunonians Under the Bed: An Alternative to University Medicine in Edinburgh During the 1780s', in W.F. Bynum and R. Porter (eds), *Brunonianism in Britain and Europe* (London: Wellcome Institute for the History of Medicine, 1988), 22–45.

S. Baur, *Hypochondria: Woeful Imaginations* (Berkeley: University of California Press, 1988).

J.H. Bayliss, 'Epidemiological Considerations of the History of Indigenous Malaria in Britain', *Endeavour*, 9 (1985), 191–4.

G. Bell, *Day and Night in the Wynds of Edinburgh and Blackfriars Wynd Analyzed*, 2nd edn (Edinburgh: Johnstone and Hunter, 1849).

T.N. Bonner, *Becoming a Physician: Medical Education in Britain, France, Germany and the United States, 1750–1945* (New York: Oxford University Press, 1995).

A. Borsay, '"Persons of Honor and Reputation": The Voluntary Hospital in an Age of Corruption', *Medical History*, 35, 3 (1991), 281–94.

A. Borsay, *Medicine and Charity in Georgian Bath: A Social History of the General Infirmary, c. 1739–1830* (Aldershot: Ashgate, 1999).

J. Brewer, '"The Most Polite Age and the Most Vicious": Attitudes Towards Culture as a Commodity, 1660-1800,' in A. Bermingham and J. Brewer (eds), *The Consumption of Culture, 1600–1800*, (London: Routledge, 1995), 341–61.

A. Brodie (ed.), *The Cambridge Companion to the Scottish Enlightenment* (Cambridge: Cambridge University Press, 2003).

J.H. Brotherston, 'The Decline of Malaria', in *Observations on the Early Public Health Movement in Scotland* (London: H. K. Lewis & Co, 1952), 26–36.

C.G. Brown, *The Social History of Religion in Scotland since 1730* (London: Methuen, 1987).

L.J. Bruce-Chwatt *et al.*, *The Rise and Fall of Malaria in Europe* (Oxford: Oxford University Press, 1980).

V.L. Bullough and B. Bullough, 'The Causes of the Scottish Medical Renaissance of the Eighteenth Century', *Bulletin of the History of Medicine,* 45 (1971), 13-28.

W.F. Bynum, 'Cullen and the Study of Fever in Britain, 1760–1820,' in W.F. Bynum and V. Nutton (eds), *Theories of Fever From Antiquity to the Enlightenment* (London: Wellcome Institute for the History of Medicine, 1981), 135–47.

C. Camic, *Experience and Enlightenment: Socialization for Cultural Change in Eighteenth-Century Scotland* (Chicago: University of Chicago Press, 1983).

A. Campbell, *The Lanarkshire Miners: A History of their Trade Unions, 1775–1974* (Edinburgh: J. Donald, 1979).

N. Campbell, R. Smellie, and S. Martin, *The Royal Society of Edinburgh (1783–1983)* (Edinburgh: The Society, 1983).

R.H. Campbell and A.S. Skinner (eds), *The Origins and Nature of the Scottish Enlightenment* (Edinburgh: J. Donald, 1982).

A. Carlyle, *The Autobiography of Dr Alexander Carlyle of Inveresk, 1722–1805,* ed. J.H. Burton (Edinburgh: Foulis, 1910).

E.F. Catford, *Edinburgh: The Story of a City* (London: Hutchinson, 1975).

S. Cavallo, 'The Motivations of Benefactors: An Overview of Approaches to the Study of Charity', in J. Barry and C. Jones (eds), *Medicine and Charity Before the Welfare State* (London: Routledge, 1991), 46–62.

A.C. Chitnis, 'Universities: Medicine and Science', in *The Scottish Enlightenment* (London: Croom Helm, 1976), 124–94.

A.C. Chitnis, 'Provost Drummond and the Origins of Edinburgh Medicine', in R.H. Campbell and A.S. Skinner (eds), *The Origins and Nature of the Scottish Enlightenment* (Edinburgh: J. Donald, 1982), 86–114.

J.R.R. Christie, 'The Origins and Development of the Scottish Scientific Community', in *History of Science,* 12 (1974), 122–41.

J.R.R. Christie, 'The Rise and Fall of Scottish Science', in M. Crosland (ed.), *The Emergence of Science in Western Europe* (London: Macmillan, 1975), 111–26.

W. Coleman, 'Health and Hygiene in the Encyclopédie: A Medical Doctrine for the Bourgeoisie', *Journal of the History of Medicine,* 29 (1974), 399-421.

J.D. Comrie, *History of Scottish Medicine,* 2 vols (London: Wellcome History of Medicine Museum, 1932).

W.S. Craig, *History of the Royal College of Physicians of Edinburgh* (Oxford, Blackwell, 1976).

W.J. Couper, *Edinburgh Periodical Press,* 2 vols (Stirling: E. Mackay, 1908).

D.L. Cowen, 'The Edinburgh Pharmacopoeia', *Medical History,* 1, 2 (1957), 123–39.

P. Crawford, 'Attitudes to Menstruation in Seventeenth-Century England', *Past and Present,* 91 (1981), 47–73.

A. Cunningham, 'Medicine to Calm the Mind: Boerhaave's Medical System and Why it was Adopted in Edinburgh', in A. Cunningham and R. French (eds), *The Medical Enlightenment of the Eighteenth Century* (Cambridge: Cambridge University Press, 1990), 40–66.

0D. Daiches, *The Paradox of Scottish Culture: The Eighteenth-Century Experience* (London: Oxford University Press, 1964).

D. Daiches, P. Jones and J. Jones (eds), *A Hotbed of Genius: The Scottish Enlightenment 1730–1790* (Edinburgh: Edinburgh University Press, 1986).

T.M. Devine and R. Mitchison (eds), *People and Society in Scotland, 1760–1830* (Edinburgh: J. Donald, 1988).

T.M. Devine and J.R. Young (eds), *Eighteenth-Century Scotland: New Perspectives* (East Linton: Tuckwell Press, 1999).

A. Digby, *Making a Medical Living: Doctors and Patients in the English Market for Medicine, 1720–1911* (Cambridge: Cambridge University Press, 1994).

H. Dingwall, *A History of Scottish Medicine: Themes and Influences* (Edinburgh: Edinburgh University Press, 2002.

M.J. Dobson, *Contours of Death and Disease in Early Modern England* (Cambridge: Cambridge University Press, 1997).

A. Doig *et al.* (eds), *William Cullen and the Eighteenth-Century Medical World* (Edinburgh: Edinburgh University Press, 1993).

G. Donaldson and R.S. Morpeth, *Who's Who in Scottish History* (Oxford: Blackwell, 1973).

G. Donaldson, *Church and Nation Through Sixteen Centuries*, 2nd edn (Edinburgh: Scottish Academic Press, 1972).

A.L. Donovan, *Philosophical Chemistry in the Scottish Enlightenment: The Doctrines and Discoveries of William Cullen and Joseph Black* (Edinburgh: Edinburgh University Press, 1975).

A.M. Douglas, *Church and School in Scotland* (Edinburgh: St Andrew Press, 1985).

A. Drummond and J. Bulloch, *The Scottish Church 1688–1843* (Edinburgh: Edinburgh University Press, 1973).

K. Duncan, 'The Possible Influence of Climate on Historical Outbreaks of Malaria in Scotland', *Proceedings of the Royal College of Physicians, Edinburgh,* 23 (1993), 55–62.

A.I. Dunlop, *The Kirks of Edinburgh: The Congregations, Churches and Ministers of the Presbytery of Edinburgh, Church of Scotland, 1560–1984* (Edinburgh: Scottish Record Society, 1988).

J. Dwyer, R.A. Mason and A. Murdoch (eds), *New Perspectives on the Politics and Culture of Early Modern Scotland* (Edinburgh: J. Donald, 1980).

J. Dwyer and R.B. Sher (eds), *Sociability and Society in Eighteenth-Century Scotland* (Edinburgh: Mercat Press, 1993).

J. Dwyer, *Virtuous Discourse: Sensibility and Community in Late Eighteenth-Century Scotland* (Edinburgh: J. Donald, 1987).

A. Eccles, *Obstetrics and Gynecology in Tudor and Stuart England* (Kent, Ohio: Kent State University Press, 1982).

R.L. Emerson, 'Science and the Origins and Concerns of the Scottish Enlightenment', *History of Science,* 26 (1988), 333–66

R.L. Emerson, 'The Enlightenment and Social Structures', in P. Fritz and D. Williams (eds), *City and Society in the Eighteenth Century* (Toronto: Hakkert, 1973), 99–124.

R.L. Emerson, 'The Philosophical Society of Edinburgh, 1737–1747', *British Journal of the History of Science* 12 (1979), 154–91.

R.L. Emerson, 'The Founding of the Edinburgh Medical School', *Journal of the History of Medicine,* 59 (2004), 183–218.

J.F. Enders, 'Francis Home and his Experimental Approach to Medicine', *Bulletin of the History of Medicine,* 38 (1964), 101–12.

J.W. Estes, 'Making Therapeutic Decisions with Protopharmacologic Evidence', *Transactions and Studies: College of Physicians, Philadelphia,* 1 (1979), 116–37.

J.W. Estes, *Dictionary of Protopharmacology, Therapeutic Practices, 1700–1850* (Canton, Mass.: Science History Publications, 1990).

J.W. Estes, 'The Medical Properties of Food in the Eighteenth Century', *Journal of the History of Medicine,* 51 (1996), 127–54.

T. Ferguson, *The Dawn of Scottish Social Welfare: A Survey from Medieval Times to 1863* (Edinburgh: T. Nelson & Sons, 1948).

E. Fischer-Homberger, 'Hypochondriasis of the Eighteenth Century – Neurosis of the Present Century', *Bulletin of the History of Medicine,* 46 (1972), 391–401.

M.E. Fissell, 'The Disappearance of the Patient's Narrative and the Invention of Hospital Medicine', in R. French and A. Wear (eds), *British Medicine in an Age of Reform* (London: Routledge, 1991), 92–109.

M.E. Fissell, 'Charity Universal? Institutions and Moral Reform in Eighteenth-Century Bristol,' in L. Davison *et al.* (eds), *Stilling the Grumbling Hive: The Response to Social and Economic Problems in England, 1689-1750* (New York: St Martin's Press, 1992), 121–44.

M.E. Fissell, *Patients, Power and the Poor in Eighteenth-Century Bristol* (Cambridge: Cambridge University Press, 1991).

A. Fleck, 'The Industrial Development of Scotland in the Cullen-Black Period', in A. Kent (ed.), *An Eighteenth-Century Lectureship in Chemistry* (Glasgow: Jackson, Son & Co, 1950), 107–25.

A. Forty, 'The Modern Hospital in England and France: the Social and Medical Uses of Architecture', in A. D. King (ed.), *Buildings and Society: Essays on the Social Development of the Built Environment* (London: Routledge & Kegan Paul, 1980), 61–93.

M. Foucault, *The Birth of the Clinic: An Archeology of Medical Perception,* trans. A. M. Sheridan Smith (New York: Pantheon, 1973).

M. Foucault, *The History of Sexuality: An Introduction,* trans. R. Hurley (New York: Vintage Books, 1980).

M. Foucault, *The Order of Things: An Archeology of the Human Sciences*, trans. from French (London: Tavistock Publications, 1970).

R.K. French, *Robert Whytt: The Soul and Medicine* (London: Wellcome Institute for the History of Medicine, 1969).

R. French, and A. Wear (eds), *British Medicine in an Age of Reform* (London: Routledge, 1991).

R. Goldberg, 'Charity Sermons and the Poor: A Rhetoric of Compassion', *The Age of Johnson*, 4 (1991), 171–216.

J. Golinski, *Science as Public Culture: Chemistry and Enlightenment in Britain, 1760–1820* (Cambridge: Cambridge University Press, 1992).

A. Grant, *The Story of the University of Edinburgh During its First Three Hundred Years*, 2 vols (London: Longmans, Green & Co., 1884).

J. Gray, *History of the Royal Medical Society 1737–1937*, ed. D. Guthrie (Edinburgh: Edinburgh University Press, 1952).

A. Guerrini, *Obesity and Depression in the Enlightenment: The Life and Times of George Cheyne* (Norman, Okla.: Oklahoma University Press, 2000).

D. Guthrie, 'William Cullen MD and his Times', in A. Kent (ed.), *An Eighteenth-Century Lectureship in Chemistry* (Glasgow: Jackson, Son & Co, 1950), 49–65.

D. Guthrie, *Extramural Medical Education in Edinburgh and the School of Medicine* (Edinburgh: Livingstone, 1965).

L. Haakonssen, *Medicine and Morals in the Enlightenment: John Gregory, Thomas Percival and Benjamin Rush* (Amsterdam: Rodopi, 1997).

D. Hamilton, *The Healers: A History of Scottish Medicine* (Edinburgh: Canongate Publishing, 1981).

J.E. Handley, *The Agricultural Revolution in Scotland* (Glasgow: Burns, 1963).

D. Harley, 'Honour and Property: The Structure of Professional Disputes in Eighteenth-Century English Medicine', in A. Cunningham and R. French (eds), *The Medical Enlightenment of the Eighteenth Century* (Cambridge: Cambridge University Press, 1990), 138–60.

H.W. Hart, 'Some Notes on the Sponsoring of Patients for Hospital Treatment under the Voluntary System', *Medical History*, 24, 4 (1980), 447–60.

W.S. Harvey, *Lead and Labour: The Story of the Miners of Leadhills and Wanlockhead* (Internet publication).

A. Herron, *Kirk by Divine Right: Church and State: A Peaceful Coexistence* (Edinburgh: St Andrew Press, 1985).

D.B. Horn, *A Short History of the University of Edinburgh 1556–1889* (Edinburgh: Edinburgh University Press, 1967).

R.A. Houston and J.D. White (eds), *Scottish Society 1500–1800* (Cambridge: Cambridge University Press, 1989).

R.A. Houston, *Social Change in the Age of Enlightenment: Edinburgh, 1660–1760* (Oxford: Clarendon Press, 1994).

W.B. Howie, 'Finance and Supply in an Eighteenth-Century Hospital, 1747–1830', *Medical History*, 7, 2 (1963), 126–46.

J. Jenkinson, *Scottish Medical Societies, 1731–1939. Their History and Records* (Edinburgh: Edinburgh University Press, 1993).

N. Jewson, 'Medical Knowledge and the Patronage System in 18th-Century England', *Sociology*, 8 (1974), 369–85.

R.W. Johnstone, 'William Cullen', *Medical History*, 3, 1 (1959), 33-46.

M. Joyce, *Edinburgh: The Golden Age, 1769–1832* (New York: Longmans, Green, 1951).

L.S. King, *The Medical World of the Eighteenth Century* (Chicago: University of Chicago Press, 1958).

L.S. King, 'Rationalism and Empiricism', in *The Philosophy of Medicine: The Early Eighteenth Century* (Cambridge, Mass.: Harvard University Press, 1978), 233–58.

A.C. Kors (ed.), *Encyclopedia of the Enlightenment*, 4 vols (Oxford: Oxford University Press, 2003).

C. Lawrence, 'The Nervous System and Society in the Scottish Enlightenment', in B. Barnes and S. Shapin (eds), *Natural Order: Historical Studies of Scientific Culture* (Beverly Hills: Sage Publications, 1979), 19–40.

C. Lawrence, 'William Buchan: Medicine Laid Open', *Medical History*, 57, 1 (1983), 22–42.

C. Lawrence, 'Ornate Physicians and Learned Artisans: Edinburgh Medical Men, 1726–1776', in W.F. Bynum and R. Porter (eds), *William Hunter and the Eighteenth-Century Medical World* (Cambridge: Cambridge University Press, 1985), 153–76.

C. Lawrence, 'The Edinburgh Medical School and the End of the "Old Thing" 1790-1830', *History of Universities*, 7 (1988), 259–86.

S. Lawrence, *Charitable Knowledge: Hospital Pupils and Practitioners in Eighteenth-Century London* (Cambridge: Cambridge University Press, 1996).

R. Leonardo, *History of Gynecology* (New York: Froben Press, 1944).

A. Lord, '"The Great Arcana of the Deity": Menstruation and Menstrual Disorders in Eighteenth-Century British Medical Thought', *Bulletin of the History of Medicine*, 73 (1999), 38–63.

M. Lynch, *Mining in World History* (London: Reaktion, 2002).

F.A. Macdonald, 'Reading Cleghorn the Clinician: The Clinical Case Records of Dr Robert Cleghorn, 1785–1818', in C.W.J. Withers and P. Wood (eds), *Science and Medicine in the Scottish Enlightenment* (East Linton: Tuckwell Press, 2002), 255–79.

D.D. Mc Elroy, *Scotland's Age of Improvement. A Survey of Eighteenth-Century Literary Clubs and Societies* (Pullman, Wash.: Washington State University Press, 1969).

A.H. Maehle, 'Pharmacological Experimentation with Opium in the Eighteenth Century', in R. Porter and M. Teich (eds), *Drugs and Narcotics in History* (Cambridge: Cambridge University Press, 1995), pp. 52-76.

A.H. Maehle, *Drugs on Trial: Experimental Pharmacology and Therapeutic Innovation in the Eighteenth Century* (Amsterdam: Rodopi, 1999).

G. Marshall, *Presbyteries and Profits: Calvinism and the Development of Capitalism in Scotland, 1560-1707* (Edinburgh: Edinburgh University Press, 1992).

R. Mitchison and L. Leneman, *Sexuality and Social Control: Scotland 1660-1780* (Oxford: Blackwell, 1989).

R. Mitchison, 'Poor Relief and Health Care in Scotland, 1575-1710', in O.P. Grell and A. Cunningham (eds), *Health Care and Poor Relief in Protestant Europe 1500-1700* (London: Routledge, 1997), 220–33.

A. Moffat, *Kelsae: A History of Kelso From the Earliest Times* (Edinburgh: Mainstream Publication Co., 1985).

J.B. Morell, 'The University of Edinburgh in the Late Eighteenth Century: Its Scientific Eminence and Academic Structure', *Isis,* 62 (1971), 158–71.

J.B. Morell, 'Reflections on the History of Scottish Science', *History of Science,* 12 (1974), 81-94.

J.B. Morell, 'The Edinburgh Town Council and its University, 1717-1766', in R.G. Anderson and A. D. Simpson (eds), *The Early Years of the Edinburgh Medical School* (Edinburgh: Royal Scottish Museum, 1976), 46–65.

O. Moscucci, *The Science of Woman: Gynecology and Gender in England, 1800–1919* (Cambridge: Cambridge University Press, 1990).

J. Murray, *Life in Scotland a Hundred Years Ago as Reflected in the Old Statistical Account of Scotland, 1791–1799* (Paisley: A. Gardner, 1900).

P.H. Niebyl, 'The Non-Naturals', *Bulletin of the History of Medicine,* 45 (1971), 486–92.

D. Owen, *English Philanthropy, 1660–1960* (Cambridge: Belknap Press, 1965).

W.Perry (ed.), *Two Hundred Years of Materia Medica at Edinburgh* (Edinburgh: University of Edinburgh, 1968).

N.T. Phillipson, 'The Scottish Enlightenment', in R. Porter and M. Teich (eds), *The Enlightenment in National Context* (Cambridge: Cambridge University Press, 1981), 19–40.

N.T. Phillipson and R. Mitchison, *Scotland in the Age of Improvement* (Edinburgh: Edinburgh University Press, 1970).

M. Plant, *The Domestic Life of Scotland in the Eighteenth Century* (Edinburgh: Edinburgh University Press, 1952).

D. Porter and R. Porter, *Patient's Progress: Doctors and Doctoring in Eighteenth-Century England* (Stanford, Calif.: Stanford University Press, 1989).

D. Porter and R. Porter, *In Sickness and in Health: The British Experience, 1650-1850* (London: Fourth Estate, 1988).

R. Porter, 'The Gift Relation: Philanthropy and Provincial Hospitals in Eighteenth-Century England', in L. Granshaw and R. Porter (eds), *The Hospital in History* (London: Routledge, 1989), 149–78.

R. Porter, 'Reforming the Patient in the Age of Reform: Thomas Beddoes and Medical Practice', in R. French and A. Wear (eds), *British Medicine in an Age of Reform* (London: Routledge, 1991), 9–44.

R. Porter, 'Civilization and Disease: Medical Ideology in the Enlightenment', in J. Black and J. Gregory (eds), *Culture, Politics and Society in Britain, 1660-1800* (Manchester: Manchester University Press, 1991), 154–83.

R. Porter, 'Consumption: Disease of the Consumer Society?', in J. Brewer and R. Porter (eds), *Consumption and the World of Goods* (London: Routledge, 1993), 58–81.

R. Porter (ed.), *Medicine in the Enlightenment* (Amsterdam: Rodopi, 1995).

R. Porter, *The Creation of the Modern World: The British Enlightenment* (New York: Norton, 2000).

R. Porter, *Bodies Politic: Disease, Death and Doctors in Britain, 1650-1900* (Ithaca, NY: Cornell University Press, 2001).

R. Porter, *Flesh in the Age of Reason* (New York: W.W. Norton, 2003).

S.J. Reiser, 'Examination of the Patient in the Seventeenth-and Eighteenth Centuries', in *Medicine and the Reign of Technology* (New York: Cambridge University Press, 1978), 1–22.

G.B. Risse, 'The Brownian System of Medicine: Its Theoretical and Practical Implications', *Clio Medica,* 5 (1970), 45–51.

G.B. Risse, '"Doctor William Cullen, Physician, Edinburgh": A Consultation Practice in the Eighteenth Century', *Bulletin of the History of Medicine,* 48 (1974), 338–51.

G.B. Risse, '"Typhus" Fever in Eighteenth-Century Hospitals: New Approaches to Medical Treatment', *Bulletin of the History of Medicine,* 59 (1985), 176–95.

G.B. Risse, *Hospital Life in Enlightenment Scotland: Care and Teaching at the Royal Infirmary of Edinburgh* (New York: Cambridge University Press, 1986).

G.B. Risse, 'A Shift in Medical Epistemology: Clinical Diagnosis 1770-1828,' in *History of Diagnostics, Proceedings of the 9th International Symposium on the Comparative History of Medicine-East and West* (Osaka: Tanaguchi Foundation, 1987), 115–47.

G.B. Risse, 'Clinical Instruction in Hospitals: The Boerhaavian Tradition in Leyden, Edinburgh, Vienna, and Pavia', *Clio Medica,* 21 (1987–8), 1–19.

G.B. Risse, 'Hysteria at the Edinburgh Infirmary: The Construction of a Disease, 1770–1800', *Medical History*, 32, 1 (1988), 1–22.

G.B. Risse, 'Britannia Rules the Seas: The Health of Seamen, Edinburgh 1791–1800', *Journal of the History of Medicine,* 43 (1988), 426–46.

G.B.Risse and J.H. Warner, 'Reconstructing Clinical Activities: Patient Records in Medical History', *Social History of Medicine,* 5 (1992), 183–205.

G.B. Risse, 'Medicine in the Age of Enlightenment', in A. Wear (ed.), *Medicine in Society: Historical Essays* (Cambridge, Cambridge University Press, 1992), 149–95.

G.B. Risse, 'Cullen as Clinician: Organization and Strategies of an Eighteenth-Century Medical Practice', in A. Doig *et al.* (eds), *William Cullen and the Eighteenth-Century Medical World* (Edinburgh: Edinburgh University Press, 1992), 133–51.

G.B. Risse, 'Before the Clinic was "Born": Methodological Perspectives in Hospital History', in N. Finzsch and R. Jütte (eds), *Institutions of Confinement: Hospitals, Asylums, and Prisons in Western Europe and North America, 1500-1950* (Cambridge: Cambridge University Press, 1997), 75–96.

G.B. Risse, 'Enlightenment: Medicalization of the Hospital: Edinburgh 1750-1800', in *Mending Bodies – Saving Souls: A History of Hospitals* (New York: Oxford University Press, 1999), 231–56.

J. Ritchie, 'Ague in Scotland', in *The Influence of Man on Animal Life in Scotland: A Study in Faunal Evolution* (Cambridge: Cambridge University Press, 1920), 508–13.

M.M. Roberts and R. Porter, *Literature and Medicine During the Eighteenth Century* (London: Routledge, 1993).

L. Rosner, *Medical Education in the Age of Improvement* (Edinburgh: Edinburgh University Press, 1991).

L. Rosner, 'Eighteenth-Century Medical Education and the Didactic Model of Experiment', in P. Dear (ed.), *The Literary Structure of Scientific Knowledge: Historical Studies* (Philadelphia: University of Pennsylvania Press, 1991), 182–94.

G. Rousseau, 'A Strange Pathology: Hysteria in the Early Modern World, 1500-1800', in S.L. Gilman *et al.*, *Hysteria Beyond Freud* (Berkeley: University of California Press, 1993), 91–221.

D.J. Rowe, *Lead Manufacturing in Britain: A History* (London: Croom Helm, 1983).

S. Shapin, 'The Audience for Science in Eighteenth-Century Edinburgh', *History of Science,* 12 (1974), 95–121.

S. Shapin, 'Property, Patronage and the Politics of Science: The Founding of the Royal Society of Edinburgh', *British Journal of the History of Science* 7 (1974), 1–41.

R.B. Sher, *Church and University in the Scottish Enlightenment: The Moderate Literati of Edinburgh* (Princeton, NJ: Princeton University Press, 1985).

R.B. Sher, 'Science and Medicine in the Scottish Enlightenment: The Lessons of Book History', in P. Wood, *The Scottish Enlightenment: Essays in Reinterpretation* (Rochester: Rochester University Press, 2000), 99–112.

N. Smith, 'Sexual Mores and Attitudes in Enlightenment Scotland', in P.G. Bouce (ed.), *Sexuality in Eighteenth-Century Britain* (Manchester: Manchester University Press, 1982), 47–73.

V. Smith, 'Prescribing the Rules of Health: Self-Help and Advice in the Late Eighteenth Century', in R. Porter (ed.), *Patients and Practitioners: Lay Perceptions of Medicine in Pre-Industrial Society* (Cambridge: Cambridge University Press, 1985), 249–82.

T.C. Smout, 'Lead Mining in Scotland, 1650–1850', in P.L. Payne (ed.), *Studies in Scottish Business History* (London: Cass, 1967), 103–35.

M. Steven, *Parish Life in Eighteenth-Century Scotland: A Review of the Old Statistical Account* (Aberdeen: Scottish Cultural Press, 1995).

C. Stevenson, *Medicine and Magnificence: British Hospital and Asylum Architecture, 1660–1815* (New Haven: Yale University Press, 2000).

D. Stevenson, *The Origins of Freemasonry: Scotland's Century, 1590–1710* (Cambridge: Cambridge University Press, 1988).

A.H. Stirling, *A Sketch of Scottish Industrial and Social History in the Eighteenth-and Nineteenth-Centuries* (London: Blackie, 1906).

R.M. Stott, 'Health and Virtue: Or, How to Keep out of Harm's Way. Lectures on Pathology and Therapeutics by William Cullen c. 1770', *Medical History,* 31, 2 (1987), 123–42.

R.M. Sunter, *Patronage and Politics in Scotland, 1707-1832* (Edinburgh: J. Donald, 1986).

R. Thin, 'The Old Infirmary and Earlier Hospitals', *The Book of the Old Edinburgh Club,* 15 (1927), 135–65.

J. Thomson, *An Account of the Life, Lectures and Writings of William Cullen, MD,* 2 vols (Edinburgh: Blackwood & Sons, 1859).

J.L. Trainer, *The Doctors of Kelso: A History of Medical Care in the Town and District* (Berwick: Martin's, 1987).

U. Tröhler, 'To Improve the Evidence of Medicine: Arithmetic Observation in Clinical Medicine in Eighteenth and Early Nineteenth Centuries', *History and. Philosophy of the Life Sciences,* 10 (1988), 31–40.

A.L. Turner, *Story of a Great Hospital: The Royal Infirmary of Edinburgh* (Edinburgh: Oliver and Boyd, 1937).

E.A. Underwood, 'English–Speaking Medical Students at Leyden', *Nature,* 221 (1969), 810–4.

H. A., Waldron, 'The Devonshire Colic', *Journal of the History of Medicine,* 25 (1970), 383–413.

C. Warren, *Brush With Death: A Social History of Lead Poisoning* (Baltimore: Johns Hopkins University Press, 2000).

F.W. Watkeys, *Old Edinburgh*, 2 vols (Boston: Page, 1908).

J. Watson, *The Scot in the Eighteenth Century: His Religion and his Life* (London: Hodder & Stoughton, 1907).

A. Wear, 'The History of Personal Hygiene', in W.F. Bynum and R. Porter (eds), *Companion Encyclopedia of the History of Medicine*, 2 vols (London: Routledge, 1993), Vol. 2, 1283–1308.

A. Wilson, 'Conflict, Consensus and Charity: Politics and the Provincial Voluntary Hospitals in the Eighteenth Century', *English Historical Review*, 111 (1996), 599–619.

K. Wilson, 'Urban Culture and Political Activism in Hannoverian England: The Example of Voluntary Hospitals', in *The Transformation of Political Culture: England and Germany in the Late Eighteenth Century* (New York: Oxford University Press, 1990), 165–84.

C.W.J. Withers and P. Wood (eds), *Science and Medicine in the Scottish Enlightenment* (East Linton: Tuckwell Press, 2002).

P. Wood, 'The Scientific Revolution in Scotland', in R. Porter and M. Teich (eds), *The Scientific Revolution in National Context* (Cambridge: Cambridge University Press, 1992), 263–87.

P. Wood, 'Science, the Universities and the Public Sphere in Eighteenth-Century Scotland', *History of Universities*, 13 (1994), 99–135.

P. Wood, *The Scottish Enlightenment: Essays in Reinterpretation* (Rochester: Rochester University Press, 2000).

J. Woodward, *To Do the Sick No Harm: A Study of the British Voluntary Hospital System to 1875* (London: Routledge & Kegan Paul, 1974).

D.E. Wooley, 'A Perspective of Lead Poisoning in Antiquity and the Present', *Neurotoxicology*, 5 (Fall 1984), 353–61.

D. Young, and A.J. Youngson, *Edinburgh in the Age of Reason* (Edinburgh: Edinburgh University Press, 1967).

A.J. Youngson, *The Making of Classical Edinburgh: 1750–1840* (Edinburgh: Edinburgh University Press, 1966).

Index

L

M